THE 120-YEAR DIET

"Dr. Walford is a highly respected scientist, regarded by his peers as a pioneer of the life-span revolution. His diet and health plan is packed full of sound advice and useful information for those of us who plan to be around for a long, long time."

—Senator Alan Cranston

"The healthful recipes are . . . creative and appealing . . . Readers will appreciate the critical examination of current medical trends (antioxidants, vitamin supplements, exercise, bodybuilding), as well as an explanation of food-related causes of potentially fatal diseases (excessive salt and hypertension; fat and breast and prostate cancer, for example)."

—*Publishers Weekly*

ROY L. WALFORD received his [illegible] gree from the University of Chicago an[illegible] essor of Pathology at the UCLA [illegible] since 1966. The author of [illegible] and five previous bo[illegible] erous awards of rec[illegible] delegate to the last W[illegible] Aging, and a member of the [illegible] Sciences Committee on Aging, [illegible] one the the leading researchers in the [illegible] tes in the field of aging.

THE·120·YEAR DIET

HOW TO DOUBLE YOUR VITAL YEARS

Roy L. Walford, M.D.

PUBLISHED BY POCKET BOOKS NEW YORK

Important Note: Always consult with your personal physician before starting any diet or exercise program.

POCKET BOOKS, a division of Simon & Schuster, Inc.
1230 Avenue of the Americas, New York, N.Y. 10020

Library of Congress Catalog Card Number: 86-11826

For information address Simon & Schuster, Inc.,
1230 Avenue of the Americas New York, N.Y. 10020

ISBN: 0-671-64904-3

First Pocket Books printing January 1988

10 9 8 7 6 5 4 3 2 1

Printed in the U.S.A.

In memory of my distinguished ancestor,
the barrister, biologist, and antiquarian,
Cornelius Walford, F.R.H.S., London.

Acknowledgment

I am grateful to Susan Ritman and Kristine von Jutrczenka for expert secretarial and library research assistance and for their comments on various aspects of the manuscript; to Susan Ritman in particular for her thorough putting together of widely scattered nutritional data and for a number of the menus; to Dennis Mock for the outstanding computer programming underlying the food combinations; to Gwen Dangerfeld for arranging of tabular material; to John Thomas, Richard Weindruch, Sheldon Ball, and Steve Harris for their criticisms of the manuscript; to my editor at Simon and Schuster, Bob Bender, for his extremely useful organizational suggestions; to my agent, John Brockman, for his fierce representation; and finally to my colleagues, students, and technicians for their interest and encouragement in our joint research into the biology of aging.

Preface

My previous book *Maximum Life Span* presented an overview of gerontology, the science of aging research. In it I described the 5,000-year history of observations and experiments dealing with the aging process, the different scientific theories about how we and other animals age, and how the rates of aging can be measured in the different organ systems of the body. I gave some very general advice about what we can do right now to slow down our rate of aging. And finally, I discussed the implications for us as individuals and for our society if life span is greatly extended, as I believe it soon will be.

Maximum Life Span was intended as a general book of science, history, and philosophy, a popular introduction to the ancient but newly vigorous science of gerontology, rather than a "how-to" book. But the chapter "Practical State of the Art of Life Span Extension" evoked the strongest public interest—more, in fact, than I had bargained for.

This book is a response to that interest. This time I've written a complete how-to book aimed at helping you stay healthy and free of the main killer diseases, while you take the only steps known that with a high order of probability will retard your own aging, keep you functionally young, and (depending on how old you are when you start) stretch out your potential life span to well over a hundred years—

indeed, very possibly to longer than anyone has ever lived in mankind's countless generations.

We are all on the verge of entering the era of the long-living society. I present in this book the first detailed scientifically sound explanation of what you can do to become a member of that society.

Roy L. Walford, M.D.
Professor of Pathology
School of Medicine
University of California at Los Angeles

Contents

I cannot accept the way in which we fix the duration of our life.

—Montaigne

My desire is to save them from nature.

—Christian Dior

CHAPTER 1

Better Health and Greater Longevity

Let's Get Oriented

Not many years ago, about all a physician asked himself when he saw a new patient was "What disease does this patient have, that I can *cure* it?" Today's physicians are beginning to add the question "What diseases will this patient have, that I can *prevent* them?" In early Chinese medicine, the patient paid the doctor only as long as he (or she) stayed well. When the patient got sick, the doctor paid. Imagine how different American medicine would be today if such a system prevailed!

Whoever you are, reading this book, I can tell you with more than 75-percent accuracy that you will die of heart attack, hypertension, stroke, cancer, diabetes, kidney failure, or complications arising from osteoporosis. It's sad but safe to make this prediction because three out of four Americans do indeed succumb to these major killer diseases. Fortunately, you can do a great deal to cut your chances of being struck down by any of them. But avoiding them is just *part* of what you must do to live longer and better.

Even if every one of the killer diseases is prevented or cured, still you will grow old, and at about the same old rate. Your skin will dry out and wrinkle, your hair will thin and turn gray, your sight will dim, your hearing capacity will decline. You'll get heavier and shorter. Your muscles will shrink; your joints will stiffen. Your heart will pump blood less well; your lungs will take in less oxygen, and your tissues will use the oxygen less efficiently. Your kidney function will diminish and your endocrine glands secrete a lower level of hormones. Your breasts will sag or your erection flag; your resistance to infection will be less than a fourth what it was in your youth. There will be slowing of your reaction time to a stimulus, such as the sight of a car hurtling toward you. Some phases of your learning process will slow down, with a lapse in memory for recent events, such as what movie you saw three nights ago. You may not come down with a major disease, but your vulnerability to changes in your environment, the weather, and your personal life will markedly increase with age. Finally you will die from what for a young person might not be a serious problem at all: a mild attack of the flu will become the big sleep, or you won't manage to jump out of the way of that speeding red Pontiac.

> It's like a lion at the door,
> And when the door begins to crack,
> It's like a stick across your back
> And when your back begins to smart
> It's like a penknife in your heart,
> And when your heart begins to bleed
> You're dead, and dead, and dead indeed.
>
> —Nursery rhyme

Even if we avoid disease, we age just about as I've described, because aging is not itself a disease but the last stage of development. I am going to tell you how this unpleasant process of aging can be slowed down and even postponed to a much later time in life than it would otherwise occur. The method mainly involves losing weight gradually on a carefully selected diet that is high in nutrition but low in calories, or what I shall refer to as the "high/low" diet.

In conservative scientific circles, what I recommend will be regarded as more or less "controversial." That's another way of saying "not completely verified." Whether one should recommend measures to prevent disease and retard aging for which there is strong evidence that they do indeed work, but which are not 100 percent verified, will evoke different and sometimes (in fact, usually) heated opinions from biologists and medical doctors.

Proof and Probability

For many years firm but not conclusive evidence suggested that lowering the amount of cholesterol in the blood would help prevent heart disease.

Populations with high blood cholesterol levels experienced more heart attacks than those with low levels. But this neat correlation was not considered absolute "proof," and rightly not, because other differences between the populations might show a similar correlation but have nothing to do with susceptibility to heart attacks. The population with more attacks might be mostly blue-eyed, and the other one brown-eyed, but it wouldn't necessarily mean that to be blue-eyed was to carry a time bomb in your chest. Correlation is not the same as causation! It only tells you where to look.

Despite population data and other "correlation" evidence, the only way to obtain scientifically acceptable "proof" of the association between blood cholesterol and heart disease would be to take a large number of persons from *the same population*, put half of them on a cholesterol-lowering regimen, and see if that half developed less heart disease than the rest. This critical test was recently performed in a 7–10-year, $150-million study conducted by the National Institutes of Health. It formally proved that lowering blood cholesterol will substantially decrease the chance of a heart attack.

But for years before this "proof" was in, many very creditable physicians, including professors at major medical schools, recommended measures aimed at lowering blood cholesterol. They did so on the basis of inferential, or "probable," evidence gained from observations in humans and experiments in animals. Other equally prestigious doctors didn't agree that the evidence was enough to act upon. Until formal proof is established, such matters remain legitimate questions of judgment, which varies from one physician to another, and even between panels of experts. In 1980, for example, the Food and Nutrition Board of the National Research Council was unwilling on the basis of available data to recommend much at all in the way of nutritional changes in the American diet, whereas in the same year and *on the same body of data* a committee of the American Heart Association advised lifelong adoption of a considerably altered diet. This illustrates our situation concerning many aspects of preventive medicine, including ways to slow down the aging process. Should we wait for "conclusive" evidence which may be years away and too late for some of us? Can we in some instances accept "probable" evidence?

Physicians, patients, and bodies of experts alike should realize that *not* taking a stand, insisting on waiting until *all the evidence is in*, is itself a position and a recommendation. Not taking a stand is not really the neutral position it is made out to be.

We cannot easily run a $150-million 7–10-year conclusive study on every promising assembly of "probable" evidence about preventing disease and retarding aging, so we must either stay neutral and do nothing or take a stand on the basis of imperfect evidence. Physicians like to pretend, and many have kidded themselves into believing, that whatever they espouse has been "scientifically proved." Nonsense! A great deal of what established medicine recommends with good conscience is not formally "proved"—the health benefits of exercise, for example: the formal proof on that is not yet in, yet practically all physicians recommend it. And they are right to do so, because the "probable" evidence is excellent.

Recommendations about disease prevention and life extension are only as good as the ability of the recommending person to analyze and judge a wide assortment of important but inconclusive evidence. In this book I undertake to explain and rate the evidence, analyze it, judge it, and make specific recommendations. My credentials in relation to age retardation are among the best in the world. In the matter of disease prevention, they are less, but they reflect extensive reading on the subject, plus my experience as a teacher and practitioner at the University of California School of Medicine.

By "rating the evidence" I mean stating whether any case in point can be considered to display a very high order of probability (almost certain), a high order of probability, a moderate order, or less.

It is almost certain that a diet superhigh in nutritive quality but low in calories (the "high/low diet" described in this book) will retard your basic rate of aging, greatly extending your period of youth and middle age; postpone the onset of such late-life diseases as heart disease and cancer; and even lower your overall susceptibility to disease at any age.

Principles of the High/Low Diet

The high/low diet is based upon many years of animal experimentation in my own laboratory at the U.C.L.A. Medical School and in other laboratories in other major universities in the United States. There is no doubt at all that the life span of animals can be extended by more than 50 percent by dietary means, corresponding to humans living to be 150 or 160 years old. I don't actually expect quite to achieve this much life extension in humans. The necessary regimen would be too tough; but a less rigorous regimen will still add many years to your life, as well as life to your years. The former without the latter would not be so good, but the high/low dietary program promises both.

The diet consists of food combinations and menus arrived at by computer techniques so that the Recommended Daily Allowances of all important nutrients are approximated with *minimal caloric intake*. The program calls for *gradual* weight loss over several years until you reach and remain at a new weight point substantially below your "set point." Your set point is the weight toward which you naturally gravitate if you neither over- nor undereat. Your new weight point, if you are on the proper nutritive program, is your point of maximum metabolic efficiency, maximum health, and maximum life span.

(The high/low diet would also serve superbly well as a quick-weight-loss regimen, but I do not recommend such an undertaking, as it would be counterproductive in terms of good health and longevity.)

I will also tell you how to estimate your individual aging rate, as well as can be done with present techniques. You can then determine how well the program is working for you. And you will soon observe that you simply feel better. You will have more energy, and a clearer head, than ever before.

The high/low diet is well founded scientifically. But evidence that taking fairly large amounts of certain vitamins, drugs, and chemicals will give an added boost to health and longevity varies from moderate to less than moderate. It does exist, however, and we must at least consider supplementation as a part of our longevity program. The proper types (more than one) and amounts of exercise may yield additional advantages.

We shall thus be discussing evidence at every order of probability. In consultation with your personal physician, you must finally decide which recommendations you want to adopt.

Interacting with Your Chosen Physician

Don't use this book just to strike out on your own, regulating your diet, testing your progress, and swallowing a lot of chemicals and pills. My recommendations may apply to an average across-the-board person but still not be appropriate for a particular individual like yourself. You should discuss this book with a physician qualified to establish your current health status and supervise your longevity and health program. Unfortunately, such qualifications are more easily asked for than found. Modern medical training is weak in disease prevention, and even weaker concerning the biology of aging and antiaging therapy. Nutrition is still a woefully insignificant part of the medical-school curriculum. The average physician will be only vaguely familiar with much of the evidence I cite in this book, but will recognize that *some* of my recommendations are not in line with what establishment medicine preaches. He (or she) is apt to feel safe in hiding his ignorance of the subject behind his doctoral authority. That's not what you need.

Establishment medicine is in general excellent, but it maintains its status and its authority by two maneuvers: consensus, and the assumption of complexity.[1] By *consensus* I mean that biologists and doctors may squabble among themselves, but they try to present a unified front to the public. By the *assumption of complexity* I mean they behave as though the arguments about health care were too complicated for even a reasonably educated lay person to understand. The acceptance of doctors as all-wise authority figures (which, believe it or not, dates only from about 1920) signifies "a surrender of private judgment" on the part of patients.[2] In considering what I say in this book, I ask you *not* to surrender your private judgment.

Warped into the consensus view by a rigorous but narrow education, your physician may not be willing even to consider evidence and recommendations contained in a semi-popular book such as this one. In that case, he or she will find the hard-core scientific evidence for much of what I say here more extensively and rigorously documented in a book my U.C.L.A. colleague Dr. Richard Weindruch and I have written, *Retardation of Aging by Dietary Restriction*, to be published by Raven Press sometime in 1987. What I say here may well be debatable, but it is based upon sound scientific investigations carried out at numerous recognized universities by many different investigators. All this will become apparent as we go along.

The National Institute on Aging has recently set up a colony of more than 30,000 rats and mice, about half of which are being maintained on an animal version of the high/low diet and the other half on a traditional diet. These colonies are being established so that investigators throughout the country can test the hallmarks of this life-span-prolonging, age-retarding regimen without the enormous trouble of establishing their own animal groups, as nutritional scientists have had to do until now. The regulation of aging by diet, an area in which I and my associates have done some of the pioneering work, has become a major field of investigation into the aging process. If your doctor does not know about it, he or she should do some reading.

To establish the best interplay between yourself and your physician you must take an active participatory interest. Anyone—either layman or physician—can easily see from his two fine books *Anatomy of an Illness* and *The Healing Heart* that Norman Cousins has mastered the technique of the patient/physician interplay. Because of that, he receives more careful, informed care from his doctors than if he just blindly left everything to them and followed their authoritarian advice. His books portray a new kind of patient/doctor relationship. Be guided by their example.

Of course you should seek advice from your personal physician. Still, in preventive medicine you must assume a large measure of responsibility for your own health. This means knowing or learning how to evaluate evidence. Even respectable medical journals contain a great deal of hogwash, lay journals a lot more, and television commercials almost nothing but. But hogwash is not hard to recognize, wherever it occurs, if you have the key.

Finally, to hold up your side of the patient/physician interplay, you must acquire a basic knowledge about the major killer diseases of late life, and about certain critical aspects of the biology of aging. This knowledge is provided by the book you have in your hand.

Average and Maximum Life Spans

To begin to understand aging and how to retard it, you must understand survival curves, in particular the significance of the average and maximum life-span points on those curves. Figure 1.1 shows four curves, A, B, C, and D. Curves A, B, and C are from actual populations; D is hypothetical. The vertical axis on the left indicates the percentage of the population that is alive at any age. At birth all these population members were alive, so we start with 100 percent. In population A, half the people were dead by the age of 44; in population B, by 60; in population C, by 74; in hypothetical population D, by 100 years of age. All these 50-percent survival points express *average life spans* (also known as *life expectancies at birth*) for the four populations. Curves A, B, and C are the survival curves for the United States in 1900, 1950, and 1982. The *average life span* has been increasing since the turn of the century. This

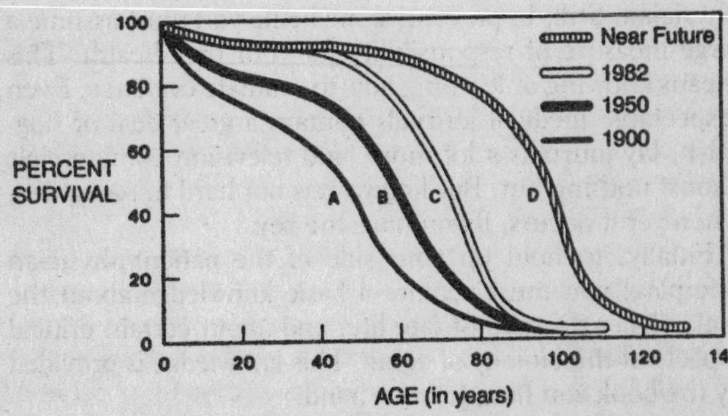

Figure 1.1: Survival curves for the United States in 1900 (curve A), 1950 (curve B), and 1982 (curve C) and for a near-future subpopulation (people on the high/low diet) whose aging rate has been slowed (curve D).

largely reflects the virtual conquest of infectious diseases and to some extent other diseases in First World societies. But it can be shown mathematically that if *all* known diseases were cured—no heart disease, no stroke, no cancer, no diabetes—the average life span would move up to 85 years of age, *but no further*, unless the aging process itself were brought under control. *The remarkable increase in average life span since 1900 does not reflect any retardation of the basic aging process!*

Notice in Figure 1.1 that the *maximum life spans* are the same for curves A, B, and C. *Maximum life span* reflects the genetically determined longevity potential for our species. At the same time, it's a good measure of the basic aging process. It has remained at about 110 years not only since 1900 (Two persons have lived to 113, and one to 119), but even since the time of ancient Rome—and even before that. Indeed, according to Genesis 6:3, "man . . . also is flesh: yet his days shall be an hundred and twenty years." That's close enough to the observed 110-year maximum! No matter how off-base His devotees have portrayed Him with respect to evolution, God shines through, at least in this passage, as an excellent gerontologist.

The survival curves teach us that we cannot influence maximum life span just by curing diseases. Even if absolutely all the major diseases were eliminated, the disease-free older-growing population would just become vulnerable to smaller and smaller environmental assaults, and still die off by 110 years. Only measures that truly retard biologic aging and stretch out the periods of youth and middle age will budge the boulder of this maximal survival point and create a long-living society like the one represented in curve D. That's what the high/low diet will do.

I shall tell you not only how you can jump from curve A onto B or C, or from B onto C—thus increasing your average survival potential—but how you can jump onto curve D itself, becoming a member of the longest-living society that has ever existed.

So we have two goals in this book. They are related, but

not quite the same. We want to learn how to improve our survival chances in terms of average life span. That means preventing as much as possible those diseases most of us would otherwise die of. Second, we want to learn how to slow down the rate of aging, so that while we avoid the diseases, we also do not age so rapidly. In other words, we will not only *live* longer, we will stay *younger* longer. We will neither sag nor flag nor forget where we are or where we have been or where we are going in this fast-moving and exciting world.

Questions and Answers

I expect by now you have a lot of questions. I've encountered some of them in connection with my previous book *Maximum Life Span*. The more specific and practical questions will be answered as we go along, but it will help if I answer some of the more common ones right here.

Question 1: Who wants to live to be 120 years old anyway?

Answer: I find I can evoke an "I do" or a "Not me" answer from most people, depending on how the question is phrased. The very fact that it *is* often asked reflects the negative attitude about aging so common today. This attitude prevents people from properly imagining what a long-living society will be like when it arrives.

Do you ever hear a positive joke about the elderly? Most jokes about aging are nasty or condescending, like "Her face is so wrinkled, when she wears long earrings she looks like a venetian blind." That tasteless quip brings a terrible image to the mind. With such an image, people don't think rationally. Of course they say, "No, I don't want to live to be 120."

Who can blame them? But this image of decrepitude is not the true picture at all. The 120-year (or even much longer) survival curve cannot be produced by addition of old years to old years, but only by stretching out the period of youth and middle age. In the new society I envision, an 80-year-old person will look and act and feel like a 40-year-old person of today. That allows us to ask the question differently. "Who wants to be younger longer and middle-aged longer, and in full possession of his faculties?" Who wouldn't say "I do" to that one?

In thinking about a 120–140-year society, we musn't be influenced by the mentality and outlook of the 110-year society we live in now. In a long-living society, for example, people will have multiple careers. How many times have you heard a friend exclaim, "If I could just do it over again, with what I know now"? But we become old, worn out, and even one career is exhausting enough.

Intensely creative people sometimes die soon after their one career reaches its end. James Joyce succumbed two years after finishing *Finnegans Wake*, Marcel Proust not long after completing *Remembrance of Things Past*, and poet Robert Lowell did not outlive his muse. Novelist Romain Gary wrote in his final note that the reason for his suicide was "I have explained myself fully."

These abrupt terminations would be less likely to happen if the persons involved were *functionally* only 30–35 years old. They would just roll over and arise from the other sides of their lifestyle beds, in a sense reborn. Young people don't realize at gut level that they'll ever become old. Older people forget the energy, tirelessness, and vitality of youth, that wonderful sustaining feeling of physical well-being. But keep that energized vitality and you'll *want* to reach 120 or 140, want to go from one career to another, be able to "do it again with what I know now."

Of course some people will get stuck. They're the ones to feel sorry for. How would you like the elegantly boring job of being Queen Elizabeth II for 120 years?

I don't believe one grows older. I think that what happens early in life is that at a certain age one stands still and stagnates.

—T. S. Eliot[3]

Question 2: The search to retard aging is an old one. After thousands of years of fruitless effort in the life-extension game, why do you think we've arrived now, or at least are close to some major breakthroughs?

Answer: For four good reasons. One: We can with a high order of probability extend maximum human life span by means of the high/low diet right now, so at least one breakthrough has already taken place.

Two: Like the Red Army in 1945, biology is advancing rapidly on a broad front. This is not only the day of the "information revolution," with computers going full blast around the country, but also the day of the "biological revolution." An enormous fallout cascades into the sphere of gerontology, the science of aging. Rapid advances can be expected. In 1933 Albert Einstein, Niels Bohr, and Lord Rutherford, three of the greatest physicists of the early 20th century, all predicted that man would never achieve power from the atom.[4] How wrong they were! Science often advances faster than many of its own experts predict.

Three: For a long time people looked upon major extension of maximum life span as a pipe dream, and life extensionists as impractical visionaries. My own experience shows that this view is changing rapidly. In 1983 I was invited to testify before the U.S. Senate Finance Committee.[5] It seemed that government statisticians had been underestimating the numbers of old people accumulating in the population, making it difficult for the Finance Committee to anticipate Social Security requirements. My task was not to discuss these statistics but to portray the possibilities of a true retardation of aging, and its socioeconomic effects. I noticed that when I spoke of the prospect that a long-living society, or at least a long-living subpopulation, might evolve in the near future, I got no skeptical feedback from the senators, or even the assembled statisticians. They did not think I was merely indulging in a science-fiction fantasy. The prospects were accepted as serious possibilities. If I had said the same thing five years before, everyone would have thought: "Dr. Walford may have impressive credentials, . . . but the poor man has obviously gone over the hill."

Recently the Population Reference Bureau in Washington, D.C., predicted that eliminating cancer and heart disease will prolong millions of lives but add burdensome costs to society in caring for the elderly, whose average life spans have been extended into the period of being "functionally old." The Bureau urged the government to focus research on slowing the aging process . . . *because a chronologically old but "functionally young" elderly population would be not a burden but a great social asset.*[6]

Public consciousness is changing, and acceptance of the possibility of progress greatly facilitates actual progress. If people still thought going to the moon a pipe dream, the great ships would not be streaking up off their launch pads in Florida, even if the technology were available. Belief and confidence foreshadow practical action.

Four: Here my reason for optimism is fanciful and romantic, I admit. Throughout its long history mankind has dreamed three classic dreams: to go to the moon and other planets; to change one element into another, like lead into gold (the old alchemical dream of the philosopher's stone); and to be immortal, or at least to live a lot longer than we do. Of these three great dreams, the first two not only have been realized, but in our own lifetimes. We have already been to the moon. No one doubts we are bound for the planets. With the techniques of modern physics we can change one element into another. Is it too fantastic to believe we shall also realize the third dream, the longevity dream, within the lifetimes of many of us now alive?

Question 3: Dr. Walford, a lot of the research you cite as "evidence," especially for the life-extending benefits of the high/low diet, was done in animals. How do you know it applies to humans?

Answer: We don't know absolutely, but I believe the order of probability is very substantial that the high/low diet will extend maximum life span in humans just as it does in all animal species so far tested. The small amount of data in humans supports this belief. If you want to be still around, hale and hearty, when other, more powerful methods become available, you'd better start with this one.

Many front-rank gerontologists agree that the high/low diet will very probably work in humans: for example, Dr. Leonard Hayflick, past president of the Gerontological Society of America and a major figure in world gerontology;[7] Dr. Alexander Leaf, professor of medicine at Harvard University;[8] and Dr. Robert Good, former director of the Sloan-Kettering Institute for Cancer Research in New York.[9] Some scientists have adopted a "wait and see" attitude. Of course if they wait too long, they won't see.

We are dealing with the question of "translatability." What is the probability that a phenomenon observed in animals can be translated to humans? Well, it depends on the phenomenon. Fertilization, growth, development, and aging are basically much the same across large species differences. There may be an occasional uniqueness in the mechanism of aging. Salmon and octopi, for example, age almost overnight as the result of a programmed hormonal outpouring. But these are easily recognized exceptions. Nobody doubts that most animals—for example, mice, rats, horses, chimpanzees, and humans—age by essentially identical mechanisms. Any general process that retards aging in one such species ought to do so in another. The high/low dietary regimen is such a process.

My comments about *general* processes can be illustrated by reference to *nongeneral*—that is to say, narrower and more specific—processes. These often cannot be translated between species. Humans, guinea pigs, apes, and monkeys, for example, do not manufacture vitamin C in their bodies. They have to get it in their diet. Other mammals, like rats, mice, dogs, and goats, synthesize vitamin C in their own bodies. It would obviously be hazardous to assume that a vitamin C experiment in rats had any direct applicability to humans.

Question 4: But suppose that despite the higher order of probability, the animal work on extending maximum life span turns out in fact not to apply to humans? What then?

Answer: In that case, all I can promise you is that your susceptibility to cancer, heart disease, diabetes, and perhaps osteoporosis will be only about half that of the other people in your car pool. Your *average* survival chances will be better even than those of the people in curve C—and certainly better than those in A or B if you happen to belong to one of those less fortunate curves (Figure 1.1), even if your maximum survival chances are no better. Nontranslatability still adds about 10 more years to your life, and healthier years at that, as a "worst case" estimate.

Question 5: Do I have to give up all that good food?

Answer: No, just some of the bad food. You do have to change your attitude toward food. But you didn't write your own attitude program anyway. It has been written into you by a lifelong daily barrage of slick advertising, which tries to make you believe you are somehow *deprived* if you are not eating junk food, or that it's deliciously decadent and chic to be dining on the precursors of atherosclerotic plaque. Indulge! they tell you. Have a fabulous time! Die young!

Of course, this notion of deprivation is simply a prejudice. People who don't smoke do not feel deprived; they just don't smoke. Vegetarians (not that I particularly advocate vegetarianism) don't feel deprived; they just don't eat meat. But even scientists aren't immune to these notions. In commenting on the potential role of high-fat diets in causing arteriosclerosis, Rockefeller University's Dr. Edward Ahrens was quoted by *Time* magazine[10] as saying, "To deny everyone red meat could mean taking away the joy of life unnecessarily"—thereby denying joy to millions of Hindus, Jains, Seventh-day Adventists, and at least 3 million American vegetarians. And Dr. Suzanne Oparel, a scientist at the University of Alabama Medical Center studying the role of salt in causing high blood pressure, was quoted as saying,[11] "Not being able to eat [a lot of] salt is losing one of the pleasures of life."

It's not that hard to reprogram yourself, and it's worth it. Besides lowering your disease susceptibility, the high/low diet will give you better eyesight and hearing at every age; a sharper, more alert problem-solving mind; an increased feeling of well-being; enhanced sexuality and fertility at a more advanced age. True, you may have to give up angel-food cake, but to those for whom sight, sense, and sexuality are less important than angel-food cake, I have nothing to offer. "Let them eat cake!"

You might also remember that there are seven deadly sins: pride, greed, lust, envy, gluttony, anger, and sloth. If you must have a certain measure of sin, I suggest you give up gluttony and accentuate one of the others: lust, for example. Edward Ahrens, Suzanne Oparel, and all you other sinners, give up gluttony and double your lust!

Question 6: What do you think about the Pritikin Program?

Answer: On the positive side, I believe the Nathan Pritikin program is excellent, and with a fairly high order of probability will live up to most of his promises. The program has been disparaged by establishment medicine because Pritikin was not a trained health professional and the documentation in published articles from his center (although appearing in reputable biological journals) lacks good control data; but his evidence is still quite impressive. The Pritikin Program knowledgeably addresses itself to general health problems and to prevention of the killer diseases. The strongest aspect of the program is that it *reprograms* those who go through it, into a more healthful lifestyle. I give it high marks on most counts.

On the questionable side, Pritikin was quite naive on the subject of life extension. He mixed up ideas about disease susceptibility and the basic biology of aging. Also, he was totally against supplementation, which seems to me too severe. Finally, he based his program on what he thought "primitive man" consumed, since that would be what humans are genetically "programmed" to eat, digest, and metabolize. But he erroneously considered primitive man to be represented by the early agricultural societies, or their modern equivalents like the Tarahumara Indians. In fact primitive man was not agricultural man, who has existed for only about 10,000 years, but hunter/gatherer man, who existed for 1½ million years (*Homo erectus* and early *Homo sapiens*).[12] Cereals and grains, which form a high proportion of the Pritikin diet, were only a small part of the diet of Paleolithic hunter/gatherer man. Early man subsisted largely on meat, vegetables, nuts, roots, and fruits, with not much grain or cereals and virtually no dairy products.[13] Despite his naïveté, however, Pritikin lucked in: the wild animals eaten by a hunter/gatherer were only about 5 percent fat, compared with the 35–40 percent body fat of modern cattle. So the important low-fat recommendations of Pritikin do hold up, although his insistence that less than 10 percent of calories be derived from fat seems arbitrary. Much less than 10 percent could be too low, since vitamins A, D, E, and K are fat-soluble and require fats in order to be absorbed from the intestines.

The Pritikin Program is excellent, but ultimately it is not founded upon a thoroughgoing scientific analysis, and can be improved upon.

Question 7: What do you think of the books of Durk Pearson and Sandy Shaw, including their 1-million-copy best-selling book *Life Extension: A Practical Scientific Approach*?

Answer: In *Maximum Life Span* I gave examples showing that gerontology has always been the happy hunting ground for faddists, charlatans, pseudoscientific fringe characters, and just misinformed enthusiasts with ready "cures" for aging. Self-proclaimed "experts" spring up on all sides. Pearson and Shaw are just the latest of this long line of opportunists. The fact that they wrote a best-seller means nothing. Judy Mazel's *The Beverly Hills Diet* was a best-seller and it's probably the most ignorant diet book ever written. The only worse health advice I know of is that of Pearson and Shaw themselves. They argue that it's quite all right to lead a sedentary life and eat a high-fat, sugar-rich diet as long as you consume their formulation of vitamins, chemicals, drugs and nutrient supplements. This is simply nonsense.

Pearson and Shaw are colorful television performers, but scientifically they are a joke. While presenting themselves in person and in writing as "scientists," so far as I know they have never done any regular biological research; never published an article in any reputable biological journal; never been on the faculty of any college, university, or biological research institution. As Dr. Ed Schneider, Deputy Director of the National Institute on Aging, has remarked of the fabulous twosome, "They're fun, but I wish they weren't in aging."

Okay, I can hear you ask: so they have no credentials and misrepresent themselves—but are they totally wrong? After all, they've been *reading* about the field of life extension for years, and they are basically intelligent people. They must know *something*.

True enough, but remember that in preventive medicine and life extension we are for the most part obliged to deal with inferential evidence. Absolute answers are few. The best we can do is assess the degree of probability that different procedures will be effective. Every year several hundred articles are published in the world's scientific literature about, for example, vitamin E. You can shuffle that many articles together and come up with any answer that suits your prejudice. Pearson and Shaw lack the training and experience in science, the constant intimate contact with actual working scientists, the firsthand experience of having even one's own seemingly proved experiments explode into error to *judge* and *analyze* the validity of the enormous body of constantly outpouring literature of biology. What they say is therefore a mixture of fact, fantasy, and fallacy. They are wishful thinkers and self-propagandists who do not really understand the nature of evidence.

The Nature of Evidence

Throughout much of this book I'll be presenting you with evidence followed by recommendations. I want you to be informed and then to make up your own mind, remembering that you should seek guidance from your own doctor but not be dominated by his or her assumption of authority. The frequent bamboozling of the public by health faddists is partly the fault of medicine itself, which has taught people to rely on someone else's judgment, rather than how to examine evidence.

Evidence falls into four categories: testimonial, argumentative ("make the case for"), correlational, and experimental. Testimonial evidence is the principal type coming from the faddists, charlatans, and know-nothings. They will give you a list of people who took the treatment and say it did them good. If the list includes movie stars and professional athletes, so much the better.

Testimonial evidence is highly unreliable. The list never includes people who took the treatment and did *not* receive any benefit. It never includes people who did not take the treatment but got better anyway, spontaneously. And testimonial evidence is abundantly available for almost every claim, from the benefits of Christian Science to experience with spiritualism, herbalism, black magic, faith healing, ghosts, Scientology, UFOs, Bigfoot . . . you name it. If you accept testimonial evidence, you will end up believing just about anything and everything. Testimonial evidence isn't necessarily and inherently wrong, but it's almost impossible to evaluate.

Interestingly enough, establishment medicine is also sometimes guilty of too much reliance on testimonial evidence, but it gives it another name: the "clinical anecdote." Dr. X has seen 35 patients with a certain malady and on the basis of his experience thinks that treating them with drug Z has been beneficial. He has no controls. His opinion represents a subjective guess. He will usually say, "My impression is. . . ." or "My clinical experience is. . . ." and then give the guess. This medical version of testimonial evidence is often wrong.

Argumentative evidence consists in marshaling known facts or experimental results and reasoning from them that something else ought to be so. Exercise, for instance, increases the level of high-density lipoproteins (HDL) in the blood, and these are usually associated with a lower degree of arteriosclerosis, so exercise *ought* to increase resistance to heart attacks. That's a logical argument. But do people who exercise actually experience fewer heart attacks? You cannot just stop with a plausibility argument! You have to test your hypothesis in the real world of what is happening.

The best example of argumentative evidence in gerontology concerns the antioxidants—substances like vitamin E and the mineral selenium. These, it is argued, neutralize the damaging so-called "free radicals" which are by-products of normal metabolism. You can make an excellent case for the idea that free radicals cause aging, and that including antioxidants in the diet ought to retard it. But sad to say, when this glamorous argument is tested, antioxidants do not seem to retard the basic aging process, or only marginally do so. Making a plausible case for something is not enough! Most of the Pearson/Shaw book relies upon this lower-order category of evidence, and upon the testimonial posturing of Pearson and Shaw themselves. Sandy Shaw takes antioxidants and bends horseshoes on television, thus proving that antioxidants retard aging!

The two final types of scientific evidence, and the only really solid ones, are correlational and experimental. Correlation implies that when two things occur together all or most of the time, there may be a direct causal relationship between them, or that perhaps both are caused by some third (not necessarily apparent) phenomenon. Correlation can be seductive, but it's not actual proof. Nations whose citizens eat a high-fat diet generally display a higher incidence of heart disease than low-fat nations. That sounds reasonable, but it's not proof. When the Santa Ana wind blows in California, a lot of people develop hay fever. The wind also causes an elevation in barometric pressure. Does elevated barometric pressure, then, cause hay fever? Of course not. The wind blows pollens around; that's what leads to the hay fever. Barometric pressure is irrelevant. Yet the correlation exists.

In this book we shall be concerned a great deal with correlational evidence. Although it's very useful, we have to be careful. It has been observed on examination of the data from a large number of insurance companies that people who are slightly overweight seem to enjoy a better average survival. This observation is true, but the biological interpretation may be quite different from what the data *seem* to indicate—that is, that it's intrinsically healthful to be slightly overweight. Here's another interpretation, just to illustrate possibilities: perhaps the modern U.S. processed-food and junk-food diet is so poor that the average eater must consume excess calories just to get enough vitamins and essential nutriments to remain healthy and not be *mal*nourished.

The only kind of scientific evidence acceptable as genuine "proof" of a hypothesis is that of repeatable experiment, usually accompanied by what are called "control" data. Under appropriate conditions you do something, and that changes something else. And this something/something-else always happens! When another investigator repeats the experiment on the other side of town or in Uttar Pradesh, the same result obtains. Experiment, if done well, establishes the causal nature of a relationship between two phenomena.

Repeatedly confirmed experiments in my laboratory and in many other laboratories have proved that cutting down calories plus increasing the quality of the diet produces very lean, extremely healthy animals, greatly extends their maximum life spans, and keeps them young both in appearance and in physical and intellectual performance.

Correlation, if extensive enough, and experiment, if well conceived and carried out, constitute good evidence. Argument, or plausibility, constructs are the building blocks of hypothesis. They are good for pointing the investigator in what he hopes is the right direction and for suggesting how to proceed in testing his hypothesis. Testimony and "clinical anecdote" are not very reliable at all.

Having *categorized* the evidence, you have to *interpret* it. What does it mean biologically? American insurance-company statistics seem to indicate that it's better to be slightly overweight; experiments in animals, that it's better to be underweight. The correlational evidence in one instance and experimental evidence in the other are both correct, but they seem contradictory. Why? I've just given you one hint, and we'll be discussing these matters at some length in a later chapter. But when two sets of data both seem valid in fact but directly opposed in meaning, it often turns out in science that both are correct, and you have just not found the right interpretation.

I cannot teach you the fine points of interpretation of scientific evidence. That takes years of training and lots of experience. But you should be able to recognize the *category* of the evidence being presented to you: by me, in discussions with your friends, by other writers or lecturers, by popular health magazines, by newspapers, and of course by the 30-second flash-ad media blitzes. If your barber, hairdresser, or favorite celebrity tells you, "I went to Mexico and they shot me up with XYZ and I feel great. My cancer melted away, my arches rose, my bunions decamped, and lights went on in my head," you can recognize the statement as testimonial evidence.

I hope you will look just as critically at all the evidence in this book. That's your first step toward a superhealthy and extended life.

CHAPTER 2

Gauging Aging: What Is Your Biologic Age?

The Concept of Biomarkers

Tests You Can Do on Yourself

Tests Your Doctor Can Do or Arrange to Have Done

Biomarkers Not Readily Available

How Often to Get the Biomarker Tests Done

The Concept of Biomarkers

We can place animals or people on the high/low diet or some other regimen we think may slow their rates of aging and/or increase their resistance to cancer, heart attack, and other diseases, but how can we tell if it is working? If you take a pill for a headache, you know soon enough. The headache goes away or it doesn't. But if you take six packages of cholestyramine a day to lower your chance of having a heart attack, how do you know if it's working? Are you just going to a lot of trouble—every time you're in a restaurant asking for a glass of water without ice, pouring the packet of orange cholestyramine into the water, and drinking it up like some hypochondriac fool in a movie? How does one know if *preventive* medicine is working, since the sign that it works is that something doesn't happen?

Finding the answer is much easier in short-lived species than in man. A mouse or a rat lives for about 24 months. Its maximum life span is about 36 months. Put fifty of the animals on an experimental regimen and if the average reaches 40 months and the maximum 48 months, the regimen is a success. Aging has been retarded. And by performing autopsies on all that die, and sacrificing some of them at various times before natural death, you can see how the frequency of disease has been influenced. Are there fewer lung cancers among animals on the regimen? Are cancers that do occur postponed until a later time in life?

This kind of information is hard to get in long-lived species. The maximum authenticated life span of rabbits is 15 years; of dogs, 20; cats, 25; horses, 40; chimpanzees, 50; and man, 113 to 119 years. If we put fifty 6-year-old spaniels on what we hope is an antiaging program, we must wait more than 14 years to see if any exceed the maximum life span for dogs. In humans, the time required would be almost totally prohibitive. Not many investigators are willing to initiate a 50-year experiment.

Who could blame them, in their "publish or perish" academic community? True, they might live longer (if they were part of the test group), but academically they'd be dead, and better things would almost certainly be coming along to render their dedication a waste of time, as in the science-fiction story in which the young fellows take off in the primitive slow rocket, heroically resigned to growing old and gray in their cramped craft as it plows through infinite boring space, carrying the legends of man. Finally, just as they—now old men—are heading into the far star system of their youthful dreams, along comes a *new* and infinitely faster starship built 50 years after they had left Earth on their old workhorse. It hurtles by full of blond young ladies and gentlemen tinkling glasses of iced champagne as they come *as tourists* to visit the star system the old fellows have given their lives to reach.

No, thank you—lifetime experiments are out.

Then how do we determine in a long-lived species like man, but in a reasonably short stretch of time, whether our program is working? For that we need "biomarkers," determinants of "functional" age, ways of measuring age besides just how many years our subjects have been alive. To calculate functional age, we can use a battery of different tests whose average values change with age in the population. This battery provides a checkpoint against which to measure an individual relative to the expectation for his years. We can assess his reaction time *and* vision *and* lung capacity *and* a range of other easily measured functions, combine the results, and provide a measure of his functional age. Though he is 60, his biomarker "score" may be that of a 45-year-old man, or a 70-year-old man.

Functional age, you see, is not the same as chronologic age. Since 1850, for example, only one British Prime Minister has died before the age of 70. Seven passed the age of 80. Churchill was over 90 when he died. The Prime Ministers would probably have tested younger on a "functional" age battery than, say, steelworkers of the same chronologic ages. In men, a younger functional age and longer life are associated with a longer period of education, higher income, and more interesting work; for women, the important factors seem to be longer education and physically active leisure time.

What criteria must a useful biomarker satisfy? What should we measure? It's not good enough just to choose anything that changes substantially with age. The biomarker must make biological sense. For example, people eat fewer calories as they grow older, but obviously it would not make good sense to use caloric intake as a measure of a person's "functional" age. Old gluttons would score young on such a test.

Nor is blood cholesterol a good marker for aging! True, it increases with aging in the U.S. population, but in many societies it does not. A good biomarker ought to reflect a universal species characteristic. Even in the United States, the increase in blood cholesterol with age is much greater among the rich, who eat richer food. Blood cholesterol is an excellent marker of susceptibility to arteriosclerotic heart disease, but disease susceptibility, as our study of average survival from 1900 to 1982 has taught us (Figure 1.1, p. 22), is not the same as intrinsic aging.

The best biomarkers of *aging* will reflect changes that are not susceptible to major influence by environmental factors. Exercise enhances cardiovascular fitness and increases average life span, but it has not, perhaps surprisingly, been shown to have much influence on maximum life span in either humans or long-lived strains of animals.

Markers that change with age but are greatly influenced by exercise, physical fitness, occupation, or economic class may confuse the issue. On the other hand, they may, like blood cholesterol, be good markers for disease susceptibility. We shall want to employ them because *the high/low diet influences* both *the aging rate and disease susceptibility.*

In Table 2.1 I've listed a number of human biomarkers, dividing them into those which at least in part reflect true, intrinsic "functional" age; those which may have predictive value for how long you have left to live, whatever your cause of death; and those which reflect either susceptibility to a particular disease or perhaps accelerated aging of one organ system.

Predictive value is important but difficult to achieve. It refers to the ability of the biomarker to indicate on the average how much longer you are likely to live, barring accidents. Having antibodies in your blood that react with your own tissues (autoantibodies) predicts a shorter average survival.[1] Many tests correlate well with chronologic age but have no predictive value at all. For example, graying of hair shows a high correlation with age, but premature graying does not indicate accelerated aging, except perhaps of the hair.

Remember that in *Alice in Wonderland* the White Queen says, "It's a poor sort of memory that only works backward." In the same vein, biomarkers that tell you only how old you are, when of course you know that already, and not how long you may expect to live might be considered of limited practical use. But in fact this is not quite the case. In laboratory animals the high/low diet both extends maximum life span and postpones graying of hair. If

Table 2.1 Three categories of human biomarkers.

1. "Functional" Age
   Vital capacity, breath-holding time, maximal oxygen consumption (VO_2 max), kidney function (creatinine clearance), diameter of pupil of eye, visual accommodation, hearing, level of DHEA hormone in blood, tests of mental function.
2. Predictive Value for Remaining Life Expectancy
   Vital capacity, heart size, systolic blood pressure, hand grip strength, presence or absence of autoantibodies in blood, immune-function tests, reaction time.
3. Disease Susceptibility and/or Segmental Aging
   Glucose-tolerance test; levels of blood cholesterol, LDL, and HDL; systolic blood pressure.

you decelerate aging in the whole body, the hair goes along.

The field of human biomarker testing is now receiving top priority from the National Institute on Aging, and I expect rapid advances in the near future. As you embark upon a life-extension program, stay abreast of this field as much as possible. The present book will give you the background. A more sophisticated account of both human and animal biomarkers of aging may be found in the forthcoming book for professional scientists I have written with Dr. Richard Weindruch, *The Retardation of Aging by Dietary Restriction.*[2,3] †

Despite certain problems with the reliability of biomarkers, we can hope, at least in the future, to use them for all of five purposes: (1) to determine our "functional" age, (2) to see if the rate of change in the biomarkers over a 1–5-year period has been slowed by our antiaging regimen, (3) to predict on the average how long we might expect still to live, (4) to estimate our resistance to the major killer diseases, and (5) to see if what we are doing to increase our resistance to specific diseases is having an effect.

It may be instructive to compare your personal biomarker values against the averages for your age. More important, however, is how your values change from the time you start an antiaging program to 6–12 months later, and every year thereafter. Is the program working?

I'll divide human biomarker tests into two categories: those which you can do yourself, and those which your doctor can do or arrange for you to have done.

† References to scientific studies begin on page 374. An asterisk after a reference number indicates a discussion in the notes which might be of interest to the general reader.

Tests You Can Do on Yourself

These are skin elasticity, the falling-ruler test (for reaction time), static balance, and a simple test for visual accommodation.

Contributing to the development of wrinkles and loose skin (in the neck, for example), loss of skin elasticity begins showing significant changes at about 45 years of age, with large deviations in individual subjects.[4] It reflects deterioration of connective tissue under the surface of the skin. Animal experiments have shown that this type of deterioration can be substantially delayed by the high/low diet.

To perform the elasticity test, pinch the skin on the back of your hand between thumb and forefinger for 5 seconds, then time how long it takes to flatten out completely. Up until 45–50 years of age, only about 5 seconds is required for the skin to flatten out. But by 60 it will on the average require 10–15 seconds; and by 70, 35–55 seconds. Because of the large individual variation, the initial test should not be taken too seriously. You are more interested in the rate of change thereafter. Figure 2.2 will give you an idea of how rapidly skin elasticity does change after age 45. This is a good test if you start the high/low dietary regimen in mid or late life. It won't show much change at the younger ages whether you are on the diet or not.

The falling-ruler test measures your reaction time—that is, how long it takes to respond to an outside stimulus, like that red Pontiac which almost clipped you in Chapter 1. Buy a thin 18 inch wooden ruler. Let a friend suspend the ruler vertically by holding it at the top. Hold the thumb and middle finger of your own right hand 3½ inches apart, equidistant from the 18-inch mark on the ruler. As your friend drops the ruler without warning, you must catch it between your two fingers. Your "score" is whatever inch mark you catch it at. Do this three times and take an average. If you catch it at the 3", 6", and 6-inch marks, your "score" is $(3+6+6)/3 = 5$. On the average, the score decreases progressively from the 11-inch mark at age 20 to the 6-inch mark at age 60.

The third test is that of static balance. How long can you stand on one leg with your eyes closed before falling over? (As a matter of standardization: left leg if you are right-handed, right leg if left-handed.) This test is clearly the best among the do-it-yourself biomarker measurements. On the average, a fully 100-percent decline occurs from age 20 to age 80. Most young people can hold a one-legged eyes-closed stand for 30 seconds or more, whereas few old persons can hold the pose longer than a few seconds.

Perform the test either barefoot or wearing an ordinary low-heeled shoe. Stand on a hard surface (not on a rug) with both feet together, close your eyes, and lift your foot about 6 inches off the ground, bending your knee at about a 45-degree angle. Don't move or jiggle your foot; just stand on it with your eyes closed. How many seconds can you stand this way before you have to open your eyes or move your foot to avoid falling over? Have a friend close by to catch you in case you do in fact fall over. Do the test three times and take an average. Values for different ages are illustrated in Figure 2.1.

The fourth and final test estimates the effect of age on visual accommodation, although it should not replace the more accurate visual tests your eye doctor can do. At 21, an average person can bring a newspaper to within 4 inches of his eyes before the regular-sized print starts blurring; at 30 years, to within 5½ inches; at 40, no closer than 9 inches; at 50, 15 inches; and at 60 years, about 39 inches. Do this either without glasses or with glasses corrected for distance—that is, not reading glasses. It's not how well you can actually read the print (You may have astigmatism) that counts, but at what point it suddenly starts to blur.

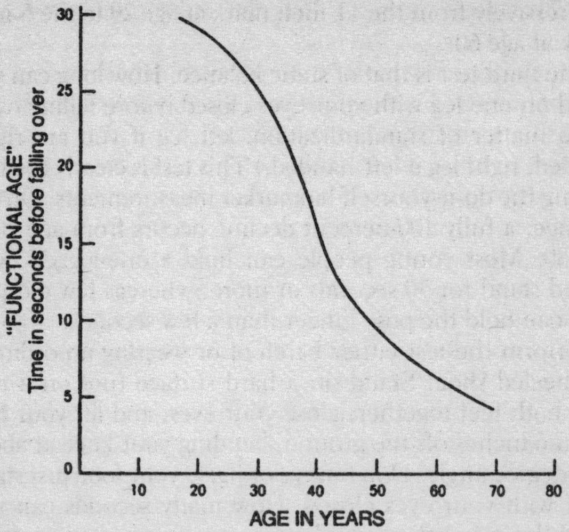

Figure 2.1 Static balance as a biomarker of age. Close eyes, stand on one leg (left if you are right-handed), don't move foot. How long before you fall over?
Score = average of 3 trials

Tests Your Doctor Can Do or Arrange to Have Done

Probably the best biomarker now available is the measurement of lung function called "vital capacity." This is the amount of air that can be taken in and breathed out in one very deep breath. It reflects the integrity of the whole respiratory system, the muscles, their central-nervous-system control mechanisms, and the elasticity of the lungs. The vital capacity, or VC, of an individual must be adjusted for his or her height in inches. How VC decreases with age is illustrated in Figure 2.2A.

VC has been the most powerful single predictor of subsequent life span in the large, very famous, and still-ongoing study involving most of the population of Framingham, Massachusetts. People with low VC for their age did not live as long on the average as those with high VC, and as we have learned, predictability is the most important indicator that a biomarker is measuring true "functional" age. Furthermore, in the Framingham study there was no difference between athletic and sedentary individuals. This means that the VC is not much influenced by physical fitness—an advantage in assessing the basic process of aging, since physical fitness influences average but probably not maximum life span.

Two measures of heart function often used as biomarkers seem to be indicators more of physical fitness and resistance to several diseases than of the basic aging rate. The first is the "maximum oxygen consumption," also known as VO_2 max. It measures the ability of the cardiovascular system to respond to stress. This ability declines with age and/or poor physical fitness, reflecting a lower maximal attainable heart rate combined with a diminished capacity of the tissues to extract oxygen quickly from the blood bathing them.

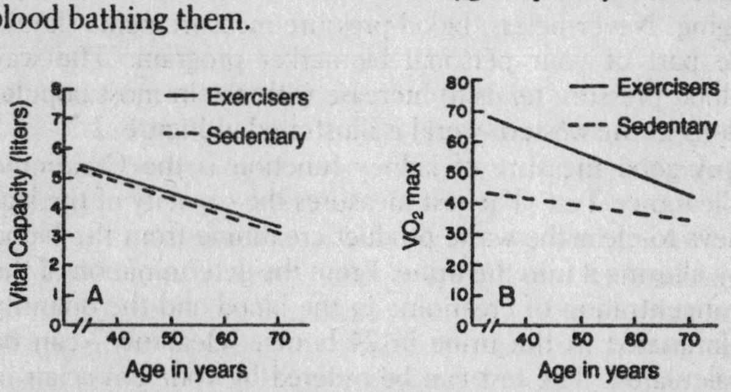

Figure 2.2 Effect of age on vital capacity (A) and on maximum possible oxygen consumption (VO_2 max) (B) in men who do frequent aerobic exercise, and in sedentary men (adapted from H. Suominen *et al., Scandinavian Journal of Social Medicine,* Suppl. 14, 1980, p. 225).

To measure your VO_2 max, your physician will have you exercise at peak rate on a treadmill or stationary bicycle. The amount of oxygen you use per minute is then divided by your body weight. How this ratio varies with age for sedentary men and for those in good physical condition is shown in Figure 2.2B. We see quite clearly by comparing the A and B panels of Figure 2.2 that whereas the vital capacity (VC) is relatively independent of physical fitness, the maximum oxygen consumption, or VO_2 max, is greatly influenced by it. For middle-aged sedentary men, the average VO_2 max is about 45 ml. of oxygen per minute for every kilogram (2.4 pounds) of body weight; for those men on a good aerobic-exercise program, who jog 15 to 30 miles per week, the value is about 58; for world-class athletes, it's about 75. Because VO_2 max is so greatly influenced by physical fitness, it is a good biomarker for *age* only if the value for the person being tested is compared with control values from people who do the same amount of exercise.

Systolic blood pressure is a second cardiovascular biomarker. Individual variation is great, and the influence of hereditary background, degree of stress, and especially diet (See Chapter 5) makes it less than optimal as a marker for aging. Nevertheless, blood-pressure measurements should be part of your personal biomarker program. The way blood pressure tends to increase with age in most populations in the western world is illustrated in Figure. 2.3.

A good measure of kidney function is the Creatinine Clearance Test. The test measures the capacity of the kidneys to clear the waste product creatinine from the blood by filtering it into the urine. From the determination of the concentration of creatinine in the blood and the quantity eliminated in the urine in 24 hours, "clearance" can be calculated. The test can be ordered by your physician in any hospital or clinical laboratory. The steep decline of creatinine clearance after age 30 is illustrated in Figure 2.4. The test is a useful biomarker.

A good marker of your blood-sugar metabolism is the Glucose Tolerance Test. When you take glucose (sugar) by

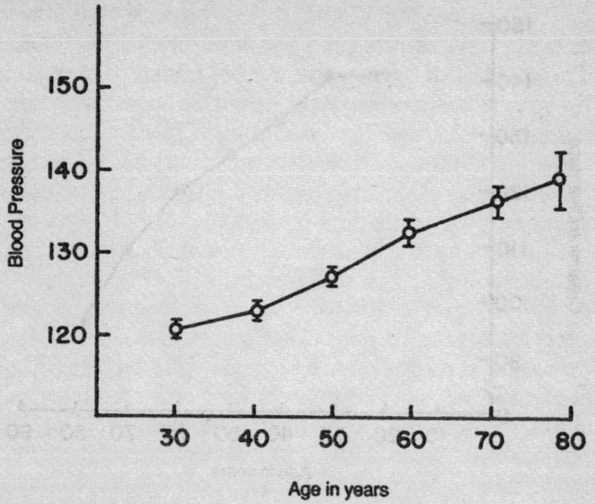

Figure 2.3 Effect of age on blood pressure. (adapted from J. D. Tobin, in *Aging: A Challenge to Science and Society, Vol. 1. Biology,* ed. D. Danon *et al.* [New York: Oxford University Press, 1981]).

mouth, your body absorbs it from your intestines and your level of blood sugar rises. Your pancreas then secretes the hormone insulin, which stimulates the utilization or storage of the sugar. With age these pathways become less effective;[5] instead of being used or stored, the sugar remains in the blood.

The Glucose Tolerance Test consists in measuring the level of blood sugar 2 hours after you have taken a standard amount of sugar on an empty stomach in the morning. This 2-hour level is very high in diabetics, and is higher in older "normal" persons than in young normal persons. Examples of the rise and decline of blood sugar (glucose) are given in Figure 2.5 and clearly document the age-related differences. But physical fitness also influences glucose tolerance. A fit person will generally have a lower overall

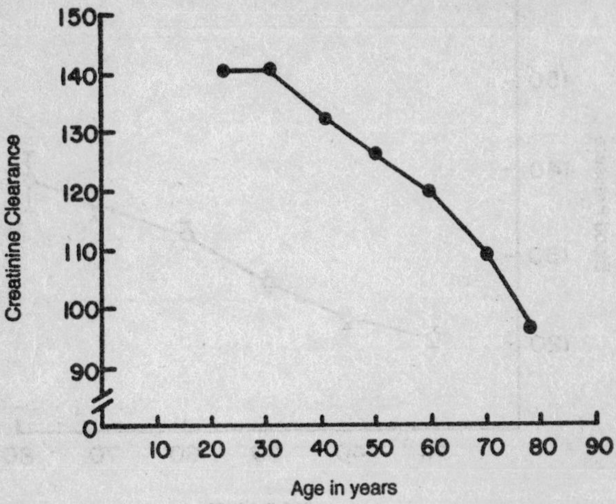

Figure 2.4 The effect of age on the important measure of kidney function known as Creatinine Clearance (adapted from J. W. Rowe *et al.*, *Journal of Gerontology*, 31:155, 1976).

curve and 2-hour value than a sedentary person of the same age.

Some of the biomarkers listed above are not very useful at young ages because the rates of change do not accelerate until late middle age. Fortunately, tests of vision and hearing are useful at young ages.

Visual accommodation is a good biomarker up to about age 50, after that not so good because the decline levels off. Accommodation—the ability of the lens of the eye to change its shape—is measured in units called "diopters." It declines in straight-line fashion from about 13 diopters at age 13 to 1–2 diopters at age 50, then remains relatively constant for the rest of your life. I outlined a simple do-it-yourself accommodation test using a newspaper, but your eye doctor can measure the diopters much more exactly.

Beginning at about age 30, a progressive decline develops

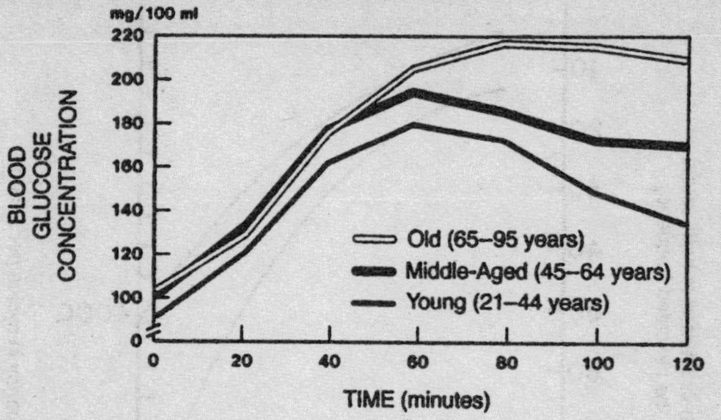

Figure 2.5: Glucose Tolerance Test curves for three age groups of normal individuals. Levels of blood glucose are shown at different time intervals after ingestion of a standard amount of glucose in the morning on an empty stomach.

in hearing ability. The hearing threshold at a fixed frequency is one of the best ways of estimating this decline, and indeed has a mild predictive value for later life expectancy. The threshold test measures how loud a sound must be at a certain frequency for you to be able to hear it at all (Figure 2.6). At 4,000 cycles per second, an 18–24-year-old person can hear a sound as low in intensity as 14 decibels, whereas a 60–70-year-old person generally requires 30–50 decibels. At 8,000 cycles per second the young person requires about 18 decibels, whereas the older person needs 50–80; this is the best frequency to show the age-related loss.

The only immune-function biomarker tests that your physician can readily order are those for antiself antibodies, called "autoantibodies." This class of protein molecules react deleteriously with the body's own tissues. Particularly useful are the tests for antibodies to DNA, the well-known "double helix" of hereditary material coiled in each cell, and for the rheumatoid factor. Positive test results increase with age, up to 50–70 percent in advanced age. People with autoantibodies in their blood have a

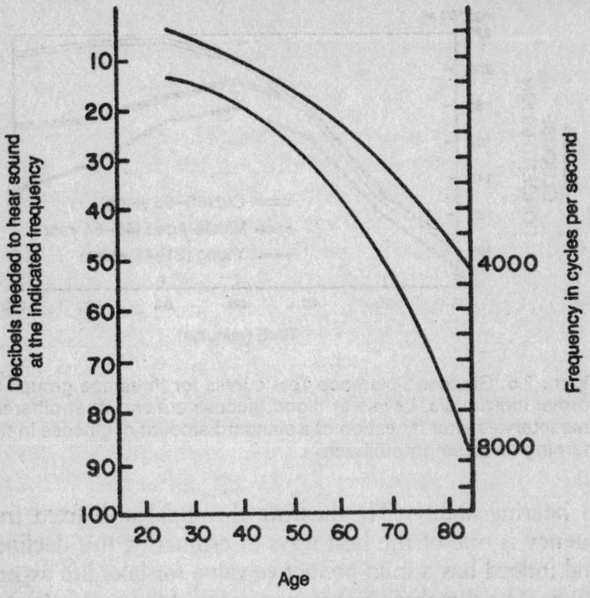

Figure 2.6 Auditory threshold in decibels in relation to age in women, at sound frequencies of 4000 and 8000 cycles per second (adapted from J. F. Corse, in *Lectures on Gerontology, Vol. 1, part B., Biology of Aging*, ed. A. Viidik [New York: Academic Press, 1982], p. 441).

shorter life expectancy than those who don't, as was shown by a study involving 10,000 individuals in the town of Busselton, Australia.[6] In animals on the high/low diet, the frequency of autoantibodies is greatly diminished with age, indeed to the point of their being wholly absent.[7]

When and How Often to Get the Biomarker Tests Done

Have as many of these tests done as possible, either before or a few months after starting the high/low dietary antiaging, health-enhancement program. Of course, the do-it-yourself tests are easy. The other first-time-around tests include a blood-pressure determination, the Glucose Tolerance Test, and the tests for the presence of autoantibodies, creatinine clearance, and the more strictly disease-related biomarkers like blood cholesterol and HDL and LDL (part of the blood-fat picture, which I will describe more fully in Chapter 5). You can delay running the other biomarker tests until you are a few months into the program. Table 2.2 outlines my suggested biomarker battery, along with average values for three age groups. Of course "average" is not good enough, and my program is designed to make you much better than average, either by altering your values toward those of a younger age group ("Rejuvenation" is possible for some biomarkers), or at least by slowing the age-related rate of decline.

There are a number of other proved or promising biomarkers, but as many of these are available only in research laboratories, I have not included them here except for the DHEA hormone levels (Table 2.2), a very promising test that may become more generally available soon. In the next 2 to 3 years, I shall be hosting the First International Biomarker Workshop, to be held at the UCLA School of Medicine. At that workshop, scientists from many laboratories will gather to try to select and standardize the best biomarker battery for human application. Many tests not now readily available may become more widespread following the workshop and thanks to the growing popularity of the life-extension movement.

Table 2.2 Biomarker battery and average values for three age groups.

Test		Age Group 20–30	40–50	60–70	Units and/or Comments
Skin elasticity		0–1	2	15	seconds
Reaction time (falling-ruler test)		12	8	5	inches
Static balance		28	18	4	seconds
Visual accommodation (self-test)		4.5	12	39	inches
Vital capacity		5.5	4.5	3.5	liters
VO_2 max:	exerciser	70	60	48	liters/min.
	sedentary	44	40	38	liters/min.
Systolic blood pressure:	men	130	138	148	mm. Hg
	women	120	136	155	mm. Hg
Creatinine clearance		140	126	112	liters/24 hrs.
Glucose tolerance		118	127	140	mg./100 ml. at 2 hrs.
Blood cholesterol:	men	175	210	213	mg./100 ml.
	women	171	203	231	mg./100 ml.
HDL:	men	45	48	50	mg./100 ml.
	women	55	60	60	mg./100 ml.
LDL:	men	110	135	145	mg./100 ml.
	women	108	125	147	mg./100 ml.
Visual accommodation		13	2	1–2	diopters
Hearing threshold at 4,000 Hz		4	16	30–50	decibels
at 8,000 Hz		15	24	50–80	decibels
Autoantibodies:	men	10	35	50	% of population
	women	10	45	65	having (+) test
DHEA hormone level	men	3400	1800	900	ng./ml. plasma
	women	2200	1100	800	ng./ml. plasma

CHAPTER 3

Scientific Background of the High/Low Diet: The Animal Evidence

Effects of the High/Low Diet on Life Span
Effects of the High/Low Diet on Disease
Effects of the High/Low Diet on Biomarkers
The High/Low Diet and Brain Function
Summary

This will be the toughest chapter of the book. But it does contain the critical evidence for the high/low diet, and even so presents only a brief survey of a much larger body of information. If you find the going too slow, skip to the next chapter and come back to this one later. But do come back. Do *not* simply rely on my authority.

Before we escalate to humans, it's important that you be convinced beyond any reasonable doubt that in experimental animals the high/low diet works dramatically at slowing the aging process and preventing disease.

We scientists now have hard evidence: not testimonial evidence, not clinical anecdote, not "make the case" evidence based on plausibility arguments, and not even correlational evidence—but hard, well-controlled *experimental evidence* that a high/low diet will greatly extend average and maximum life spans, postpone the times of onset and decrease the frequencies of most or all of the "diseases of aging," maintain biomarkers at levels younger than the chronologic age, maintain sexual potency into advanced age, and delay deterioration of the brain.

In 1935 Dr. Clive McCay at Cornell University first demonstrated that if rats from the time of weaning were fed a calorically restricted but healthful diet supplemented with vitamins and minerals, they would live remarkably longer than normally fed rats.[1] By 1,000 days of age, all the normally fed rats had died, but most of the calorie-restricted ones were still alive and active. Their growth rate and body size had been retarded by the severe restrictive regimen, but in other ways they seemed superhealthy. If they were allowed a full diet at 1,000 days, they actually began to grow again. The females were sexually active and could reproduce far beyond the normal age. And we now know that chronologically old high/low-diet male animals have higher testosterone levels than normally fed old males.[2]

The maximum life spans of McCay's restricted rats reached out to 1,800 days—equivalent to 150 to 180 human years. Of course McCay's regimen could hardly be applied to humans. The severity of restriction maintained since the time of weaning kept the rats from reaching full body size, and would do the same for humans. But the experiment definitely proved that maximum life span can be greatly extended! The rate of aging is not irretrievably fixed by some unyielding law of nature, as people had tended to think until then. And if maximum life span can be extended at all, perhaps it can be extended more easily, or with a less undesirable side effect on the size of the individual. This has proved to be the case.[3*]

In recent years the work of McCay and other early pioneers has been confirmed, extended, modified, and carried forward by investigators at the Sloan-Kettering Cancer Research Institute in New York, the University of Texas at San Antonio, the Gerontology Research Center of the National Institute on Aging in Baltimore, the University of Hull in England, the University of Sydney in Australia, my own laboratory at the University of California in Los Angeles, and still elsewhere. A great body of careful documentation now exists about the effects of the high/low diet on animals. I can only touch on the highlights here. For detailed information, see the forthcoming book for professional biologists by Dr. Richard Weindruch and me, *The Retardation of Aging by Dietary Restriction*.[4]

Effects of the High/Low Diet on Life Span

We'll consider two broad categories: caloric restriction begun during childhood, and that begun at various stages in adult life after full growth has been reached.

Look first at the survival information for mice and rats on the high/low diet. Figure 3.1A is from a study conducted in my laboratory at the UCLA School of Medicine. The life extension achieved here is especially important because we were dealing with naturally long-lived strains of mice, not strains rendered short-lived by hereditary susceptibility in young adulthood to some particular disease. The fully fed mice displayed a maximum life span of close to 38 months. That by itself is quite long for a mouse. At 10-percent caloric restriction the supplemented diet extended the maximum life span to 43 months, and at 50-percent restriction (corresponding to something close to a 1,500-calorie high/low diet in a human male of average size) to more than 54 months (corresponding to a living human who could remember the Mexican War, the Alamo, and the Gold Rush!).

Figure 3.1B expresses life extension in another but equally fascinating way. Starting at any age, the bars show *remaining life expectancies* for fully fed compared with high/low-diet rats. Those animals represented in the first bar, 0 to 100 days of age, could expect to live another 625 days if fully fed, but *1,125 days if on the diet*. At the 1,000-to-1,100-day bar, *all* the fully fed animals had died, but the diet ones could still expect 320 days of life. And a few of the vigorous and venerable diet rats lived their amazing 1,800 days.

These experiments with naturally long-lived strains of animals have been confirmed many times.[5]* It's as though, referring to Figure 1.1 (p. 22) for humans, curve C were being converted into curve D. And with short-lived strains even more impressive results can be obtained. Here one is not only retarding the rate of aging but inhibiting the development of those diseases which render these strains short-lived. In such strains (and for hereditary reasons you might well belong to the human equivalent of such strains), average life spans have been more than doubled and maximum life spans extended three- to fourfold.[6]

Restriction since time of weaning is not a feasible option for human use because it decreases ultimate body size. But fortunately, the high/low diet prolongs life span and retards aging even if begun in adult life. Studies at the University of Texas have shown that restriction begun at 6 months of age (young adulthood) in the rat is *just as effective* in extending life span as weaning-initiated restriction.[7] Using the intermittent (every-other-day) feeding technique in

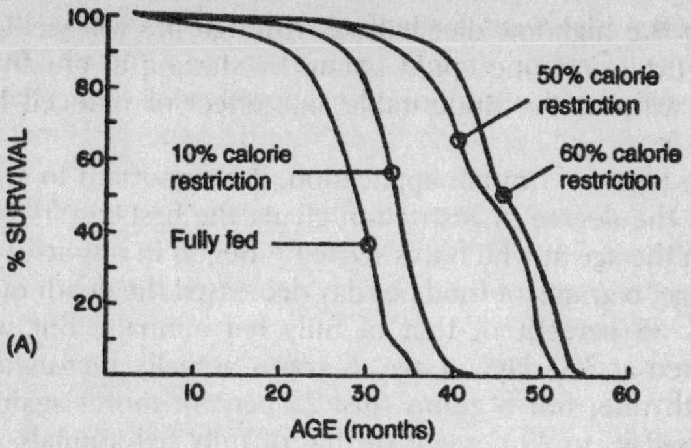

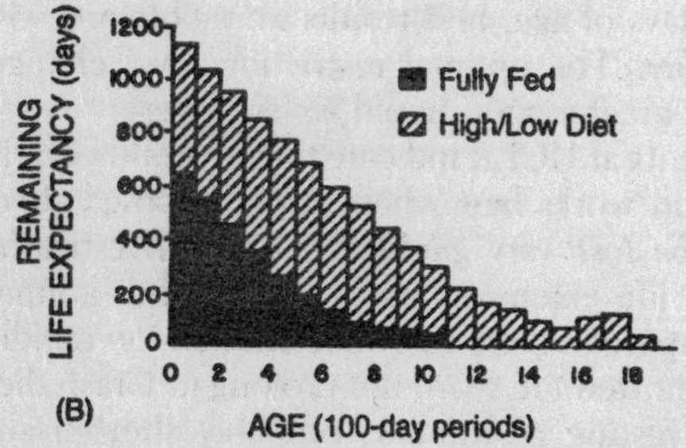

Figure 3.1: Life Extension by the High/Low Diet in Mice (A) and Rats (B). Mouse data are expressed as survival curves, with average survival going from 28 months in fully fed out to 47 months in the most restricted group. Rat survivals (B) are expressed as remaining life expectancy at any age. Thus, at 600 days of age, fully fed rats can expect to live another 120 days; high/low-diet rats, another 700 days (adapted from R. Weindruch *et al.*, *Journal of Nutrition*, 116:641, 1986, and M. Ross, in *Nutrition and Aging*, ed. M. Winick [New York: John Wiley & Sons, 1976], p. 43).

rats, and beginning at either 11 or 18 months of age (equivalent to mid-adulthood and fairly late middle age in humans), scientists at the National Institute on Aging obtained significant average and maximum life-span extensions—from 20 to 40 percent if begun at 11 months;[8] and *in short-lived strains* restriction imposed *even late in life* greatly extended the life span.[9] Roughly speaking, beginning the high/low diet halfway through life will yield half the extension one could obtain by starting in childhood, but without the undesirable side effect of reduced body size.[10]

In terms of human application, it is important to realize that the degree of restriction giving the best results varies with the age at which it is started.[11] Begun in rats at 70 days of age, 6 grams of food per day decreased the death rate to only 35 percent of that of fully fed animals. But when started at 300 days of age, 6 grams actually *increased* the death rate, but 8 grams (just 25 percent more) again *decreased* it, to 49 percent of that of fully fed animals. And starting at 365 days of age, best results were obtained with 10 grams per day. The optimal restriction level changes with age, and at greater ages should be less severe.

Our experiments at UCLA indicate that in adulthood the caloric restriction works best when slowly imposed. *Body weight should be lost very gradually.* Early investigators failed to obtain life extension starting with adult animals because they imposed severe caloric restriction too rapidly. That seems to shorten life span, not prolong it. Crash diets and prolonged fasting in humans probably shorten survival. Your body needs time to adapt, even to a more healthful lifestyle.

A final important observation about high/low diets and life span is that the amount of weight to be gradually lost depends on the "set point." The set point is the characteristic weight for the particular strain of mouse or rat, or the individual human. It is the weight toward which one naturally drifts if he neither under- nor overeats. Set point experiments have been done at several major laboratories.[12] In the strain of mouse fetchingly called "ob/ob," all mice are enormously fat, for hereditary reasons, and their life span is short. When placed on a high/low diet, they lose weight until they stabilize at about what a fully fed mouse of a *non*obese strain normally weighs. They are not at all lean in comparison with the usual high/low diet mouse, but they are lean *in relation to their own body pattern.* And *they live 50 to 85 percent longer!* So what counts is not the absolute weight or the absolute degree of leanness, but the weight relative to the set point of the strain or individual. This finding will be very important when we come to human applications of the high/low diet.

Effects of the High/Low Diet on Disease

All forms of chronic disease and "diseases of aging" are (in most cases dramatically) postponed in time of onset and decreased in overall frequency by the high/low diet. Let's look at a few main categories of disease.

Cancer

In the very first pioneering studies, caloric restriction of rats led to a significant delay in development of all cancers.[13] Soon, a second study by another investigator, using mice this time, confirmed that restriction substantially reduced susceptibility to cancer of the breast, lung, liver, skin, and subcutaneous tissues.[14] Lung tumors occurred in 58 percent of fully fed animals of one mouse strain, but in only 32 percent of high/low-diet animals. The incidence of breast cancer was knocked right down to zero in this and also in a much later, modern study.[15] And sharp reduction in breast cancer was confirmed in still another independent investigation.[16] Tumors of the testes,[17] pituitary gland, and lymphatic system[18] are all reduced in frequency by the high/low diet.

Although less dramatically, these effects also hold for animals first placed on the diet in adulthood. In studies in my own laboratory, putting mice on the diet at 12 months of age (equal to 30–35-year-old human) reduced lung-cancer incidence from 16 percent in fully fed animals down to 6 percent.[19] And for all types of tumors, the age at which they occurred was from 2 to 5 months later in dietary than in fully fed animals (or 5 to 13 *years* later in terms of human life span).

Many more studies could be cited, but they all give the same message. The high/low diet is a powerful and effective cancer-prevention and cancer-delaying regimen. If there is a high incidence of cancer in your family, particularly breast cancer, you should certainly consider being on this diet. But to keep some cancer-stricken patient from going off on a foolish self-imposed starvation tangent, I should add that there is no evidence that caloric restriction will help cure cancer once that cancer has occurred, only that it will help prevent the cancer in the first place.

Diseases of the Heart, Blood Vessels, and Kidneys

Here again we can start with McCay.[20] He noted that the calcification occurring with age in the hearts of normal rats was much less severe in high/low-diet animals. Furthermore, their pulse rates, normally a rapid 340 beats per minute, were only 240 beats per minute. Other early studies showed that a 33-percent restriction in calories markedly decreased the occurrence of diseases of the heart, blood vessels, and kidneys.[21] High/low diets lower blood pressure in animals in which it is high,[22] diminish the thickening of blood-vessel walls that occurs with age,[23] and reduce the severity of arteriosclerosis.[24]

Most mammals, including rats and humans, gradually develop kidney disease with age. They lose protein in the urine and sustain a progressive scarring of the multiple small filtration sacs in the kidney, which purify the blood. In humans this lowers the creatinine clearance, which, as we saw in the last chapter, can serve as a biomarker of aging. The high/low diet markedly slows this progressive and deleterious kidney change.[25]

Other Age-Related Diseases

The immune system functions to protect the body. It manufactures antibodies and killer cells against invading bacteria or viruses, and with its armamentarium seeks to recognize and eliminate aberrant cells (like cancer cells) arising from mutation or cellular injury. But it must distinguish "self" from "nonself," and destroy only the latter!

With age the normal immune response declines markedly, down to only 10–30 percent of its youthful capacity. The immune machinery becomes perverted, the self/nonself recognition markers failing to work well. And the destructive power of the immune system gradually turns against the body itself, leading to "autoimmunity," an antiself destructive process mediated by an immune system gone haywire.[26]

There is compelling evidence that this decline in normal response and upswing in self-destructive autoimmunity can be greatly reduced by the high/low diet.[27] And the diet even retards formation of antibrain-reactive antibodies[28]—an intriguing finding if you want to keep your wits about you.[29]*

Important in disease control, the immune system is also one of the "pacemakers" of aging, one of the main systems through which changes programmed at a more fundamental level exert their effect, resulting in what we recognize as aging. It's doubly encouraging, therefore, from the standpoints of both disease susceptibility and basic aging, to know that *the integrity of the immune system can be maintained by the high/low diet*.

Osteoporosis is yet another age-related and troublesome disease, widespread in humans. Its hallmark is loss of bone calcium, with weakened bone structure and tendency to easy fractures. Here too the high/low diet may be protective. In animals on calorie-restricted diets beginning in adulthood, the ratio of the strength of the thighbones to body weight is much greater than for fully fed controls.[30] We know that the hormone secreted by the parathyroid glands influences bone and calcium metabolism. And in normal animals we know that the blood levels of this hormone increases with age, and even more so in those animals which sustain the greatest age-related bone loss. However, in animals *on the high/low diet*, *there is no marked increase in this hormone with age and little or no senile bone loss.*[31]

Effects of the High/Low Diet on Biomarkers

For purely practical reasons, biomarkers used for studying aging in animals are different from those applied to humans. It's not easy to estimate vital capacity in a mouse because he won't give you his last breath, and he certainly can't stand on one leg, or tell you at what distance the newsprint is blurring. On the other hand, you cannot sacrifice a human in order to snatch his connective tissue or his spleen, look at the microscopic structure of his kidney, or remove the lens of his eye. So the biomarker batteries are different, although they may overlap (Both mice and men can be tested for intelligence, blood pressure, glucose tolerance, and other factors).

Perhaps the most striking example of slowdown in the age-related change of a biomarker comes from work done at the U.C.L.A. Medical School using mice from our high/low-diet colony.[32] The study concerned a protein in the lens of the eye called gamma-crystallin. This is a nonturnover protein. Once full growth is attained, no more gamma-crystallin is formed. If any deteriorates and is lost, it is not replaced. In that sense it resembles brain or heart cells, which, once formed, are not broken down and replaced in the normal course of life. What you have now is what you got early on, and that's all!

In the eye lenses of both mice and humans, the amount of gamma-crystallin declines progressively with age, sometimes in conjunction with cataract formation. We compared the amounts of the protein in the lenses of fully fed and high/low-diet mice at 2 months, 11 months, and 30 months of age. The results were impressive. The gamma-crystallin was markedly decreased by 11 months in the fully fed mice, and was wholly gone by 30 months, whereas in the diet mice the loss was much less at 11 months, and some was still present even at the advanced age of 30 months. Thus, the aging of this nonturnover protein was remarkably retarded by the high/low diet, and cataract formation was inhibited.

Another useful biomarker is "age pigment." Insoluble brown granules accumulate with age in cells of the heart, brain, adrenal gland, and liver. The pigment comes from damaged membrane material within the cells. The high/low diet will greatly retard its accumulation.[33]

Collagen, which makes up 30 percent of the body's total protein, is the main constituent of connective tissue, the tissue that holds the organs together. Your Achilles tendon, just above your heel, is almost pure collagen. The cartilage in your joints is mainly collagen. A nonturnover protein like gamma-crystallin, collagen forms itself into long parallel fibers. With age these fibers undergo what is called cross-linking. Metabolic products with two hyperactive chemical groups, like a pair of hands, grab onto one collagen molecule with one group and another with the other group, and hold them together. Obviously, having your collagen molecules handcuffed like this is not so good. But aging of collagen is substantially retarded by a high/low diet.[34] This finding is especially important because cross-linking occurs not only in collagen but in other molecules, including DNA, the hereditary material.

Other biomarker tests, and there are many, follow the same positive pattern. The high/low diet prevents the usual rise in blood insulin and blood sugar that occurs with age. It prevents the insulin-resistance of the tissues that develops with age.[35] It delays degenerative changes that take place in skeletal muscles with age.[36] It prevents the age-related rise in serum cholesterol in rats and holds the blood's LDL and HDL factors at a younger level.[37] And it greatly delays the age-related loss in sensitivity of the body's fat cells to several hormones.[38, 39]*

The youthful preservation of these and many other

biomarker values by the high/low diet program is *unequaled (and not even approached) by any other form of antiaging or preventive health therapy.*

The High/Low Diet and Brain Function

In normal aging, fully fed animals (and also humans) undergo a considerable decline in what are called "dopamine receptors" on brain cells. Concerned with passage of the nerve impulse, these receptors are necessary for motor behavior, like walking, running, or swimming. The diminished ability with age to perform tasks that require coordination and muscle strength comes in part from gradual loss of these receptors. A *high/low diet greatly slows the loss.* The concentration of receptors in 24-month-old high/low-diet rats is the same as that of 3-to-6-month-old fully fed rats.[40]

Nerve cells in the brain have projections on their surfaces called "dendritic spines," which are used to communicate with other nerve cells across the spaces between cells. With age these spines flatten out and become nubby. This change seems greatly inhibited by the high/low diet, even if not begun until 19 months of age in rats (= 55 years old in a human).[41]

In the "passive avoidance test" for intelligence, a mouse or rat is placed in a lighted chamber connected to a dark chamber. Instinctively, the animal runs immediately into the dark chamber, to hide. But in the test, when he enters the dark chamber he receives an electric shock. If you test him again in 24 hours, he will (because he remembers the shock) hesitate longer before instinct propels him into the safe gloom. Younger mice, with better memories, hesitate longer before entering. Mice 38 months old that have been on the high/low diet since youth perform in this test as though they were only 24 months old.[42] Recent studies at the National Institute on Aging indicate that caloric restriction very favorably influences the ability of rats to navigate a complicated maze.[43] Dieting rats that were 30 months old performed *as well as* 6-month-old fully fed rats, and *much better than* 22-month-old fully fed rats. High/low-diet mice from our UCLA colony also show enhanced skill at solving maze problems.[44] The high/low diet preserves brainpower!

Summary

Beyond any reasonable doubt, a high/low diet extends maximum life span in animals, retards their rate of aging, and inhibits and delays the onset of the major "diseases of aging." It holds the biomarkers younger than the chronologic age of the animals, and it keeps their brains functioning at a younger age level. Not only do the animals live a lot longer, they live younger! And these are not the fuzzy concoctions of fringe philosophers and faddists, but evidence from the world's top scientific laboratories engaged in aging research.

We are now ready to consider human application.

CHAPTER 4

The High/Low Diet for Humans: First Principles

As we have seen, much highly specific and sophisticated information has accumulated about the effects of a high/low diet in animals. I am convinced that with a high order of probability the same kind of diet will produce the same beneficial results in humans. It will retard the rate of aging whenever in life it is begun, and even "rejuvenate" the functions of some (not all) of our bodily systems. It will greatly extend maximum as well as average life span, and cut disease susceptibility by at least half. My application of the high/low diet principles to humans is based in part upon extrapolation from years of extensive work with nutritional modulation of the aging process in animal populations, and upon data from a few human studies. But just going on a hit-or-miss long-term low-calorie diet would not work at all. It might actually shorten life span.

Parameters of the High/Low Diet for Humans

The high/low diet program calls for gradual weight reduction over a period of 4 to 6 years, avoiding the danger of *mal*nutrition inherent in any other weight-loss regimen that continues this long. The plan is to proceed until you reach, stabilize, and remain at a weight 10 to 25 percent below your personal "set point."

The eventual degree of leanness required depends on where you begin. When fully fed, the genetically "ob/ob" obese mice I described in Chapter 3 (p. 60) weigh on the average, 60–65 grams. A fully fed genetically normal mouse weighs only 35 to 45 grams. If we put normal mice on a severe calorie-restriction program and cut their weights down to 25 gm., their life spans will be greatly extended. On the high/low diet an "ob/ob" mouse will not become obese but will level off at about 40 grams. It will have a very extended life span, because it is weighing in at less than its set point, even though it weighs as much as or more than a normal fully fed mouse. Below their set point, normal mice look razor-thin; "ob/ob" mice, below *their* set point, just look normal, or even slightly obese.

Heredity and early feeding experience fix a set point for each individual, which is then defended by adaptive processes within the body. These involve the central nervous system, the levels of metabolic enzymes, the amount of "brown fat" in the body (a kind of furnace fat, for generating heat), and alterations in insulin and thyroid-gland metabolism. Unless he or she grossly overeats or undereats, each person tends to maintain a particular characteristic weight. This may be considerably above or below the actual "average weight" for that person's height. The body defends its set point by cleverly shifting the efficiency of its metabolic machine. Take in fewer calories and your body increases its metabolic efficiency; up your intake and your efficiency decreases. This tends to stabilize your weight, although your set point can gradually change (increasing with age, for example).

"Efficiency" refers to the percentage of your caloric intake that goes into making *usable* energy. The rest is simply burned off as wasted heat. "Usable" means providing energy for manufacturing proteins and other bodily constituents, doing muscular work, or performing fundamental processes like transporting calcium or sodium atoms across cell membranes. Normally metabolic efficiency is about 33 percent. The top efficiency that we can possibly reach is 50 percent. We can approach this upper limit by holding our weight 10 to 25 percent below our "natural weight," or set point. Like an "ob/ob" mouse on the high/low diet, one can be well below one's personal set point and still not be razor-thin.

A study of 54 farmers in Java revealed that metabolic efficiency, expressed as work done in relation to energy intake, was actually 80 percent *higher for the 10 farmers with the lowest intake* (1,535 calories) than for those with the highest intake (2,382 calories).[1] Heights and weights did not differ, and the two groups performed the same amount of work. The basal metabolism of the farmers on the lower intake was about half that of the rest. They had "adapted" to the lower intake and were *metabolically more efficient*.

A major secret of health and longevity is to be always below your set point, maintaining yourself on a high-enough-quality diet that you are not deficient in any essentials, and to operate at maximum metabolic efficiency. This is, in fact, the central idea of my longevity program.

Reaching for Maximum Metabolic Efficiency

From the most primitive cell to the most advanced organism, living matter needs energy to do its work and to make and maintain the structures giving form to life. It also needs energy to move itself about, to procreate, and to compete with other life forms. Life depends upon energy.

In the early days of our planet, before oxygen was freely available in the atmosphere, life forms derived energy from what is called glycolysis—the conversion of sugar into lactic acid in the tissues. We still derive part of our energy this way. When you become sore and ache from vigorous exercise, it's because lactic acid has built up in your muscles.

Chemically, glycolysis is not a very effective way to generate energy, so when oxygen started percolating into the earth's early atmosphere, mutant organisms were selected by evolution which could derive energy from oxygen by means of "respiratory metabolism." Properly, this term does not refer to breathing, but to a collection of processes, mostly taking place within the energy factories (mitochrondria) of our cells and resulting in the formation of a high-energy oxygen-phosphorus compound known as ATP (short for adenosine triphosphate). This basic life process has come down more or less unchanged since remote geologic time.

Thus our human bodies do not obtain energy *directly* from food, but from ATP formed by "respiratory metabolism" (as well as by residual glycolysis). And we must manufacture ATP from carbohydrates, fats, and proteins before our cells can use the ingested food for energy.

A specific amount of energy is locked up in the chemical bonds of carbohydrates and fats. Only some 50 percent of this "potential" energy can be converted into ATP. The rest is dissipated as wasted heat or stored as fat. When you overeat, *less* of the energy from your food is channeled through the body-building ATP, and *more* when you undereat. For an average adult American or European male, the 50-percent maximum of "potential" energy that can be converted, or the *energy efficiency*, is probably reached at about 1,900 calories daily. At 2,500 calories, the so-called "caloric RDA" for average adult males, the efficiency drops to 37 percent; at 3,300 calories, to 30 percent.

The existence of so-called "futile cycles" is also important in energy regulation. A futile cycle is one in which the ATP stored in the body can be degraded without actually providing any body-building energy. It produces heat without work (that is, without usable energy), and metabolic efficiency is lowered. Of course, futile cycles can be useful! If it is cold and we need to generate body heat, increasing the futile cycles will act like an internal furnace. Futile cycles are also turned on when we overeat on junk food, serving as additional safety valves to drain off excess food energy.

Maximum energy efficiency means achieving the highest possible conversion of carbohydrates and fats into ATP and minimizing both fat storage and the breakdown of ATP by futile cycles. The high/low diet is designed to achieve both these goals.

The Concept of Nutrient Density

An important feature of the high/low diet is that every calorie must be nutrition-packed. Otherwise, gradual weight loss on a long-term basis may cause deficiencies in essential nutrients, and of course that will not prolong life span but shorten it. And do not suppose we can reach our goal by eating a low-calorie mediocre or even nutritionally bad diet supplemented with vitamins and minerals. That would be dangerous and foolhardy. Too much remains unknown about essential nutriments—what forms they should be in, how they interact, whether any are still undiscovered . . . but you can bet you are not going to find acceptable combinations simply in refined white flour, hot dogs, and cola drinks plus a handful of pills. Calcium in the form of a calcium carbonate pill, for example, has value as a supplement, but it exerts a partially suppressive effect on bone remodeling; the same amount of calcium in milk has no suppressive effect.[2] Certain forms of fiber in the diet will help lower blood cholesterol, but only if it is a component of the actual food or else carefully mixed with it. Just taking the fiber as an extra supplement may have no effect. According to a 1981 *Consumer Reports* study of vitamin-fortified cereals,[3] the added vitamins' availability to the body was questionable. Supplementation has a place in the high/low diet program, but good nutrient-dense food selection is essential.

The average American diet is anything but nutrient-dense. The calorie level is inflated—2,400 to 3,200 for men (depending on age) and 1,650 to 2,150 for women—but it is often deficient in essentials. Large surveys have been run of what Americans eat: the National Food Consumption Survey of 7,500 families conducted by the U.S. Department of Agriculture, and the National Health and Nutrition Examination by the Department of Health and Human Services. They found that meat, fish, or poultry was consumed daily by 90 percent of the families, dark green vegetables by only 9 percent, yellow vegetables by 8 percent, fruit by 33 percent, and whole-grain cereals by 16 percent. Fully half of the 7,500 families were below what the National Academy of Sciences has set as the Recommended Daily Allowances (the RDAs) of one or more nutrients, especially calcium, vitamin A, vitamin C, iron, thiamine, and riboflavin. The RDA for magnesium was reached by only 25 percent of individuals; of vitamin B_6, 20 percent; of iron, 43 percent; of vitamin A, 50 percent.[4] Magnesium levels in the average diet have dropped from 475 mg. per person per day in 1900 to 245 mg. today. One survey revealed deficiencies in iron, copper, zinc, and chromium.[5] According to another, the vitamin B_6 content of meals served in 50 American colleges averaged 1.43 mg. per person per day; thus, over 80 percent of the colleges were below the vitamin B_6 RDA of 2.0 mg. per day.[6] It is shocking to realize that even on the high-calorie diet of the richest nation in the world, our own United States, borderline nutritional deficiency is widespread. The average American diet is not nutrient-dense, but the opposite.

Simply eating less of the same old things would restrict calories, but it would also bring on malnutrition as a potentially devastating side effect. This is the danger of many weight-loss diets, including some of the popular ones.[7*]

Even well-educated, financially comfortable people may show nutritional deficiencies. Protein, vitamin C, and various B vitamins (folic acid, niacin, pyridoxine, riboflavin, thiamine, and vitamin B_{12}) emerged as the nutrients most often deficient in 5 to 10 percent of a population of 256 affluent individuals surveyed by scientists at the University of New Mexico.[8] And those persons deficient in water-soluble vitamins tested lower than nondeficient partners on tests for abstract thinking and memory! Either borderline malnutrition affects brain function, or else dumber people select worse diets.

Vitamin and mineral deficiency is even more common among the elderly. In one study, fully 50 percent of elderly patients consumed less than two-thirds of the RDA for zinc.[9] Iron and possibly chromium have also been found deficient in the diets of the elderly. Intake of vitamins C and A and niacin has been reported to be less than two-thirds of the RDAs in over 25 percent of subjects in more than 50 percent of published reports on nutrition in the elderly. Even as conservative an authority as pioneer physiologist Dr. Nathan Shock of the National Institute on

Aging has recommended for the elderly supplementation with RDA amounts for vitamins and trace elements.

The Parable of Ross's Rats

Many people suppose that animals would instinctively select what is good for them nutritionally if given the chance, and that humans would too, if they were not heavily influenced by advertising and cultural and ethnic conditioning. This is a delightful idea. Rousseau would have loved it. But Dr. Morris Ross's introduction of dietary self-selection into the study of aging and disease[10] showed it to be quite naive. Among four populations of rats, one received a diet of 10 percent protein throughout life; a second, 22 percent protein; a third, 51 percent. The rats of the fourth population were allowed to select what they wanted from among the three available diets. Dr. Ross measured growth rates, body sizes, and frequencies of different diseases in all four populations. The rats that self-selected—that is, the fourth population—grew more rapidly and attained a greater body size than all the rest. They instinctively self-selected food combinations that would *optimize growth and development*; but—and here is what made the experiment unique and fascinating—that very self-selection resulted in a *far higher incidence of tumors and other diseases*. As shown in Table 4.1, the actual data are striking. Note that the prevalence of disease was considerably greater than 100 percent if you add up most of the columns. By the time of death many animals had multiple afflictions. Indeed, 66 percent of those on the self-select diet had at least three of the four diseases listed. The same multiplicity of diseases is of course found in autopsies of elderly humans.

Now here's my parable. Given free choice, an animal will instinctively choose a diet that leads to quick growth and development and to reaching sexual maturity as soon as possible. This tendency promotes *survival of the species*

Table 4.1 The frequencies, by percentage, of diseases in male rats kept on either fixed or free-choice (self-selected) diets (adapted from M. H. Ross and G. J. Bras, *Nature* 250:263, 1974).

Disease	Fed throughout life on one diet containing either 10%, 22%, or 51% protein			Free choice daily from 10%-, 22%-, or 51%-protein diets
	10%	22%	51%	
Cancer	26	29	28	62
Kidney disease	38	56	73	90
Heart disease	11	42	48	67
Prostate disease	5	10	12	62

in the wild, but is at the same time *highly counterproductive for individual long life*. In terms of innate self-selection hungers, the welfare of the species and of the individual are in murderous conflict. Animals are instinctively programmed to choose what will make them grow fast and have lots of offspring, even if that choice brings them frequent disease later on. This direct conflict between species and individual survival may be unprecedented in biology.

The behavior of Ross's rats suggests that some of the crazy and self-destructive things we do are the result of species-survival instincts acting through us without our knowing what is really going on. These instincts were of course formed in prehistoric times, during the process of evolution, and they may not be appropriate at all in today's world, even for species survival itself, much less our long-term personal survival. Whatever the value of these speculations, it seems most unlikely that we can trust our instincts to select what is good for us.

Nutrient-Dense Food Combinations

It's difficult to devise low-calorie menus that are not deficient in essential nutrients. If you think it's easy (and many dietitians and physicians do seem to think so, judging from such bland offhand advice as "Select items from the four food groups"), just try it. Using the tables in Appendix B, try to make up a 1,500-calorie one-day's menu, a menu that approximates or exceeds the RDAs for most or all nutrients. Without the right guidelines, it's not easy.

I fed nutrient information on hundreds of foods into a computer and asked for combinations containing less than 1,500 calories but approximating or exceeding the RDA levels recommended by the National Academy of Sciences for each major nutrient, with calories derived from fat between 8 and 20 percent of the total, and total protein 60 to 90 grams per day. My diet is based on these computer-optimized food combinations.

Because it permits such a ready and graphic comparison of the nutrient values of foods (without eyeballing of endless pages of tables), the computer approach can be instructive and surprising. For example, we hear a great deal these days about the nutritive value of cereals and grains, from the Pritikin Program, the macrobiotic enthusiasts, and conventionally qualified nutritionists. But calorie for calorie, and especially if you want to restrict fat intake, vegetables are far and away the most nutritious foods. Table 4.2 tells the tale. On both a weight and calorie basis, it compares nutritive values of some of the most nutritious vegetables with top candidates from the legumes, cereals, grains, red meat, fish, and even yeast.

As an additional help in your own dietary planning, Table 4.3 lists foods from all five food groups for their nutrient density, or because they have an exceptionally large amount of some essential nutrient which is not present in large amounts in other foods.

Table 4.2 Comparative nutritive components of selected high-quality foods on a weight-for-weight vs. a calorie-for-calorie basis.

Percentage of RDAs per 100 grams

	Turnip greens	Kale	Broccoli	Soybeans	Lima beans	Brown rice	Millet	Buckwheat	Liver	Beef	Salmon	Halibut	Yeast
Amino Acids													
Tryptophan	26	27	25	291	102	46	122	81	166	144	125	111	388
Isoleucine	14	20	19	279	163	41	77	55	138	159	156	149	333
Lysine	21	18	22	326	190	41	47	62	201	266	272	244	458
Valine	16	23	22	238	153	47	71	92	142	145	142	127	321
Methionine	5	6	9	87	55	30	40	30	75	90	108	98	133
Threonine	22	26	27	262	171	53	71	75	160	173	173	158	410
Leucine	21	29	18	302	177	67	160	71	182	187	176	156	333
Phenylalanine	23	17	18	348	180	70	46	76	171	171	159	134	395
Vitamins													
Vit. A	152	178	50	1	0	0	0	0	450	0	6	8	0
Vit. D	0	0	0	0	0	0	0	0	3	0	38	11	0
Vit. K	928	0	285	271	0	0	0	0	128	0	0	0	0
Vit. C	231	208	183	0	0	0	0	0	60	0	15	0	0
Vit. E	22	53	4	153	4	13	0	36	13	1	13	8	0
B,	14	0	7	78	34	24	52	42	14	6	12	5	1142

B_2	23	15	13	17	9	2	22	8	158	11	4	4	235
B_6	13	15	10	40	30	27	37	15	35	20	35	21	125
B_{12}	0	0	0	0	0	0	0	0	2000	61	133	33	0
Niacin	4	11	5	12	10	27	12	24	61	28	38	46	222
Folic acid	23	15	17	42	27	4	0	0	55	1	6	3	975
Pant. acid	9	25	30	42	25	27	0	37	200	12	32	7	300
Biotin	0	0	0	60	9	12	0	0	100	0	5	8	110
Minerals													
Calcium	20	15	8	19	6	2	1	9	0	1	6	1	17
Magnesium	15	9	6	66	45	22	40	63	0	5	7	5	57
Copper	4	4	0	5	9	18	42	21	250	2	10	11	265
Zinc	0	0	1	24	18	12	12	5	26	27	6	4	73
Chromium	0	0	60	0	120	0	0	0	120	60	0	0	320
Potassium	4	20	20	90	81	11	22	24	14	18	22	23	101
Iron	10	12	6	44	43	10	37	17	50	17	5	3	94
Manganese	56	22	2	112	21	68	76	83	6	0	0	0	16
Selenium	0	4	0	120	0	78	0	36	86	0	0	0	142
Calories per 100 gm.	28	38	32	403	345	356	327	335	140	143	217	100	283
% Calories from fat	10	19	8	40	4	5	8	6	32	38	54	11	3

Table 4.2 Comparative nutritive components of selected high-quality foods on a weight-for-weight vs. a calorie-for-calorie basis (continued).

Percentage of RDAs per 100 calories

	Turnip greens	Kale	Broccoli	Soybeans	Lima beans	Brown rice	Millet	Buckwheat	Liver	Beef	Salmon	Halibut	Yeast
Amino Acids													
Tryptophan	93	73	78	72	29	13	37	24	118	101	57	111	136
Isoleucine	52	54	59	69	47	11	23	16	98	111	71	149	116
Lysine	77	47	69	81	55	11	14	18	142	186	125	244	160
Valine	57	62	68	59	44	13	21	27	101	101	65	127	112
Methionine	19	17	28	21	15	8	12	8	53	63	49	98	46
Threonine	80	70	86	65	49	15	21	22	114	121	79	158	143
Leucine	78	76	57	75	51	19	49	21	129	131	80	156	116
Phenylalanine	84	46	57	87	52	19	14	22	122	120	73	134	138
Vitamins													
Vit. A	542	468	156	0	0	0	0	0	319	0	2	8	0
Vit. D	0	0	0	0	0	0	0	0	2	0	17	11	0
Vit. K	3315	0	894	67	0	0	0	0	91	0	0	0	0
Vit. C	827	547	573	0	0	0	0	0	42	0	6	0	0
Vit. E	78	140	14	38	1	3	0	10	9	0	6	8	0
B_1	51	0	22	19	9	6	15	12	10	4	5	5	400
B_2	83	40	42	4	2	0	6	2	112	7	2	4	82

B_6	46	39	31	10	8	7	11	4	24	14	16	21	43
B_{12}	0	0	0	0	0	0	0	0	1420	43	61	33	0
Niacin	15	30	15	3	3	7	3	7	43	20	17	46	77
Folic acid	84	39	54	10	7	1	0	0	39	1	2	3	341
Pant. acid	33	65	93	10	7	7	0	11	142	8	14	7	104
Biotin	1	1	1	15	2	3	0	0	71	0	2	8	38
Minerals													
Calcium	74	39	26	4	1	0	0	2	0	0	3	1	6
Magnesium	53	24	18	16	13	6	12	18	2	3	3	5	20
Copper	16	11	1	1	2	5	13	6	177	1	4	11	92
Zinc	0	0	5	6	5	3	3	1	18	19	2	4	25
Chromium	0	0	187	0	34	0	0	0	85	42	0	0	111
Potassium	14	53	63	22	23	3	7	7	10	13	10	23	35
Iron	35	32	19	11	12	2	11	5	35	12	2	3	33
Manganese	202	57	7	28	6	19	23	24	4	0	0	0	5
Selenium	0	12	0	30	0	21	0	10	61	0	0	0	49
Grams per 100 calories	357	263	313	25	29	28	31	30	71	70	46	100	35
% Calories from fat	10	19	8	40	4	5	8	6	32	38	54	11	3

Table 4.3 The top quality foods according to nutrient density per portion.

Range of RDA's per portion	Portion		Nutrient											
	Wt. (gms)	Cals.	vit. A	vit. C	vit. D	vit. E	vit. K	Thia-mine	Ribo-flavin	Niacin	B-6	Panto-thenic acid	B-12	Folacin
+			91–100	79–100	100	66–100	85–100	67–100	100	61–100	34–43	60–100	100	42–97
Food ●			30–50	55–71	31–55	25–60	30–62	26–52	15–37	33–46	20–31	25–42	58–73	15–32
Beef (lean)	100	143									●		●	
Chicken (dark)	100	130								●		●	●	
Chicken (light)	100	117								+	+			
Liver	100	140	+	●			+		+	+	+	+	+	+
Pork (lean)	100	165						+			●			
Veal	100	156			●					●				
Cod	100	78												
Mackerel	100	191			+				●	●	●		+	
Oysters	50	33			●								+	
Salmon	100	217			●					●	+	●	+	
Sardines, fresh	50	78			+								+	
Sardines, canned	100	200												
Squid	100	84												
Tuna	100	127			+					+	●		+	

Skim milk	1 cup 244	85							●					
Buttermilk	244	100							●					
Yogurt	244	156							●			+		
Ricotta cheese (part skim)	½ cup 124	174					●							
Sunflower seeds	15	84				+								
Broccoli	200	45	+	+			+		●		●	+		●
Chard	112	28	+	●										
Kale	100	38	+	+		+			●			●		●
Mushrooms	70	20							●			+		
Parsley	100	44	+	+					●					●
Spinach	100	26	+	+			+							+
Sweet potato	180	205	+	●		+						●		●
Turnip greens	115	32	+	+		●	+		●					●
Garbanzo beans	100	360									●	●		+
Lentils	100	340						●			+	●		
Lima beans	100	345				+		●			●	●		●
Soybeans	100	403				+	+	+	●		+	●		+

Table 4.3 The top quality foods according to nutrient density per portion (continued).

Range of RDA's per portion	Portion		Nutrient											
	Wt. (gms)	Cals.	vit. A	vit. C	vit. D	vit. E	vit. K	Thia-mine	Ribo-flavin	Niacin	B-6	Panto-thenic acid	B-12	Folacin
+			91–100	79–100	100	66–100	85–100	67–100	100	61–100	34–43	60–100	100	42–97
Food ●			30–50	55–71	31–55	25–60	30–62	26–52	15–37	33–46	20–31	25–42	58–73	15–32
Banana	150	127									+			
Cantaloupe	200	60	+	+										
Papaya	100	39	●	+										
Millet	100	327						●	●		+			
Rice—brown	100	356									●	●		
Rice—wild	100	353						●	●	●		●		
Wheat germ	10	40				+	●							
Whole wheat pasta	80	266						●						
Kombu	8	19			●						●		●	
Nori	8	20	●		●						●		●	
Wakami	8	20			●					●			●	
Yeast	10	28						+	●					
Yeast	20	56						+	●	●		●		

Beef (lean)	100	143					●			●			+	+
Chicken (dark)	100	130											+	+
Chicken (light)	100	117											+	+
Liver	100	140	+			+	+	+		●	+		+	+
Pork (lean)	100	165									●		+	+
Veal	100	156					●			●			+	+
Cod	100	78								+	+		+	+
Mackerel	100	191									+		+	+
Oysters	50	33					●			+	+			
Salmon	100	217											+	+
Sardines, fresh	50	78	●								+		+	
Sardines, canned	100	200		+										
Squid	100	84						+					+	+
Tuna	100	127					●				+		+	+
Skim milk	1 cup 244	85		+									+	
Buttermilk	244	100		+									+	
Yogurt	244	156		+		●							+	
Ricotta cheese (part skim)	½ cup 124	174		+									+	

Table 4.3 The top quality foods according to nutrient density per portion (continued).

Range of RDA's per portion	Portion		Nutrient											
	Wt. (gms)	Cals.	Biotin	Ca	Mg	Potas.	Iron	Cu	Mn	Zn	Se	Cr	Lysine	Meth.
+			60–100	18–36	32–66	69–100	34–50	83–100	44–100	97–100	60–100		72–100	75–100
Food •			10–31	12–16	15–28	25–53	15–26	17–42	21–24	16–31	36–48			30–50
Sunflower seeds	15	84						•						
Broccoli	200	45		•										
Chard	112	28			•	•	•		+					
Kale	100	38		•										
Mushrooms	70	20	•		+	•	•		•				+	
Parsley	100	44		•		•	+	•						
Spinach	100	26			•	•	•		•		•			
Sweet potato	180	205							+					
Turnip greens	115	32		+	•	•			+	•	+		+	+
Garbanzo beans	100	360	•	•	+	•	+	•	+	•			+	•
Lentils	100	340			•	•	+	•		•				•
Lima beans	100	345			+	+	+		•	•			+	•
Soybeans	100	403	+		+	+	+		+	•	+		+	+

Banana	150	127				●								
Cantaloupe	200	60				●								
Papaya	100	39												
Millet	100	327			+		+	●	+					
Rice—brown	100	356	●		●				+		+			
Rice—wild	100	353			+		●			●			+	
Wheat germ	10	40												
Whole wheat pasta	80	266			●						+			
Kombu	8	19		●	●									
Nori	8	20		●	●		●		●					
Wakami	8	20		●	●		●							
Yeast	10	28	●					●					●	
Yeast	20	56	●					●					+	

When to Go on the Diet

I definitely do not recommend that anyone begin the high/low diet until fully grown. But after that, the sooner the better. Beginning the program halfway through life should yield about half the degree of life extension as starting in young adulthood, and proportionately for other time periods.

Caloric restriction beginning in childhood might yield the greatest extension of maximum life span, but is still an unacceptable option for humans. Substantial restriction in very young animals may cause an increased infant or early-age mortality, even though the survivors do go on to enjoy remarkably long lives. We could not sacrifice a small percentage of young humans to ensure long lives for the survivors. Also, restriction during the growing years in animals is often associated with a smaller final body size. In humans, this could mean being 6 to 8 inches shorter than nonrestricted persons.

Do not take this to mean that a somewhat lower-calorie, higher-quality diet would not potentially increase life span for today's children. Indeed, translating this animal data into human terms, Dr. Morris Ross[11] stated that a difference in daily intake of 100 to 125 calories during the period of human growth would influence the duration of life by 2.5 years. Empty calories for children—energy snacks and the like—are bad news for their health later on in life.

How to Lose Weight

The high/low diet works very well for rapid weight loss. In fact, because of its nutrient density, it is certainly the best and probably the easiest of all diets for that purpose. At an equivalent caloric intake, it will leave you feeling better and less hungry than other diets. But a word of caution is needed here. In Western societies, enormous subliminal and not-so-subliminal pressure is exerted on everyone to be as slim as starlets and models. We are made to feel we should be not merely "not fat" but positively slender. Responding to this pressure, people plunge desperately into quick-weight-reduction regimens. A popular diet book promising rapid, painless slenderization comes out almost every other month. No checkout-counter tabloid is without one. From the standpoint of health and longevity, quick weight loss is harmful.

It had been known since 1935 that if you kept animals on a low-calorie, supplemented diet from time of weaning, you could dramatically extend life span and decrease susceptibility to disease. But nobody could make the method work if it was started in adulthood. Indeed, in the early experiments this actually *shortened* the life span. Studying these early experiments, Dr. Richard Weindruch and I noted that the investigators had put the animals suddenly, or over a very short period, on the lower-calorie diet. This sudden switch, we reasoned, may have injured them metabolically. Then in our own investigations we found that if the high/low diet was begun very gradually, leading to a very gradual weight loss (equivalent to weight loss in humans over a 4-to-6-year period), life span could be greatly extended and disease incidence reduced.[12] If this applies to humans, then the quick weight loss promised by most modern diet books may be dandy for your immediate cosmetic appeal, but across-the-board bad for your ultimate health —and for the long-term cosmetic appeal of looking younger than you are. Anyway, almost everyone knows that all these diets don't work very well. You lose weight but then you gain it back. Then you buy another highly touted diet book, and do it again. The whole cycle is discouraging, irrational, and unhealthful.

If you adopt the high/low diet primarily to live longer, don't lose weight too fast. Allow yourself ample time for metabolic adaptation.

What calorie range suffices to enable you to lose weight slowly over a 4-to-6-year period, placing you below your set point, or very possibly resetting that point? The range will vary from person to person, but we can form a general idea. Not long after World War II, scientists at the University of Minnesota performed a very pertinent experiment with 32 young male conscientious objectors.[13] Kept on a strict 1,600-calorie-per-day diet for 6 months, the subjects lost weight fairly rapidly, and the loss leveled off to a maintenance value of 75 percent of the original weight. Once lost, the weight was not regained unless more than 2,000 calories per day were given.

Start your own program with about a 2,000-calorie high/low diet if you are an average-size man, 1,800 calories if a woman, and see if this induces gradual weight loss and at the same time improves your sense of physical well-being. If so, continue. If you are losing weight too fast or too slowly or not at all, adjust your intake accordingly. The food and menu combinations given in Appendix A are pitched to approximate or exceed the RDAs for all important nutrients at a level of 1,500 or fewer calories. Unless you have a medical reason for wanting quick weight loss, add about 300 to 500 calories of intake to any of these daily regimens. Choose whatever you like for these extra calories, but keep in mind what I shall outline in the next chapter about susceptibility to the major killer diseases.

Fasting

Caloric intake can also be cut back by frequent short fasts. Some of the animal studies have entailed "intermittent fasting"—giving the animals as much as they want of a high-quality diet, but only every other dav. On alternate days they get nothing. The overall weekly caloric intake turns out to be less, slow weight loss results, and life span is extended.

In human societies fasting has an extensive history dating back to antiquity. Many cultures and religions have incorporated it into their writings and practices. North

American Indians and Eskimos fast prior to being ordained for their priesthoods. Muslims fast for many reasons (before prayer, when ill, or when they wish to conjure). Eastern yogis fast to achieve spiritual enlightenment. Jesus fasted forty days and nights.

Technically, you are "fasting" only if you consume nothing but water. Such fasting is short-term starvation. Fasting under proper supervision (especially if long-term) differs from actual starvation in that the diet is supplemented with vitamins and minerals. Without this, symptoms of frank vitamin deficiency develop in totally fasting individuals in considerably less than two months. On the other hand, very obese people have gone without food (properly supplemented and in a hospital, where they could be observed) for as long as 249 days without apparent harm.[14, 15]*

However, except for very precise medical indications, I do not recommend long-term fasting, because only *gradual* weight reduction and metabolic readaptation extends life span. Short-term fasts of one or two days per week, with more generous amounts of high-quality foods on the eating days, are just as effective in inducing gradual weight loss as simply eating less each day. It depends on what is comfortable for you. An occasional short-term fast is also good because it will change your perceptions of hunger and energy. Hunger is partly habit. And skipping or cutting down on meals does not rob you of energy: in fact, the reverse. In one study, five men were subjected to five 2½-day fasts at 5–6-week intervals.[16] Their ability to undertake hard physical labor during the fast periods was measured. Between the first and final periods, reaction times and pattern recognition (a test of intellectual function) actually *improved*. Glucose-tolerance tests showed an increased ability to regulate blood sugar. Short-term fasts aid metabolic adaptation; however, they are not a necessary part of the high/low diet program.

Appetite and Its Control

In any long-term dietary program leading to gradual, substantial, and sustained weight loss, appetite control could be a worry. You will ask, "Am I going to be famished all the time?"

You won't feel as full as a gorged lion, but on a high/low diet you won't be as hungry as you might think. The type and quality of food itself influences appetite. Rats on a low-protein, high-carbohydrate diet voluntarily restrict their intake and live longer.[17] Rats fed a high-fat, "junk food" diet gain a great deal more weight than normally fed rats. A study at the University of Alabama[18] revealed that volunteer humans allowed to eat as much as they liked achieved full satisfaction from as little as 1,500 calories a day from whole foods, but it took 3,000 calories of refined and processed foods to satisfy them. The "whole" foods included fruit, hot cereals, skim milk, soups, salads, nonmeat sandwiches, pasta, fish, chicken, rice, vegetables, and whole-wheat toast and rolls. The "refined" foods included bacon, eggs, juice, buttered toast, fast and fried foods, roast or steak, buttered vegetables, whole milk, cake, and ice cream.

A popular hypothesis of appetite regulation maintains that unrefined foods with a low energy density will induce a feeling of fullness at a low energy intake.[19] "Low energy density" means a lot of bulk per calorie. There is no contradiction between high *nutrient* density and low *energy* density: turnip greens, for example, are packed with nutrients but are low in calories (Table 4.2, pp. 78–81).

Fiber material such as guar gum added to a meal significantly prolongs the time after eating before hunger returns. Addition of 10 grams of guar gum to meals twice daily decreased appetite by delaying gastric emptying time, with a significant weight loss over 10 weeks in obese persons, accompanied by a decrease in LDL fats in the blood and an improved glucose-tolerance curve.[20]

Refined sugar in the diet stimulates appetite. Persons eating highly refined and processed foods have been shown to take in 25 percent more calories than persons on a more natural diet.

The high/low diet is a high-nutrient-density/low-energy-density formulation. As such, it will give you greater satiety per calorie than any other diet.

Drugs that decrease appetite are not a good answer for long-term slow weight loss. A number of complex events occur in the body that result in its asking, "What's to eat?" These involve metabolic rates, the energy enzymes of the body, insulin, blood sugar, and a portion of the brain called the hypothalamus. Trying to handle all these events with a pill doesn't make sense. Like suppressing a toothache with codeine, it'll work for a while . . . but your tooth will rot.

You can make a rat eat by pinching its tail.[21] The pain causes the release of chemicals (opioids) in the hypothalamus which block the sensation of pain, but also stimulate hunger. Like opium or morphine, these opioids (also known as endorphins) are addicting. Pinch a rat's tail frequently for ten days and it will release opioids and overeat, and you will have a fat rat. Suddenly stop pinching its tail, opioids are not released, and the addicted rat will go into a fit—the same reaction as a heroin addict. Mental pain or stress may also augment endorphin or opioid release and so stimulate hunger. Avoidance of stress will aid in appetite control. In this sense, weight gain and obesity are a kind of autoaddiction.

The best answer to hunger turns out to be high-quality nutrition and rational self-restraint.

Will It Work?

Translatability

Granted that the high/low diet works well in animals, how do we know it will work in humans? It is of course not yet *proved*, but we are not forced to wait for absolute proof!

In medicine it is not uncommon to recommend measures not yet "proved" but for which substantial evidence exists. As I mentioned earlier, many doctors have for years been recommending the lowering of blood cholesterol because this would probably help prevent coronary heart disease, but this was not "proved" until 1984, and then for only a selected category of patient. And only in early 1985 did a panel of 13 experts convened as part of a National Institutes of Health "consensus conference" conclude "beyond a reasonable doubt" that lowering elevated blood cholesterol levels will reduce the risk of heart attacks. "Beyond a reasonable doubt" in fact means "with a high order of probability." Many more examples could be cited. The key question for much good medical advice is not whether "proof" is at hand, but what is the order of probability that the advice is correct.

Existing evidence indicates not absolutely but with a high order of probability that the same high/low diet which extends life span in all the varieties of nonhuman species so far tested would do the same for man. One reason for thinking so is that we are dealing with a very *general* process. Experiments involving the overall operation of the immune system, the nature of DNA repair, and the various types and causes of cancer indicate that these *general* phenomena are quite similar across the species barrier. Nutritional modulation of the aging process seems to me to be such a general phenomenon, involving common processes across wide species barriers. In my view this animal work is entirely translatable to humans.

It is occasionally asserted, as evidence against translatability of calorie-restriction experiments, that in underdeveloped countries or situations where people are underfed, there is no increase in longevity.[22] I find it astonishing that those who express this view never pause to consider that these underfed populations are also *mal*nourished. Their caloric restriction is often accompanied by inadequate vitamin, mineral, protein, and other intake. Nobody claims that undernutrition *with malnutrition* increases life span.

Direct Evidence

Aside from the question of translatability, there is in fact a modest amount of *direct* evidence that the high/low diet will have the same effect on humans as in animals.

Long-term (3–9 months) low-calorie supplemented diets have been investigated in the treatment of obesity and of diabetes.[23] These diets yield metabolic effects in humans which closely resemble those seen in animals on similar diets: a decrease in LDL, an increase in HDL, an improved insulin response, and a better regulation of blood sugar.

Anorexia nervosa is a dreadful, sometimes fatal psychological disease in which (usually) young women, often overachievers, develop a compulsive urge to control their weight. They literally starve themselves slowly, sometimes even unto death, as did the popular singer Karen Carpenter in late 1982.

Despite the disastrous nature of the disease, certain things about it are interesting for our purpose. Anorexics typically restrict their intake of fat and carbohydrates but allow themselves relatively more protein in vegetables and low-fat cheeses. They undergo drastic weight loss but with considerably less comparative *mal*nutrition than is seen in typical semistarved individuals from famine or poverty areas. So it's a bit like a high-quality low-calorie diet except that it's carried to excess. And for a while, anorexics do remain surprisingly well despite their growing emaciation. They do not usually get into serious problems until up to 30 to 40 percent of their body weight has been lost.[24] Despite an extremely low calcium intake, they do not experience an automatic increase in parathyroid-hormone level and resorb calcium from bone.[25] They do not show any increased susceptibility to infections. And quite unlike the results of malnutrition caused by famine or poverty, the immune system in anorexics is generally preserved until weight loss is far advanced. Indeed, in early stages the immune responses may be *better* than control values.[26] The same phenomenon of heightened immune response is of course found in rodents subjected to caloric restriction commencing in adulthood.[27]

In *Maximum Life Span* I discussed two populations world-famous for fabulous longevity, the people of Soviet Georgia and the villagers of Vilcabamba, Peru. They are not really long-lived. They have no secrets of longevity at all, and their maximum life span is no longer than anybody else's. Yogurt advertisements notwithstanding, in the absence of reliable birth records, no knowledgeable gerontologist believes the Georgian myth. The same is true for the villagers in Vilcabamba, who for about a dozen years got a great deal of press because they supposedly had many supercentenarians in their society. But it's just not true. According to the most recent evidence, the oldest person in Vilcabamba is only 96.

But there are two populations today who just might be breaking the maximum-life-span barrier, and they are not in mysterious places. One is on the Japanese island of Okinawa. The other (maybe!) is our own population right here in the United States.

The Okinawan Experience

In Japan, large-scale and quite accurate nutritional surveys have been conducted yearly since 1946 by the Ministry of Health and Welfare.[28] Accurate information is available about weight, body size, health, and disease incidences of the different areas of Japan. The numbers of centenarians are also known throughout Japan, since accurate legal birth records have been kept since 1872.

On the island of Okinawa and in a few other areas of Japan, there are 15 to 37 centenarians per 100,000 persons over 65 years of age (the highest incidence is in Okinawa!), whereas in most of Japan the number ranges from 1 to 9. One way to estimate maximum life span of a population besides finding the age of the oldest survivor is to calculate the average age of the last surviving 10 percent of the population. This is called the "tenth decile" of survivorship. With so many more actual centenarians in the population (and therefore also a lot more people over 90) than elsewhere,[29] it seems likely that the tenth decile is significantly higher in Okinawa than elsewhere in Japan. It's not just average age that's longer there, but maximum survival too.

Now, the daily caloric intake of Okinawan schoolchildren, though adequate in vitamins and animal protein, is only 62 percent of the "recommended intake" for Japan. Average sugar and salt intake for Okinawans is lower than the national average, while consumption of green/yellow vegetables and meats is higher. Although it is not nearly so rigorous as the one spelled out in this book, the Okinawans, compared with the rest of the Japanese, seem to be on a high/low diet.

The frequencies of cancer, heart disease, high blood pressure, diabetes, and senile brain disease are lower by 30 to 40 percent in Okinawa than elsewhere in Japan. And the average heights and weights of the population are lower.

The increased number of centenarians among Okinawans, the quality and caloric content of their diet, the lowered incidence of the major diseases of aging, and their smaller body size are exactly what one finds in laboratory animals on a high/low diet since early life. Professor Yasuo Kagawa of Jichi Medical School attributes the longevity of the Okinawan population to caloric restriction.[30]

Right Here in America

A fascinating recent study by Drs. Ed Schneider and Jacob Brody of the National Institute on Aging,[31] based on census data, suggests that in the present-day United States the "oldest" segment of the population is proportionately enjoying the greatest increase in life expectancy. We are experiencing a decrease in the death rate for both sexes at very advanced ages. From 1900 to 1960 the life expectancy for white females in the United States at age 85 increased by only 0.6 years, but from 1960 to 1978 it increased by fully 2 years. The reason for this decline is puzzling. It does not seem, for example, to be happening in the Scandinavian countries.[32] Possibly, with the increasing emphasis on good diet by at least a health-conscious, nutrition-oriented subpopulation in American society (a phenomenon not yet much evident in Europe), coupled with our now rather long-term thinness craze, some of our citizens are both eating better and operating slightly below their biological set points. Should this be true on a large-enough scale, I would predict the results that have been observed. Of course we need more evidence.

Dr. Vallejo's Experiment

The high/low-diet idea was tackled in an experiment performed in Madrid.[33] An over-65 population of 180 men and women in an old-age home were divided into two equal groups. One group was placed on a diet of 2,300 calories one day and 885 calories the next. The control group received 2,300 calories every day. Over the three years of the experiment, the subjects receiving the fewer calories spent only 123 days in the infirmary, compared with 219 days for the fully fed subjects. And their death rate was only half that of the control group. While Dr. Vallejo's experiment was not large enough, long enough, or careful enough to be regarded as definitive proof, it is still of considerable interest.

Two Venerable Gentlemen

The Renaissance Italian gentleman Luigi Cornaro, a member of the minor Italian nobility, led a gluttonous life which resulted in dangerous ill health at age 37. Then, on his doctor's advice, he adopted a very temperate dietarily restricted regimen, which seems to have been equivalent to about 1,500 calories per day. The diet was also of good quality, considering the primitive state of nutritional science at that time. We know all about Signor Cornaro because he wrote a famous autobiography called *The Art of Long Living*. He died in 1567 at the age of 103. A few hundred years later Dr. A. Guenoit, president of the Paris Medical Academy, elected to follow a similar regimen. He died in 1935 at the age of 102.

Summary

You will recognize, I hope, that the histories of Cornaro and Guenoit are merely anecdotal evidence. Does it really mean much that among historical figures who followed a (for their times) carefully selected high-quality, low-calorie diet, two out of two lived to become centenarians? No, not a great deal by itself. But note carefully where we now stand, even leaving aside the amusing histories of our venerable gentlemen.

Overwhelming evidence proves the high/low diet will increase maximum life span in animals, and the biology involved is of such a general nature it ought to apply to humans. In humans, caloric regimens showing features of the high/low diet yield biomarker changes similar to what the diet produces in animals. One existing well-documented human population on an approximation of the high/low diet appears to have extended survival. In an experimental human population, and even beginning in old age, 3 years on a similar diet seemed to decrease the rates of illness and death.

For these reasons I am convinced that a high/low diet by itself (and the one you'll find in this book is finer-tuned than any of the above) will greatly retard human aging and extend maximum survival.

CHAPTER 5

Prevent What Is Going to Kill You

You not only want to live longer, you want to remain as healthy as possible and free of disease throughout that extended time. Although the high/low diet will go a long way toward achieving this double goal, we can further target our program toward specific prevention of many of the diseases that might otherwise afflict us during the course of our 120+ years of life. I don't want to die at 100 if I'm still functionally young, still chasing the apples of desire. Neither do you. We all want to die of "old age" rather than cancer, which means we'll be healthy until our 120th+ year, and then succumb rather quickly to some minor irregularity—pneumonia from exposure to ski weather, say, or complications arising from a motorcycle spill on the way to a dance. In the poem "The Deacon's Masterpiece" by Oliver Wendell Holmes, all parts of the wonderful one-hoss shay were built to endure exactly 100 years, ever smooth and shining, and then turn to dust all together. Poof! And blow away!

I am talking now about the enhancement of *average* life span, the part of the survival curve influenced mainly by disease. The high/low diet will increase *maximum* life span, and to a considerable extent carry average life span along with it, but other measures can further square or rectangularize the survival curve. These measures deal with fat, fiber, and fitness, with having larger amounts of certain vitamins and minerals in our diet than the official Recommended Daily Allowances (RDA), adding other chemical agents to the diet (a very controversial but potentially important matter), and avoiding stress and noxious environmental agents. In this and the next several chapters, I will discuss all but the last two of these, which are out of my area of expertise.

Aging Without Sickness

As we grow older, partly because of the increasing vulnerability that comes with normal aging, and partly because poor health habits gradually catch up with us, we tend to develop a number of diseases: arteriosclerosis, cancer, high blood pressure, diabetes, osteoporosis, and others. You won't develop lung cancer from smoking for one year, but after thirty years your liability to it will be 15 to 20 times that of nonsmokers. There may be a history of hypertension in your family, but you may not have a high-pressure blowout until 20 to 30 years of eating too much salt.

A genetic predisposition to develop a disease may not show itself until played upon by environmental factors over a long period. You can express this idea as a kind of equation: genetic component + environmental component = disease. Medical science now believes that up to 75 percent of the major killer diseases in the Western world are shaped in part by environmental influences. Aside from smoking, the main influence is what we eat, or fail to eat.

The Average American Diet: Quantity Without Quality

By 1925 we had cornflakes, hot dogs, processed cheese, and bright white bread; by 1950, baby foods and cake mix; by 1975, fast foods, frozen dinners, and kids who drank more pop than milk. Today's American diet is long on quantity and sadly short on quality—much more so than health authorities admit. Until recently the major role of diet in disease susceptibility had not been appreciated. Its role in cancer for both men and women is strikingly illustrated in Figure 5.1. Add to this the fact that diet, impinging upon the aging process itself, is by all odds the main cause of arteriosclerosis and heart disease, and significantly

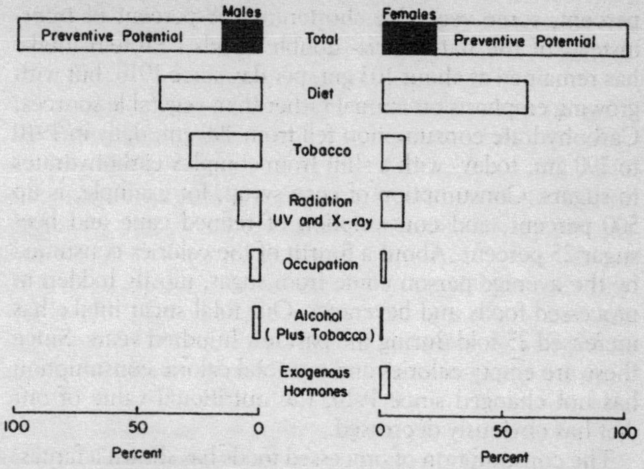

Figure 5.1 Environmental factors and cancer. Only 10–20% of cancers are genetically determined, as shown by the solid portion of the topmost horizontal bar. The rest are due to environmental influences, of which diet is by all odds the most important factor (adapted from G. B. Gori, *Cancer* 43:2151,1979).

contributes to diabetes and other late-life diseases. What a shame it is that with such abundance of food in the stores, supermarkets, and restaurants, people are not eating what is good for them, but the contrary.

From 1910 to 1980, fat consumption in the United States increased from 125 to 156 gm. per day. Today's average American diet derives 42 percent of its whopping 2,400 (for women) to 3,200 (for men) calories from fat, with a polyunsaturated-to-saturated fat ratio of 0.5:1.[1] Most authorities believe this ratio should be close to 1:1. The past 50 years have seen an increase in the consumption of processed vegetable fats: margarines, oils, and vegetable shortenings which contain significant quantities of chemically altered unsaturated fatty acids. (Some commercial vegetable oils contain up to 17 percent, some margarines 47 percent, some vegetable shortenings 58 percent of *trans-* instead of the natural *cis-* double bonds.) Protein intake has remained at about 103 gm. per day since 1910, but with growing emphasis on animal rather than vegetable sources. Carbohydrate consumption fell from 490 gm. daily in 1910 to 390 gm. today, with a shift from complex carbohydrates to sugars. Consumption of corn syrup, for example, is up 500 percent, and consumption of refined cane and beet sugar 25 percent. About a fourth of the calories consumed by the average person come from sugar, mostly hidden in processed foods and beverages. Our total sugar intake has increased 25-fold during the past few hundred years. Since these are empty calories and our total calorie consumption has not changed since 1910, the nutritional value of our diet has obviously decreased.

The consumption of processed foods has shown a fantastic increase in the past 70 years. And 18 percent of our meals and 25 percent of the money we spend on them goes for eating away from home. The annual $7 billion in sales of McDonald's, the world's largest fast-food purveyor, far outstrips the number two contender, the United States Department of Agriculture itself, which in 1980 dispensed a paltry $2.8 billion worth of food to schoolchildren and the elderly.

The big trends in our diet have been to maintain the level of calories even though as a nation we are much more sedentary than we were in the early part of the century and so don't need as many, and to increase fats and refined sugars, to increase animal and decrease vegetable proteins, to sharply decrease cereal and fiber intake, to shift from natural to processed foods, and to create nutritionally ghastly diet and food-preference habits. What is more revolting healthwise than the thought of eating a killer Twinkie? Or more criminal than feeding one to a child!

The Scale of Obesity

"Let me have men about me that are fat," pleaded Julius Caesar in Shakespeare's play. Caesar thought fat men were less dangerous. Right or wrong, if he lived in the United States today, Caesar would have his wish. We are definitely fatter than we once were. Since the American Civil War our average weight has increased fully 16 percent.

It's more important as an individual to concentrate on your personal set point than to struggle with how your weight compares with your neighbor's or your ancestor's. But to grasp the relations between fatness and disease we must understand the prevalence and measurement of obesity as it relates to the "average" body weight for sex, height, and body frame. And certain controversies about body weight and life expectancy must be cleared up.

"Obesity" means a weight 20 percent or more above average, or a body fat content exceeding 30 percent for women and 20 to 25 percent for men. About 40 million of today's citizens—25 percent of women and 12 percent of men—are 20 percent or more above the average body weight for their height. Obesity can be largely central (that is, on the trunk), peripheral (hips, arms), or both. A fatty trunk is more directly related to health risk than obesity in general.[2]

The actual proportion of the body consisting of fat can be estimated by various methods. I'll mention just two. The first is easy but not very accurate, and involves measuring skin-fold thickness. In most places the skin of the body is about 1 mm. thick, so the distance between folds in different locations is due to fat. By measuring this distance at selected sites, we can estimate body fatness from tables or equations. The proportion of body fat in young adults at what insurance companies generally regard as "desirable weight" is about 12 percent for men, 19 percent for women.

Several easy-to-use instruments are available for estimating skin-fold thickness: Slimguide, Fat-O-Meter, and Skyndex (See Readings and Resources, p. 418). Central obesity can be estimated by measurement of the skin-fold thickness between your shoulder blades, and peripheral obesity by the skin-fold thickness on the back of your upper arm (triceps).

A more accurate way to estimate body fat (Your doctor would have to arrange this) is by the density method. It was originally discovered by the ancient Greek mathematician Archimedes while sitting in his bath. Archimedes had the task of finding whether the king's crown was pure gold or whether the crown-maker had adulterated it with baser metal. Seeing how his own body caused the water level in the tub to rise, Archimedes perceived that the amount of water he displaced equaled his own volume. By the same criterion, he could measure the crown's irregular volume, and thus see if the proper weight of gold displaced exactly as much. "Eureka!" he shouted—"I have found it!"—and in his excitement leaped from his bath and ran naked through the town.

To estimate your percentage of body fat, you are submerged in a tank of water and weighed after you have completely exhaled. Just as though you were a crown of gold, dividing your weight by the amount of water you displace (that is, by your volume) will determine your density. As the density of fat is 0.9 and of the nonfat parts of the body about 1.1, the percentage of you that is fat can be read from tables. If it is substantially less than 12 percent, you will not look bad running naked through the town, although you may encounter stricter laws than Archimedes did.

Body Weight and Overall Mortality

How does obesity, relative body weight, or degree of leanness affect the overall death rates of a population? Does being fat or slim influence your survival chances? The question became highly controversial with the 1983 publication of insurance-company statistics indicating that the lowest death rates coincide with being mildly *overweight* in terms of average values. This contrasts sharply with earlier (1959) data showing that lowest mortality coincided with being about 10 percent *underweight*.

The new Metropolitan Life Insurance Company figures for weights associated with lowest death rates are given in Table 5.1. In these new data the weight range for lowest mortality looks to be 10 to 20 percent higher than it was 20 years ago. In relation to death rates, "desirable weight" now appears to be 13 lb. above the current average weights (10 percent) for short men, 7 lb. (5 percent) above average weights for medium-sized men, and 2 lb. (1 percent) above average weights for tall men than formerly. Corresponding figures for women are 10 lb. (10 percent), 8 lb. (6 percent), and 3 lb. (2 percent).

Additional studies seem to indicate that in recent years mortality has been lowest at 10 to 25 percent above average body weight for ages 40–49 years and 30 percent above average weight for ages 50–59, and that only after age 65–74 is mortality least for mildly underweight persons.[3]

What are we to make of these surprising data? They seem to show that if you want to live longer it's best to be mildly overweight. However, an enormous body of consistently confirmed experiments in animals, from 1935 right on up to today, indicates that life span can be substantially prolonged by being underweight, provided that the quality of the diet is very high. Something seems to be wrong here. What's the answer?

The answer is that *both sets of data are correct*, and that an appropriate biological interpretation can reconcile them. The data are only superficially contradictory.

To begin with, insurance-company data on the weight/mortality relationship have changed over the years. In the last half of the 19th century, insurance companies insisted that thin people pay a higher premium. At that time tuberculosis, the number one killer, caused 20 percent of all deaths. Because tuberculosis is an emaciating disease, its

Table 5.1 1983 Metropolitan Life Insurance Company height and weight tables. Weights at ages 25–29, by height and body frame, that correspond to lowest death rates (from 1979 Build Society of Actuaries and Association of Life Insurance Medical Directors of America, 1980).

MEN (in indoor clothing weighing 5 lb., shoes with 1-inch heels)					WOMEN (in indoor clothing weighing 3 lb., shoes with 1-inch heels)				
HEIGHT Feet	HEIGHT Inches	SMALL FRAME	MEDIUM FRAME	LARGE FRAME	HEIGHT Feet	HEIGHT Inches	SMALL FRAME	MEDIUM FRAME	LARGE FRAME
5	2	128–134	131–141	138–150	4	10	102–111	109–121	118–131
5	3	130–136	133–143	140–153	4	11	103–113	111–123	120–134
5	4	132–138	135–145	142–156	5	0	104–115	113–126	122–137
5	5	134–140	137–148	144–160	5	1	106–118	115–129	125–140
5	6	136–142	139–151	146–164	5	2	108–121	119–132	128–143
5	7	138–145	142–154	149–168	5	3	111–124	121–135	131–147
5	8	140–148	145–157	152–172	5	4	114–127	124–138	134–151
5	9	142–151	148–160	155–176	5	5	117–130	127–141	137–155
5	10	144–154	151–163	158–180	5	6	120–133	130–144	140–159
5	11	146–157	154–166	161–184	5	7	123–136	133–147	143–163
6	0	149–160	157–170	164–188	5	8	126–139	136–150	146–167
6	1	152–164	160–174	168–192	5	9	129–142	139–153	149–170
6	2	155–168	164–178	172–197	5	10	132–145	142–156	152–173
6	3	158–172	167–182	176–202	5	11	135–148	145–159	155–176
6	4	162–176	171–187	181–207	6	0	138–151	148–162	158–179

high frequency influenced the weight aspect of the mortality picture. It was not "thinness" itself that caused higher death rates, but that many thin people had undiagnosed tuberculosis. Today there is little tuberculosis in Western societies, so the association no longer holds.

In the first half of the 20th century, the insurance-company tables found mortality to be highest in the heavier segment of the population, who were therefore charged extra premiums for their insurance. The pattern keeps changing.

We need a biological interpretation of today's life tables. First of all, according to obesity expert Dr. Albert Stunkard of the University of Pennsylvania School of Medicine[4] most of the current data are not adequately controlled for smoking, which is second only to poor diet in damaging health. In the famous study in Framingham, Massachusetts, the proportion of smokers in the population was 55 percent in the most overweight group and over 80 percent among the most underweight.[5] So it's not that fat people are healthier and so live longer, but that thin people smoke more and so live less long. It is also true that a higher death rate among thin middle-aged men may reflect hidden disease (especially cancer) rather than leanness in itself. In one 10-year study, lean middle-aged men who maintained the same weight they had had as young men enjoyed the lowest mortality of all.[6]

Besides smoking and the possible association of undiagnosed cancer with leanness, there are three additional ways to explain the insurance-company figures without assuming that mild obesity is good for you.

First and best explanation: The Metropolitan "best weight" tables may be valid for fully fed persons but be largely *irrelevant* to the phenomenon of the high/low diet. Look at it this way: Different strains of mice are available which are genetically (that is, "naturally") very obese, mildly obese, of average weight, or quite slender when fully fed. But the life spans of *all* of these strains are greatly extended by the high/low diet. Thus, animals or persons whose hereditary makeup causes them to be mildly heavy when they eat freely may enjoy a survival advantage over others when everyone is on a full diet (because they have more efficient metabolic genes), but they and all others would live *still longer* on a reduced intake.

Second: With today's wide use of low-quality processed foods and the emphasis on fast foods, you may have to eat more calories simply to get adequate nutrition. Only overweight gourmands get enough essential nutrients when the diet quality is low.

Third: Remember our genetically obese "ob/ob" mice. When these short-lived and monstrously obese animals are placed on a high/low diet, their weight falls to a normal range (*normal*, not thin), but their life span now extends as far as that of genetically *non*obese mice on a high/low diet. So it is not merely absolute weight that determines subsequent life span but how much below your set point you are. Responding to our society's pressure to be as slim as possible, people who naturally tend to be overweight are constantly striving to lose some of it. Many people above average weight may actually be below their personal set points, and so be *biologically* underweight[7] and have an improved metabolic efficiency.[8] That would give them a survival advantage.

In view of these contrary facts and alternative interpretations, I do not believe the current life-insurance-company statistics prove that mild obesity is advantageous in and of itself. It looks that way at first glance, but the looks are deceiving. Indeed, a major conference sponsored recently by the National Institutes of Health Nutrition Committee and the Centers for Disease Control concluded that *the weights associated with the greatest longevity are below average weights of the population*, as long as such weights are not associated with illness.[9]

You might hear smug claims from the pro-obesity lobby, but don't believe them. It's *in* to be thin, and stout is still definitely *out* in terms of health.[10]

Diet and the Killer Diseases

Poor nutrition is the chief factor in most of the major diseases in First World societies. Let us single out these diseases and see how susceptibility to them can be greatly diminished by adjustment of our eating habits.

Arteriosclerosis and Heart Disease

Arteriosclerotic heart disease is the greatest epidemic mankind has ever faced, carrying off a larger percentage of the population than the Black Death in the Middle Ages (Figure 5.2). Yet it's by no means an inevitable factor of life. We almost entirely bring it on ourselves by our lifestyles. And we start young. Many of the supposedly healthy American soldiers killed in Vietnam were found, on autopsy, to have arteriosclerosis.

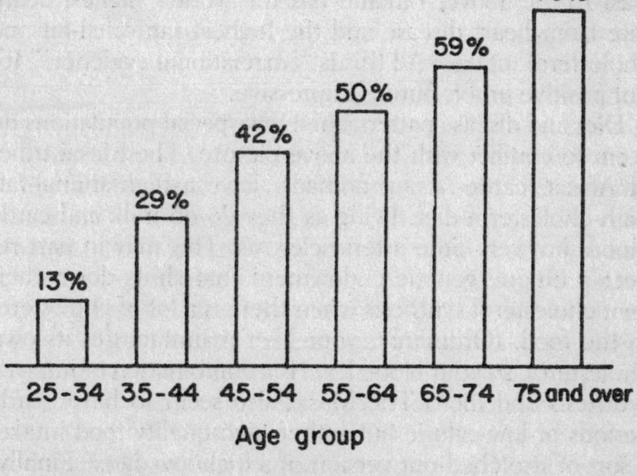

Figure 5.2 Percentage of all deaths due to heart disease according to age groups.

Worldwide population studies show that arteriosclerotic heart disease is lowest in populations eating diets high in complex carbohydrates and low in fat and cholesterol. The Japanese are a modern, industrial, high-stress, heavy-smoking society but enjoy a relatively *low* incidence of heart disease—unless they emigrate to the United States and adopt American dietary habits. The typical diet in Japan is low in fat, especially in saturated animal fat. Red meat, with its high saturated-fat content, is not a traditional Japanese dish.

The vegetarian Hunzas of India, whose diet consists of whole grains, vegetables, and fruits and is high in fiber, have very little heart disease or diabetes. The Seventh-day Adventists, also mostly vegetarians, enjoy a much lower incidence of heart disease than the average American population. The "diseases of affluence"—heart disease, large-bowel cancer, diabetes, and others—are rare in Polynesian communities until these people emigrate to New Zealand and fall victim to a Western way of life.[11] By contrast to the above, Finland has the world's highest death rate from heart disease and the highest saturated-fat and cholesterol intakes. All this is "correlational evidence." It's not positive proof, but it's impressive.

Diet and disease patterns of a few special populations do seem to conflict with the above picture. The Masai tribes of Africa, cattle-raising nomads, have a high-animal-fat, high-cholesterol diet, living as they do on milk and cattle blood, but very little arteriosclerosis. This may in part reflect a unique genetic endowment that shuts down their own cholesterol synthesis when there is a lot of cholesterol in the food. (Ordinarily, your liver manufactures its own cholesterol, so your blood level is a combination of internal synthesis and diet.) The Masai also seem to have yearly periods of low-calorie but rather-high-quality food intake, a sort of stretched-out version of a high/low diet.[12] Finally, Masai cattle are grass-fed and lean, whereas U.S. cattle are fattened with grains and high-protein feed for 4–5 months before slaughter. Free-roaming cattle have much less total body fat than domestic cattle, and probably a different blood-fat pattern. And in free-roaming cattle, up to 40 percent of the fat they do have is polyunsaturated, whereas in our U.S. domestic cattle it's only 4 percent.[13] So the fat-intake pattern in the Masai may resemble that of primitive Paleolithic man (page 31)—exactly what we in advanced countries are genetically programmed to consume but don't.

Eskimos, who subsist almost exclusively on fish, seal, whale, and caribou, with an average daily intake of 3,400 calories, including 377 grams of protein and a whopping 162 grams of fat, show little or no arteriosclerosis. But the fat in their diet is also unlike that of the typical American. It is rich in polyunsaturated fatty acids derived from fish oil, especially in eicosapentaenoic acid, which protects against arteriosclerosis.[14] (Three rich natural sources of eicosapentaenoic acid are albacore tuna, Atlantic mackerel, and pink salmon.) When Eskimos adopt a Western-style diet, they too become arteriosclerotic.

The correlational evidence has been good enough that many doctors for many years have been recommending cholesterol-lowering diets to their patients. Not every doctor agreed with this, saying that it had not been formally shown in a large, well-controlled clinical study that lowering bood cholesterol would also lower the frequency of actual heart attacks.

Direct experimental evidence became available recently. A $150-million tracking study supported by the National Heart, Lung and Blood Institute has established that lowering cholesterol in blood reduces coronary risks. A total of 3,800 men between the ages of 35 and 59, with no history of hypertension or heart disease but with abnormally high blood cholesterol levels, were divided into two groups. Both were placed on a low-cholesterol diet. In addition, one group received the cholesterol-lowering drug cholestyramine for a period of 7 to 10 years. This drug binds to the bile acids in the intestines and enhances their excretion from the body. There is a double effect here. Bile acids are needed to emulsify ingested fat so it can be absorbed in the intestines. If they are bound by the gritty cholestyramine resin, less fat is absorbed. Also, bile acids are manufactured in the liver out of cholesterol. Normally they are reabsorbed, used over again, recycled. Bound to cholestyramine, they are eliminated.

In this study, the group receiving cholestyramine averaged an 8-percent greater reduction in cholesterol and a 12-percent greater reduction in LDL than the other group —and 24-percent fewer cardiac deaths. In those individuals who faithfully took the drug (5–6 packets per day) for the whole period, with decreases of 25 percent or more in total blood cholesterol and 35 percent in LDL, the incidence of heart attacks was less by an amazing 50 percent.

Food clearly affects the levels of blood fats, particularly cholesterol, LDL (low-density lipoproteins), and HDL (high-density lipoproteins). In the body, cholesterol is packaged in envelopes of protein for moving through the blood and tissues. The packages are the LDL and HDL molecules. LDL is like an oil truck. It carries 70–80 percent of the cholesterol in the blood plasma, and delivers fat and cholesterol to the cells. The cells manufacture "receptors" on their surfaces which serve as docks for the LDL trucks to make their deliveries. When cells contain an excess of cholesterol, reflecting too much animal and dairy fat in the diet, they manufacture fewer receptor docks, and the undelivered loads of LDL cholesterol pile up in the blood.[15] If breaks occur in the inside lining of the vessel wall (Smoking and high blood pressure are the commonest causes of such injury), the crowded LDL oil trucks drive through them and dump their cargo into the tissues, as industrial polluters do on the back roads of our fair land. That's the beginning of arteriosclerotic plaques. HDL trucks, on the other hand, go in the opposite direction. They help remove cholesterol from the blood and tissues, reducing the risk of arteriosclerosis. A ratio of total blood cholesterol/HDL of 5 carries an average risk of heart disease; a ratio of 3.5 only half the average risk.

The National Institutes of Health now strongly recommends that you reduce your dietary fat and cholesterol. Average cholesterol levels in the U.S. population by age groups are shown in Table 5.2. In the famous Framingham study in Massachusetts, the risk of coronary disease was fairly low if the cholesterol was under 200 (and the lower the better). Keep yours below 180 and you very likely will never have a heart attack. Unless you have a strong genetic predisposition toward a high blood cholesterol level, the high/low diet will bring you into that range. But do not go overboard. Excessively low cholesterol levels have been associated with some increase in cancer risk.[16]

Table 5.2 Blood cholesterol levels in American men and women. Average values for the total population at each age group are shown, also the average values for the 5% of the population with the lowest and the 5% with the highest cholesterol levels (adapted from *Hospital Practice*, May 1983).

	MEN			WOMEN		
Age (years)	Average Values (all persons)	Average Values lowest 5%	Average Values highest 5%	Average Values (all persons)	Average Values lowest 5%	Average Values highest 5%
0–4	155	114	203	156	112	200
5–9	160	121	203	164	126	205
10–14	158	119	202	160	124	201
15–19	150	113	197	157	120	200
20–24	167	124	218	164	122	216
25–29	182	133	244	171	128	222
30–34	192	138	254	175	130	231
35–39	201	146	270	184	140	242
40–44	207	151	268	194	147	252
45–49	212	158	276	203	152	265
50–54	213	158	277	218	162	285
55–59	214	156	276	231	173	300
60–64	213	159	276	231	172	297
65–69	213	158	274	233	171	303
70+	207	151	270	228	169	289

Changing your blood-fat factors for the better: Many authorities now recommend a diet lower than 300 mg. per day in cholesterol (1 egg contains 275 mg.) and with less than 30 percent of calories derived from fat. That's wise for the cholesterol, but the 30 percent fat is merely a compromise between what the authorities think people will insist on and what is healthful.[17] Actually, the lower the fat the better, at least down to about 8 percent. You do need enough to provide the essential fatty acids and to support absorption of fat-soluble vitamins; but lowering dietary fat and cholesterol will lower blood cholesterol.[18] Total fat may even be more important than total cholesterol in controlling cholesterol levels.[19]* The high/low diet calls for 8 to 20 percent of calories derived from fat.

The type of fat is also important. Saturated fats promote arteriosclerosis and polyunsaturated fats inhibit it. Remember that even though Eskimos eat an enormous amount of fat, their diet is high in polyunsaturated fish-oil fats; they have low LDL, high HDL, and very little heart disease.

Vegetable oils such as corn oil, and seed oils such as sunflower-seed oil, are more or less polyunsaturated. About 2 gm. of polyunsaturated oils is required to neutralize the cholesterol elevation caused by 1 gm. of saturated fats.[20] In one study, adding polyunsaturated fats to the diet in the amount of 20 percent of total energy (a polyunsaturated-to-saturated-fat ratio of about 1 to 1), led to 20–23-percent drop in cholesterol, with the main effect being on LDL.[21]

The fatty acids called linolenic and eicosapentaenoic acid (again the Eskimos) are especially important as they influence the metabolism of some remarkable body chemicals called prostaglandins, which in turn influence blood-vessel contraction and blood clotting. The prostaglandins PGE1 (made by your body from linolenic acid) and PGE3 (from eicosapentaenoic acid) are the ones you want to have more of; and PGE2 (made from arachidonic acid), less of. Cod-liver oil and mackerel contain large amounts of eicosapentaenoic acid. In clinical trials, adding fish oil rich in eicosapentaenoic acid to the diet has decreased blood viscosity, decreased blood clotting, increased bleeding time, increased HDL, and somewhat decreased LDL.[22] All these changes are to the good. One of the available products, if you decide to take eicosapentaenoic acid as a supplement, is called MaxEPA. Ten grams of MaxEPA contains about 3 gm. of eicosapentaenoic acid. One to 2 gm. of MaxEPA per day would be a conservative dose. Salmon oil is also acceptable. Neither of these contains the excessive amounts of vitamins A and D present in fish-liver oils.[23] Recent evidence reported in the *New England Journal of Medicine*[24] strongly supports the idea that high-fish diets may help prevent coronary heart disease. The consumption of as little as one or two fish dishes per week may be of preventive value.

Other dietary components besides actual fats and oils will influence your levels of blood fats and susceptibility to arteriosclerosis. These include the kinds of protein you eat, as well as carbohydrates, sugars, minerals, trace elements, and fibers. And a small amount of aspirin, such as one baby aspirin every second day, may favorably affect the prostaglandin pattern.

Replacement of animal with vegetable protein in the diet will lower plasma cholesterol and LDL and favorably influence both the onset and the course of arteriosclerosis. This effect is not merely due to the greater fat intake associated with animal protein, since it can be seen (in animals) with low-fat, cholesterol-free semipurified diets in which milk and soybean proteins are compared.[25] Figure 5.3 dramatically shows the effects on blood cholesterol of feeding various types of protein for 28 days to rabbits maintained on cholesterol-free diets. We see that *all* plant proteins are better than *any* animal proteins, and that within the two classes some influence the bunnies' cholesterol more than others. But don't let these data necessarily scare you off animal proteins. They are just one more item in the balance.

With regard to carbohydrates: refined sugars, especially sucrose (the sugar in your sugar bowl), may increase blood cholesterol. As I have said, a significant part of your blood

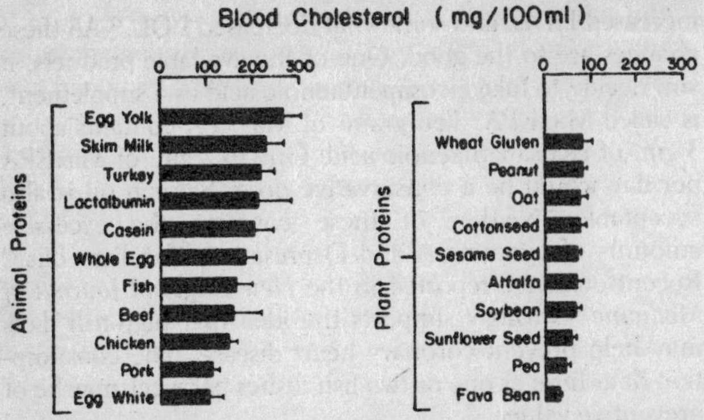

Figure 5.3 Effects on blood (plasma) cholesterol levels of feeding various protein preparations to rabbits maintained on cholesterol-free diets (adapted from K. K. Carroll, *Federation Proceedings*, 41:2792, 1982).

cholesterol is synthesized by your liver, while the rest comes from the diet. Refined sugar increases the internal synthesis. It also lowers HDL in animals and humans, and animals that receive sugar as part of their carbohydrate source don't live as long as partners fed cornstarch (a complex carbohydrate) at the same calorie level.

Dietary changes in zinc, copper, chromium, and magnesium may influence susceptibility to arteriosclerosis. Copper deficiency increases blood cholesterol, and the average copper intake in the United States is only about 1 mg. per day, well below the RDA of 2 mg. per day. An excess of zinc in the diet (unlikely unless the diet is oversupplemented) will further increase the cholesterol-raising effect of copper deficiency.

Chromium deficiency may play a role in both arteriosclerosis and diabetes. In rats, when the diet is low in chromium, the levels of both blood cholesterol and glucose are abnormally high. The tissues of American adults show on the average only about 2.4 micrograms of chromium per 100 grams of tissue, whereas in other North American mammals—cattle, sheep, rats, squirrels, foxes, and so on

—the level averages 21 micrograms. In a recent study of 10 adult American males and 22 females, 90 percent habitually ate less than the minimum suggested "safe and adequate" amount of chromium.[26]

Why are we Americans deficient in chromium? *Raw* sugar contains 36 micrograms of chromium per 150 grams of sugar, *refined* sugar only 3 to 4 micrograms. On the average we consume 200 grams of refined sugar a day, including the large amount in many processed foods. Whole wheat contains 175 micrograms of chromium per 100 grams, refined white flour only about 22. The high intake of refined sugar and white flour in today's average American diet simply does not supply enough chromium. This forces the body to use its own stores in order to help insulin handle the rise in blood sugar that follows a sugar-rich meal. Part of this mobilized chromium is then excreted through the kidneys, and our deficiency increases. A good way to stimulate chromium deficiency is to drink tea and coffee all day long with plenty of refined sugar and eat toast with jam on it, processed breakfast food with sugar, white bread, and sugary desserts. And taking chromium in pill form may not help: less than 1 percent is absorbed unless you take it as Glucose Tolerance Factor pills. Shellfish and chicken as well as some forms of brewer's yeast are good sources of usable chromium.

Long-term inadequacy of magnesium in the diet will contribute substantially to heart disease.[27] Those parts of the United States where the drinking water is low in dissolved minerals experience a higher death rate from heart disease than where the ground water is hard. The responsible element seems to be magnesium. Magnesium balances the effects of calcium on the heart. Calcium keeps the heart in a highly electrically stimulated state, and increases the heart rate; magnesium relaxes and slows the heart. Patients with coronary heart disease tend to have lower blood magnesium levels than well persons.[28]

Magnesium intakes in the United States have been declining since 1900 in the face of sharp rises in nutrients that increase the need for it, such as vitamin D (in fortified milk) and phosphorus (high in soft drinks). Alcohol decreases magnesium absorption and increases magnesium excretion. A factor in the long average life spans of the Hunzas may be their drinking of "glacial milk," essentially an aqueous extract of rocks. The moving glacier grinds up rocks in its bed and percolates its melting waters through the mineral-rich mush.

Studies of fiber intake in relation to fat metabolism have given interesting but variable results. In part this is due to there being many different kinds of "fiber."[29] Just as "vitamin" was treated as a single entity when first discovered, so today with "fiber." Strictly speaking, dietary "fiber" refers only to cell-wall material, including nondigestible cellulose and such noncellulose sugars as the galactomannans. Pectin, gum tragacanth, gum arabic, guar gum (a galactomannan extracted from the Japanese konjac root, a member of the yam family), locust bean gum, and carrageenin are chemically similar to components of the plant cell wall, and pectin is an actual component of the cell wall (although it is water-soluble and gelatinous); but some of these materials are produced by secretory cells. In truth the "gums" are not "fibrous" at all.

Most brans and other particulate fibers in cereal grains (the fibers in All-Bran, for example—which, however, contains 19 percent sugar[30]) are high in nondigestible cellulose. They increase fecal bulk and fluidity, but they have no effect at all on blood cholesterol.

The other kinds of fibers, the gel-forming pectins and gums, lower LDL and blood cholesterol[31] by interfering with fat absorption from the intestines, slowing the rate of sugar absorption, and binding with and increasing the secretion of bile acids. Table 5.3 compares how wheat bran, guar gum, and the cholestyramine used in the National Heart, Blood, and Lung Institute study bind bile acids, cholesterol, and fat. In general, vegetable but (excepting oat bran) not cereal fibers exert an anti-blood-fat effect.

Guar gum and other vegetable gums are often used in

Table 5.3 Percentage of binding of bile acids, cholesterol, and fat by dietary "fibers" and by the drug cholestyramine (adapted from K. K. Carroll, *Federation Proceedings* 41:2792, 1982).

Dietary substance (40 mg)	% binding of Bile acids	Cholesterol	Fat
Wheat bran	4	0	11
Alfalfa meal	7	1	19
Guar gum	36	23	23
Cholestyramine	82	95	92

low-fat salad dressings. They impart an oily sensation but are not oils. You can make your own gum-rich Creamy Russian Dressing using the following formula:

Creamy Russian Dressing

In a blender add 25 gm. gum arabic* to ½ cup water and blend until clear, then add ½ cup vinegar, 2 tbsp. lemon juice, 1 tbsp. chopped green onion, 1 tsp. dry mustard, ½ tsp. garlic powder, ¼ tsp. paprika. Blend until there is no separation into 2 layers (about 5 minutes). Store in refrigerator.

* If not available in health-food store, write to TIC Gums, Inc., 144 East 44th Street, New York, N.Y. 10017.

Because of the vinegar, this dressing keeps well in the refrigerator. Take a small bottle of it with you when you eat out and pour copiously onto salad. Besides providing an oil-feeling but oil-free dressing, the gum arabic will partially inhibit absorption of fat from the rest of your dinner —if you are having steak or roast beef, for example.

Many oil-free salad dressings on the market contain guar gum. That's fine as a taste substitute for real oil, but guar gum makes up into such a thick, viscous solution that the actual amounts in these prepared dressings are too low to interfere much with fat absorption. Gum arabic doesn't do this, so you can add more to get a double effect. I should warn you not to take large amounts of gum in unhydrated powder form, as it will swell in the digestive tract and may cause blockage.

The average-sized person should be (but usually isn't) consuming at least 40 grams of total "fiber" per day, including cereal, pectin, and gums. Few people do, and 60 grams in even better. High-fiber-combined-with-low-fat diets very favorably affect the blood lipid picture, with an average 32-percent lowering of blood cholesterol in long-term usage.[32] Table 5.4 gives fiber contents of different foods in normal-size portions. These values are only approximations as different sources vary widely, depending on just what has been included under the designation "fiber."

Table 5.4 Fiber content of some common foods expressed as grams of fiber per 100 grams (3½ oz.) of food, and as amount of fiber in one average, uncooked portion.

	Gm. fiber per 100 gm.	Portion	Gm. fiber per portion
FRUITS			
Apple	3	1 med.	4
Apricot	2	3 med.	2
Banana	2	1 med.	4
Blackberries	7	½ cup	5
Cherries	2	10	1
Orange	2	1 med.	3
Peach	2	1 med.	3
Pear	2	1 med.	4
Pineapple	1	½ cup	1
Plums	2	3 med.	2
Prunes, dry	14	3–4	5
Raisins	7	¼ cup	3
Strawberries	2	½ cup	2
VEGETABLES			
Asparagus	3	4 spears	2
Beets	3	½ cup	2
Broccoli	3	½ cup	4
Brussels sprouts	3	4	2
Cabbage	2	½ cup	4
Carrots	4	1 med.	2
Cauliflower	2	½ cup	1
Celery	2	1 stalk	1
Corn	5	½ cup	3

	Gm. fiber per 100 gm.	Portion	Gm. fiber per portion
Cucumber	1	½ cup	1
Onions	1	¼ cup	½
Potatoes, white	2	1 med.	3
Potatoes, sweet	4	1 med.	4
Spinach	4	½ cup	2
Tomato	1	1 med.	2
Zucchini	3	½ cup	2
LEGUMES			
Black beans	6	½ cup	6
Kidney beans	5	½ cup	5
Lentils	4	½ cup	4
Lima beans	5	½ cup	4
Pinto beans	5	½ cup	5
Peas, fresh	3	½ cup	3
Peas, split	4	½ cup	4
White beans	5	½ cup	6
Soybeans	6	½ cup	5
CEREALS & GRAINS			
Bread, white	3	1 slice	1
Bread, whole-wheat	12	1 slice	3
Barley	2	½ cup	2
Bran, wheat	53	1 tbsp.	2
Bran, oat	26	1 tbsp.	1
Oats	11	¼ cup	3
Rice, brown	6	¼ cup	3
NUTS & SEEDS			
Almonds	14	¼ cup	5
Peanuts	6	¼ cup	3
Sunflower seeds	14	¼ cup	5
Walnuts	5	¼ cup	2

Avoiding arteriosclerosis: Obesity in and of itself is a definite risk factor for arteriosclerosis. In a long-term follow-up of Framingham participants, the degree of obesity on the initial examination predicted the 26-year frequency of heart attacks in men regardless of age, cholesterol, blood pressure, or other factors.[33] Weight gain after the young-adult years brought a considerably increased risk of heart disease, with change from a slim youth to an obese adult being especially bad. By contrast, change from an obese youth to a thin adult greatly lowered susceptibility.

The amount and type of fat in your diet is the single most important risk factor. Much over 20 percent of calories from fat or oil promotes arteriosclerosis. Much under 8 percent may interfere with the absorption of fat-soluble vitamins, including anticancer vitamins like vitamins A and E and the beta-carotenes.

Half of the fats should be polyunsaturated, or at least not fully saturated. (Olive oil is monounsaturated, but its effects on cholesterol are such that you can count it in the polyunsaturated category.) If you are an average American you should increase the ratio of fish to red meat in your diet, increase vegetable protein in relation to animal protein, increase the amount of complex carbohydrates, cut back sharply on refined sugars (especially sucrose), make sure that your copper and chromium intake are not greatly below the RDA levels, raise your magnesium intake over the current average amounts, and let the ratio of your magnesium/calcium intake be 1 to 1 (instead of the 2 to 1 found in many mineral supplements currently on the market). And increase your intake of gel-forming fibers. Most of these measures are included in the high/low diet formulation. Additional measures, including vitamin and mineral supplementation and the right quality and quantity of exercise, will be described in later sections of this book. If you follow these combined protocols, you will be far less likely than the average person to be among that 50 percent of the population who end their lives with the stabbing pain of a cardiac death.

"The Big C"

Operated on for lung cancer and initially doing well, John Wayne thought he was cured. "I licked the Big C," he boasted. But he hadn't—not even the Duke. Neither did Babe Ruth, Humphrey Bogart, Yul Brynner, Julian Beck, and a long string of tough and not-so-tough other guys. After arteriosclerosis of the heart and brain, cancer is public enemy number one. And as we've seen, 80 to 90 percent of cancers are due to environmental factors, of which diet is the most important.

Overwhelming evidence shows that diet plays a role in cancer. Studies comparing worldwide cancer frequencies between cultures with different dietary patterns, of changes in frequency of different types of cancer as people migrate from one culture to another and adopt new eating habits, of cancer frequencies in particular populations within one culture that have different eating habits from the rest of the population, and of experimental animals all point to diet as a leading cancer culprit. Figure 5.4 shows the distribution of the different types of cancer and (in parentheses) the breakdown of deaths from cancer. Because some cancers can now be cured, there is a difference in distribution between percentage of occurrence and percentage of deaths. Lung cancer constitutes 22 percent of all cancers that occur, but since it is rarely curable, it makes up 35 percent of all fatal cancers. The greatest single

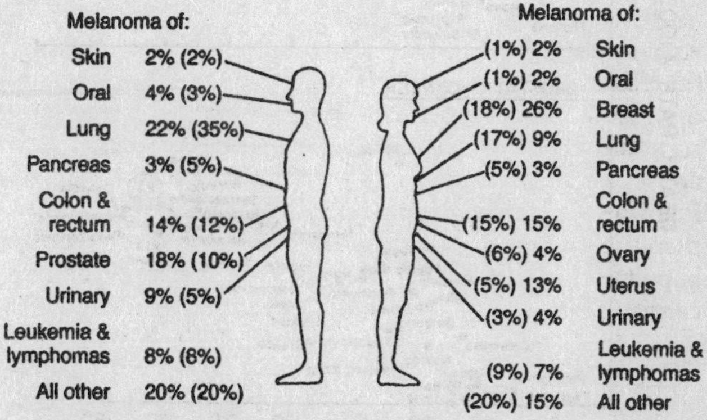

Figure 5.4 Distribution of all cancers occurring, cured or not, and (in parentheses) distribution of cancers among persons who die of cancer. The number in parentheses is greater for those cancers which cannot now be very effectively treated. All percentages, both inside and outside the parentheses, can be substantially reduced by the high/low diet.

killer cancer, it caused 121,000 deaths in 1984 alone. Cancer of the prostate constitutes 18 percent of cancers that occur, but only 10 percent of fatal cancers. It can often be cured.

The cancers in which diet plays a significant role are those of the colon, breast, and stomach for sure, probably those of the uterus and prostate, and maybe oral cancer. Frequencies of breast and prostate cancer in relation to fat intake for different world populations are shown in Figure 5.5. Total fat is a better predictor of cancer than specific

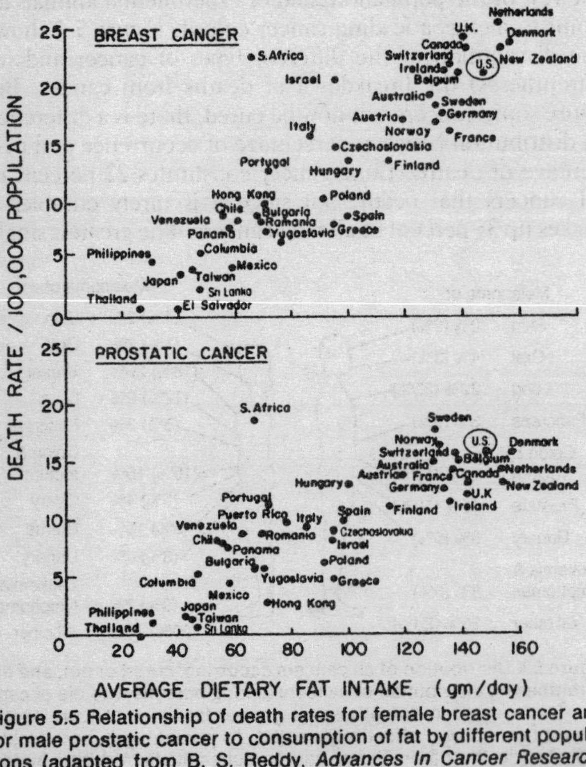

Figure 5.5 Relationship of death rates for female breast cancer and for male prostatic cancer to consumption of fat by different populations (adapted from B. S. Reddy, *Advances In Cancer Research*, 32:237, 1980).

types of fat, animal or vegetable, saturated or polyunsaturated.

When people migrate from one country to another, they or their descendants acquire the cancer pattern of their new country. Japan has one of the highest rates of stomach cancer in the world, five times the U.S. rate. This may be due to nitrates in the Japanese diet or drinking water, low consumption of fruits and vegetables, and excessive consumption of salt-cured fish. Emigrants from Japan to Hawaii continue to be at high risk for stomach cancer, but their children who adopt Western dietary habits are not. In contrast to stomach cancer, cancers of the colon, breast, and pancreas are low in frequency in native Japanese, but high in their descendants in the United States. The genetic background is the same, but the cancer pattern changes as the diet changes.

Many types of cancer require an "initiating event" that involves alteration of DNA, the genetic material inside each cell. "Initiation" is irreversible, but by itself it does not lead to cancer. It must be followed by "promotion," which *is* reversible and seems to act either by stimulating inappropriate cell division or by stimulating cells to manufacture large amounts of the injurious chemicals known as free radicals.[34] High-fat diets have a strong promotion effect.

A high fiber intake inhibits the development of colon cancer. Since bile salts are, under the right circumstances, tumor "promoters," the protective effect of fiber against colon cancer may depend on its capacity to bind bile acids in the intestinal tract. The daily fiber intake in Third World countries is over 60 gm./day, largely derived from starchy foods (insoluble cell-wall fibers), compared with only about 20 gm./day in the West, largely from fruits and vegetables (pectins and gums). The special importance of fiber intake in colon cancer is illustrated by the observation that in Finland, where the food intake is high in *both* fat and fiber, the frequency of colon cancer is in fact low. The benefit from fiber, at least for colon cancer, seems to cancel out the ill effects of fat.

The types of fibers which act against cancer in the gut (and also militate against obesity and diabetes, as we shall see) are those particularly present in cereals. Wheat fibers (bran) are among the best for these effects. In the high/low diet I include a generous amount of wheat bran in most breakfast meals.

Vitamin C intake may influence cancer susceptibility. The National Research Council[35] now specifically recommends eating plenty of vitamin C–containing materials—more, although no precise amount is stipulated, than the RDA of 60 mg. per day. Extra amounts of the element selenium and of beta-carotene may also offer protection against cancer,[36] and will be discussed later. A recent 19-year study suggested that colon cancer is increased in persons with a diet too low in calcium and vitamin D.[37]

Large amounts in the diet of brussels sprouts, cabbage, turnips, broccoli, and cauliflower, all vegetables of the Brassicaceae family, may decrease the incidence of colonic and rectal cancer. All these vegetables, when they are fresh, contain chemicals called "indols" which may raise intestinal levels of enzymes (the monooxygenase enzymes) that inactivate some of the cancer-causing agents.[38a] Women who eat 2–3 servings of fruits and vegetables per day have been reported to have less than half the risk of mouth and throat cancer of those consuming less than 1½ servings.[39]

Avoiding cancer: The lowered fat intake recommended for arteriosclerosis also holds for cancer prevention. Increased amounts of vitamin C, selenium, beta-carotene, and vegetables like cabbages and broccoli are indicated, and at least RDA amounts of calcium and vitamin D. Fiber intake should be 40 to 60 gm. or more, including both insoluble (cereal) and gel-forming fibers.

Hypertension and Stroke

On April 12, 1945, as World War II was drawing to a close, 63-year-old President Franklin D. Roosevelt was sitting quietly for his portrait during a much-needed rest at Warm Springs, Georgia. Suddenly he said, "I have a terrible headache" and fell forward, unconscious. He had had high blood pressure for a long time, and now had sustained a massive brain hemorrhage—a stroke. He was dead in a few hours.

Blood pressure is usually given in two numbers, such as 140/90. The upper number, called the systolic pressure, is the pressure the blood exerts on the walls of the arteries during the heartbeat. The lower one, the diastolic pressure, is the pressure remaining in the arteries between heartbeats. In adults a blood pressure exceeding 140/90 is abnormal, the lowest rung of hypertension. At any level of increased blood pressure, the younger the person, the greater the decrease in his life expectancy. By 65 to 74 years of age three-fourths of U.S. adults have either definite or borderline hypertension.

Intelligence itself may be influenced by hypertension. At the Duke University Center for the Study of Aging, individuals in their 60s were divided into three groups—normal, borderline, and frank hypertensives—and their intelligence levels were tested regularly for ten years. Those with normal blood pressure suffered no decline, but considerable decline occurred in those with frank hypertension.

Most authorities believe that excessive salt (sodium chloride) plays a major role in causing hypertension. While not perfect, the evidence is good enough that the American Medical Association, the American Heart Association, the National Academy of Sciences, the Food and Drug Administration, and the U.S. Department of Agriculture have all recommended a decrease in salt intake for the U.S. population.

Salt has an ancient history in its interactions with human culture. The connotations of the word in English include worthiness ("to be worth one's salt") and excellence ("salt of the earth"). The word "salary" comes from a salt allowance *salarius*, given to Roman soldiers. Jews seal covenants by exchanging salt. Desert Arabs will not attack a man whose salt they have eaten. Bread and salt are gifts in Slavic countries. Kings in countries such as Babylon, Egypt, China, Mexico, and Peru ruled by salt monopoly. One of Mahatma Gandhi's most dramatic maneuvers was against the British salt tax. He walked 200 miles to the seashore, evaporated a pan of water, ate the residue of salt, and paid no tax to the British.

Despite its romantic history, an excess of salt is unhealthful, and the average American consumes 12 or more grams a day when less than 1 gram is all he needs. Surveys of many cultures, from Greenland Eskimos to nomads of southern Iran to South Sea Islanders, indicate that hypertension is virtually absent in populations that use only small amounts of salt. Figure 5.6 shows the relation between average daily salt intake and the percentage of hypertensives in five different populations.

Why do we crave so much salt? Primitive man didn't get enough in his diet and experienced a chronic salt hunger.

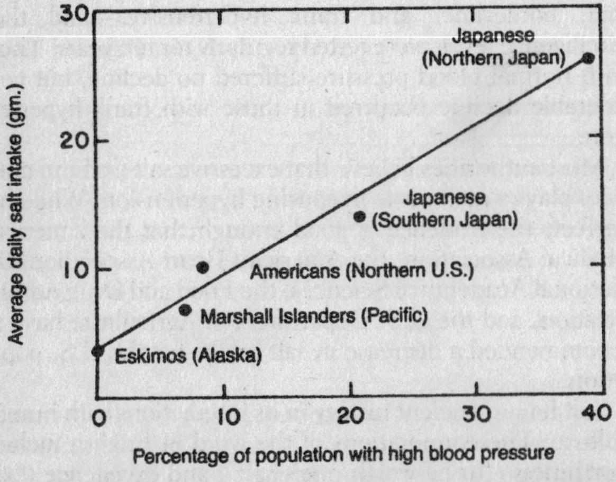

Figure 5.6 Salt intake and the frequency of high blood pressure in different populations.

He would fill up on it when it was available. Perhaps we have the same hunger even though salt is now abundant.[40] That's one possible reason. But a large part of our "salt hunger" today is no doubt culturally induced. The exposure of infants to saltiness, which is of quite recent origin, induces a taste for salt later in life. Breast milk contains much less salt than cow's milk, and before 1900 nearly all infants were breast-fed. Also, babies are now started earlier on solid foods, and are more likely to be fed salt-high commercial foods than low-salt dishes cooked at home.

Probably the sodium rather than the chloride in salt is related to hypertension. As a result of widespread use of processed and prepared foods, often high in sodium chloride, Americans commonly consume 5 to 20 times as much sodium as they need. One hundred grams of fresh peas contains only 2 mg. of sodium; canned peas, about 590 mg. A bowl of Campbell's Chicken Noodle Soup contains 1,140 mg. of sodium; 3 ounces of Chicken of the Sea tuna packed in water, 400 mg. sodium; a Big Mac, 1,510 mg.; one serving of Minute Rice's Long Grain & Wild Rice, 570 mg. (1 mg. naturally, 569 added); 1 ounce of Kellogg's Corn Flakes, 260 mg. sodium . . . and so on, and on and on.

Some processed-food companies are now putting out two versions of their products, one with the old amount of salt and a low-salt equivalent. Campbell's Chunky Vegetable Beef Soup in the "regular" variety has 935 mg. sodium; in the "low-salt" variety, 90 mg. Its low-salt Chicken Noodle Soup has only 130 mg. sodium,in contrast to the 1,140 mg. given in the above list. Unfortunately, in the low-salt products the companies have substantially increased the fat content. A can of Campbell's regular French Onion Soup contains 2.6 gm. of fat; its low-sodium equivalent contains 5 gm.[41]

Evidence of a relationship between salt and hypertension is less convincing if one compares data *within* populations rather than *between* them. In the United States, for example, some people eat a great deal of salt and others not so much, but the amount does not seem to correlate very well with who actually develops hypertension. The probable explanation has been termed the "saturation" effect, which postulates that about 20 percent of us have a hereditary tendency to develop high blood pressure *in response to increased salt intake*. The other 80 percent will not develop it regardless of intake. Under these conditions, if nearly everyone in the population consumes excess salt, no relation will be found between salt intake and hypertension because nearly everyone is far above the threshold.

Nevertheless, a reduced salt intake can lower blood pressure in humans who are already hypertensive. In fact, a low-sodium diet can lower blood pressure even among people with normal blood pressure,[42] and increasing the salt intake in middle-aged men has been shown to raise blood pressure regardless of hereditary background.[43] In the 1940s and early 1950s doctors tried using drastic reduction of sodium intake to treat hypertension, but few patients would tolerate the monotonous diets. The patient has to be talked into it—and scared enough to stick to it—but it frequently works. I recall that when I was an intern in Gorgas Hospital, in the Canal Zone, I cured a young woman who had a sudden onset of severe hypertension, with hemorrhages into the eyes, by placing her on what was then called the "rice" diet, which consisted basically of nothing but rice. I cured my patient in two weeks.

But salt is not the only factor, and the nationwide preoccupation with excessive salt has clouded the role of other factors in hypertension. Switching to a vegetarian diet may lower blood pressure. There is good evidence in both humans and animals that simple sugars like sucrose or fructose may potentiate the development of hypertension in some individuals. Weight reduction often brings significant decreases in blood pressure. Weight change from thin youth to obese adult gives a high incidence of hypertension, and from obese youth to thin adult a low incidence.[44] Reduction of fat intake can lower high blood pressure, and may even lower blood pressure in normal persons.[45] Finnish scientists[46] divided 114 subjects with normal or high blood pressure into three groups. Group 1 ate a low-fat diet for 6 weeks; group 2, a low-salt diet. Group 3 served as controls. Only group 1 experienced a decline in blood pressure.

Potassium, magnesium, and calcium deficiencies may play roles. Potassium is particularly important because the balance between potassium and sodium in the diet is intertwined and delicate.[47] Thanks to more abundant supplies of fruits and vegetables, people of Southern Europe have twice the potassium intake of those in the North . . . and less hypertension. Diets of primitive societies with low incidence of hypertension are not only low in sodium, they are high in potassium. Their intake averages 4 to 7 gm. as potassium chloride, so the *ratio* of potassium to sodium is 2 to 1 or greater, whereas in a typical American diet with its high proportion of commercially prepared and processed foods the ratio is 1 to 2—the exact reverse.

Commercial freezing and canning processes often increase the sodium-to-potassium ratio, as illustrated in Table 5.5. Frozen peas are not necessarily right out of the pod. Sometimes they are presorted by the use of sodium chloride solutions at different concentrations. Some vegetables are skinned in sodium hydroxide solutions before being frozen.

Table 5.5 Sodium and potassium contents in representative fresh, frozen, and canned foods.

Food		Portion	Sodium (mg.)	Potassium (mg.)
Corn	fresh	1 ear	1	364
	frozen	3.5 oz.	4	188
	canned	½ cup	239	144
Peas	fresh	½ cup	1	157
	frozen	3.5 oz.	88	126
	canned	½ cup	246	79
Potato	fresh	1 medium	5	587
	canned	½ cup	376	304
	instant	½ cup	280	287

Calcium deficiency may also be important in hypertension. A recent study by Dr. David McCarran of Oregon Health Sciences University analyzed data from 10,372 individuals in relation to diet and hypertension.[48] He reported that a decreased consumption of calcium rather than too much salt was the main common denominator. Some studies[49] and at least one large survey denied the calcium connection,[50] and another only partially confirmed it.[51] But Guatemalan Indians ingest about 1,200 mg. of calcium per day, as they moisten the flour for making corn tortillas with lime water, and they have a very low rate of hypertension.[52] And calcium supplementation of 1 gm./day for 22 weeks may lead to a decline in blood pressure, even in healthy young persons without hypertension.[53] So calcium seems involved in hypertension, but the situation is complex.

Avoiding hypertension: Reduce your sodium intake (from all sources, not just salt, and not just salt from the salt shaker but also from processed foods) to less than 2 gm. per day (0.3 to 0.5 gm. is all you really need). Lemon juice can replace the taste of salt in some foods: add a tablespoon to salt-free tomato juice and try it. Salt reduction will automatically also change your potassium-to-sodium ratio to a more appropriate level. If you are of normal size, consume 1 gm. of magnesium and 1 to 1.5 gm. of calcium per day, using supplements if necessary. Lose weight. Adopt the high/low diet.

Aretaeus of Cappadocia Named It "Diabetes"

"Diabetes" is Greek for "siphon," coming from a word that means "to pass through," and indeed Aretaeus of Cappadocia described it as "a strange disease that consists in the flesh and bones' running together into the urine." Severe untreated diabetes fits this imaginative description well: a copious flow of urine along with great thirst and hunger, nevertheless resulting in the wasting away of both muscle and fat to produce severe emaciation, often ending in coma and death. The untreated patient literally starves to death because his body is unable to derive energy from glucose, either because his secretion of insulin is faulty (type 1, or "juvenile," diabetes) or because the insulin receptors on the organs of his body are greatly diminished (type 2, or "late-onset," diabetes, which occurs in older persons). In both types, glucose piles up in the blood and spills into the urine. A clever medieval diagnostic trick was to see if the patient's urine was attractive to ants. Ants like the sweetness of diabetic urine.

Late-onset diabetes afflicts 5 percent of the U.S. population, including 5 million diagnosed and an estimated 2½ million undiagnosed cases. The likelihood of developing diabetes doubles with each decade of life, going from 0.1 percent for people under 20 years old to about 15 percent for those over 60. It is the third leading cause of sickness and death if one includes its many complications—arteriosclerosis, cataracts, and nerve and kidney damage.

The likelihood of developing diabetes also doubles with every 20-percent gain in body weight above average. Even among the nonobese, it is much commoner in those who are now of average weight but were previously very lean.[54]

Diabetes is of special interest to us because it shows many features of actually accelerated aging. In this sense it is unlike the diseases we've previously talked about, which occur more often in older people but are not necessarily associated with biomarker changes denoting accelerated aging. Diabetics are functionally older than their chronologic age. A decline in immune function is seen in them earlier. Changes in their connective-tissue proteins (collagen) are characteristic of older persons. They lose gamma-crystallin from their eye-lens proteins at an accelerated rate. And the number of times their connective-tissue cells will divide is considerably curtailed, just as in aging.[55]

Diabetics usually display high blood cholesterol, a decrease in the beneficial arteriosclerosis-preventing HDL factors, and greater susceptibility to arteriosclerosis. Cataracts occur earlier than normal, as do heart disease, kidney damage, and nerve disorders. Many of these adverse effects are due to the fact that the diabetic's elevated blood sugar is itself damaging to cells. High concentrations are especially detrimental to those proteins which are slow to be replaced (low-turnover proteins)—those in the lens of the eye, the lining of blood vessels, and the insulating material around nerve cells.[56] Exposed to glucose over a long period, proteins develop so-called cross links, and an insoluble brown pigment is formed.[57]

In late-onset diabetes, the intake of glucose or carbohydrates causes the blood glucose to rise, and insulin is released by the pancreas to help the tissues utilize the glucose; however, there is a deficit in tissue receptors for insulin, and this prevents a normal rate of utilization. Blood glucose and insulin both remain abnormally high. The same situation occurs in normal aging, albeit to a much lesser degree.

The high/low diet will retard these age-related defects in normally aging persons. In one experiment in humans, when mildly overweight men and women lost an average of 24 pounds, the researchers observed an improvement in glucose metabolism and an impressive decrease in the insulin levels following a glucose meal.[58] And high/low-diet–treated 12-month-old rats give glucose and insulin responses similar to those of untreated 2-month-old rats.[59]

Supplementing the diet with gel-forming fibers such as guar gum or pectin favorably affects glucose metabolism and insulin requirements.[60] But the fiber must be either a part of or intimately mixed with the food. Guar gum taken 2 minutes before or in gelatin capsules along with glucose has no effect; it must be incorporated into the meal, as in bread or cookies.[61] The way a rich supply of fiber in the meal affects the glucose curve is illustrated in Figure 5.7.

Responsible for the biological activity of the so-called "glucose-tolerance factor," or GTF,[62] the trace element chromium may play a role in late-onset diabetes. Glucose metabolism can be improved in the elderly not only by fiber but by addition of a small quantity of organic chromium,

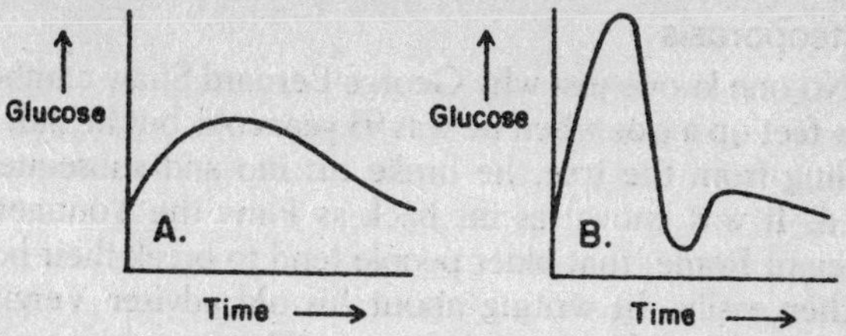

Figure 5.7 A rich supply of fiber in the meal will allow a smooth glucose curve as in A. With a low fiber, high-starch meal, a large peak and overcorrection occurs as in B.

or brewer's yeast, which contains GTF, to the diet,[63] or even inorganic chromium.[64] In one study, adding supplemental chromium to the diet of diabetics caused a drop in blood glucose levels and a significant rise in the antiarteriosclerosis HDL factors in the blood.

Avoiding diabetes: Don't let yourself be or become above average weight. If you were lean when younger, stay lean when older; don't let your weight increase to "average" as you get older because *for you*—if you were previously lean—that would be relative obesity. While late-life diabetes is partially hereditary, weight gain completes the equation and brings on the disease. Keep physically fit (See Chapter 8) and include enough of the proper kinds of fibers in your diet as well as at least RDA amounts of usable chromium. If you are genetically susceptible to developing this debilitating, troublesome, ultimately killer disease, you should certainly adopt the high/low diet. Studies of long-term low-calorie diets in humans indicate that a high/low diet should improve the insulin response and control of blood sugar not only in diabetics but in the normal elderly.[65] And the high/low diet prevents the development of diabetes in genetically susceptible mice.

Osteoporosis

No one knows just why George Bernard Shaw climbed a few feet up a tree when he was 93 years old; but he did, and falling from the tree, he broke his hip and subsequently died. It was known as far back as Pliny the Younger, in ancient Rome, that older people tend to break their bones rather easily. In writing about his old adviser Verginius Rufus, Pliny tells us in his letters, "He was rehearsing the delivery of his address of thanks to the Emperor for his election to his third consulship, when he had occasion to take up a heavy book, the weight of which made it fall out of his hands, as he was an old man. He bent down to pick it up, and lost his footing on the slippery polished floor, so that he fell and fractured his thigh."

People think of bones as inert structures, like wooden beams, but bone is a living tissue constantly being remodeled. After age 35, on the average a little more bone is lost each year than is gained during this remodeling. Between 40 and 50, men characteristically lose 0.5 to 0.75 percent of bone mass yearly, while women lose it at more than twice that rate. Bones that once were sturdy may become lighter, more fragile, their interiors resembling lacy honeycombs. The rate of natural loss increases substantially after age 50. If it's severe enough, the thinned-out bones become porous, and you develop "osteoporosis"—literally "bone porosity."

Twenty-five to 30 percent of white women and 15–20 percent of men over 50 have osteoporosis severe enough to involve compression of the vertebrae of the spinal column. Women's bone loss accelerates at menopause. Fractured vertebrae from osteoporosis produce the stoop unkindly called "dowager's hump."

Osteoporosis is one of the major problems of old age. It afflicts 20 million Americans; leads to 190,000 hip fractures yearly, 100,000 broken wrists, 180,000 "crush fractures" in which vertebrae collapse. It kills 300,000 citizens annually, and costs the nation $3.8 billion a year in medical bills.

Osteoporosis is more widespread than arthritis and about three times as common as diabetes. If you have osteoporosis, small incidents like slipping on a rug, lifting a bag of groceries, even a friendly hug can break a bone.

The causes of osteoporosis are complex. Absorption of calcium from the gut is regulated by a biologically active form of vitamin D. With age a deficiency develops in the body's ability to convert regular vitamin D to this active form. Decreased absorption results, leading to lowered blood calcium. This small drop in blood calcium triggers an increased release of a hormone from the parathyroid glands located on each side of the neck. This parathyroid hormone, or PTH, raises the blood calcium by drawing calcium from the bones, because the blood calcium has to be kept normal for the rest of the body's machinery to function. Excess PTH is then removed by the kidneys. One reason for osteoporosis in late life is that the blood level of PTH increases, secondary to a decline in kidney function that occurs with age.[66] Also, with menopause in women, the amount of estrogen in the blood decreases, and estrogen makes bone less sensitive to dissolution by PTH. Still another hormone, called calcitonin, secreted by the thyroid gland, serves to inhibit bone resorption; its level is normally greater in men than in women, but decreases in both with age. All these factors contribute to the porosity of bones.

A diet too low in calcium also contributes. Calcium requirements increase with age, whereas calcium absorption in the intestines decreases.[67] In most premenopausal women and in men, at least 800 mg. of calcium per day is required to maintain body calcium, and 30–40 percent of men require up to 1,200 mg.[68] Except for those on estrogen therapy, postmenopausal women need 1,200 to 1,500 mg. daily—about the amount contained in 1⅓ quarts of milk. More than 50 percent of American women typically consume less than 500 mg. of calcium daily, and 25 percent ingest less than 300 mg.

Protein intake affects the daily calcium requirement. An

increased intake speeds calcium excretion. The intake of sulfur-containing amino acids may be the determining factor here. These are much higher in meat than in vegetable proteins. Thus the high-meat diet in Western societies may be a factor in accelerating bone loss.

According to some authorities, the ratio of calcium to phosphorus in the diet should be greater than 1:1 to help prevent bone loss. It is often much lower, because most soft drinks contain large amounts of phosphates.

Ideally, you should have a bone-mass assessment when you are in your 30s. Heavy-boned persons are much less liable to develop osteoporosis. They still lose calcium with age, but they start with more. Weight-bearing exercise stimulates the development of heavier bones. Tennis players aged 55 to 65 have much more bone mass than the average person. And more bone in the racquet arm than in the other! At age 55, long-distance runners display a much greater bone density than semisedentary people of the same age, and osteoporosis is almost unknown in societies in which continued high levels of physical activity are customary.[69] The denser your bones are before you reach 35, the less susceptible you'll be later on. In fact, increasing your bone mass before age 35 is the single most important preventive measure against osteoporosis.

Avoiding Osteoporosis: The causes of this terrible malady are even more complex than I have outlined here. They involve interactions between calcium, phosphorus, fluoride, vitamin D, estrogens, calcitonin, parathyroid hormone, and the proteins of the bone matrix itself. Until the many complexities are better understood, these are my recommendations: Ensure an adequate calcium intake, in the diet itself if possible (milk, yogurt) or at least by supplemental calcium. There is no hard evidence that one kind of supplemental calcium salt is any better absorbed than another.[70] Calcium supplements may exert a partial suppressive effect on bone remodeling, whereas the calcium in milk does not, so milk is preferred.[71] Engage in a reasonable amount of weight-bearing exercise (Swimming, while an excellent aerobic sport, does not qualify on this score); pay some attention to your vitamin D intake; and avoid excessive phosphates in your diet. *In well-controlled animal studies a high/low diet has been shown to substantially slow down and even prevent the age-related loss of bone.*[72]

Final Comment on the Killer Diseases

If you are following an average American lifestyle, the chances are about 75 percent that you will die of one of these diseases. You can cut your susceptibility to all of them at least a third by the measures I have outlined. You can cut it by more than half by adopting the principles of the high/low diet and other forthcoming recommendations. (Not smoking is of course very important.) Among those who follow the whole program, I believe that many will break the present 110-year maximum-life-span barrier. Depending on how young they are when they start, a few should reach 140 to 150 years of age.

CHAPTER 6

The Complex Philosophy of Supplementation

One of the most confused areas we must try to make sense of is that of dietary supplementation. Vitamins, antioxidants, chemicals, hormones, minerals, minidoses, megadoses, the Recommended Daily Allowances—dietary supplementation is a battleground. The serious layman will find himself between hostile lines. The troubled air is filled with promises and dire warnings. Trumpets sound and metaphorical bullets fly. On one side, legions of lay and semilay faddists and commercial interests line up to promote their advice or their products with little understanding of or regard for real evidence. On the other side stand cadres of otherwise quite good scientists and physicians who, because establishment medicine is dead set against *any* additives in excess of the holy RDAs, accept mediocre evidence uncritically if it seems to support their views.

My current position on this controversy, and in relation to the high/low diet, can be stated briefly: (1) On the diet you should take at least small amounts of the essential vitamins and minerals, to avoid borderline deficiencies. This precaution is strongly supported by the animal studies, and has been recommended for low-calorie diets by many authorities (Nathan Shock, for example, the dean of clinical gerontology). (2) Taking substantially more than the Recommended Daily Allowances (but not really megadose amounts) of selected nutrients will, with a *moderate* order of probability (according to the evidence), enhance your average survival prospects. But (again according to existing evidence) it will *not* extend anybody's maximum life span. You will probably be doing yourself some good. You will not, except at very high doses, do yourself any harm.

If you have read my previous book, *Maximum Life Span*, you will see from what follows that I have become a bit less enthusiastic about large-dose supplementation, and about the potential antiaging benefits of antioxidants. This is simply because continuing evidence based upon survival curves (the only unassailable evidence, to my way of thinking) does not bear out the extravagant claims made by many megadose and antioxidant enthusiasts.

The chief danger of taking more than RDA amounts of any supplement is that you will be caught in a storm of controversy, be swept away, start gulping down everything on the shelf, and possibly neglect basic nutrition and good health habits. I am reluctant to become further involved in the whole supplementation area. But I think I must. If you are going to undertake a life-extension program, I want to forewarn you against overzealous promotion on the one hand and blind prejudice on the other. Let's take a fresh look.

Let's Look First at the Faddists and Commercializers.

Almost every bodily process changes with age. Among the vast, constantly outpouring medical literature, it's not hard to select an article or articles which suggest that a particular vitamin, drug, chemical, or lifestyle will prevent or slow down a particular change. If you are not too critical about the evidence in these articles and if you neglect or underplay *nonconfirming* articles, you can build what sounds like a strong argument for any hot-topic product or procedure. But that's endless and foolish. "Make the case for" evidence can unroll forever. You can bet it sells a lot of products! But if we insist on *hard evidence* that the vitamin or drug extends maximum life span in long-lived strains of animals (the only positive proof of an antiaging effect), we shall find that *none* of them have been shown to do so to any great extent in any mammals, including man.

For specific examples, let's take the antioxidants, by all odds the most-touted antiaging chemical remedy. They are supposed to prevent or neutralize those damaging agents spontaneously produced in the body and called "free radicals."

What Are Free Radicals?

Described as "great white sharks in the biochemical sea," they are fragments of molecules that have become unstuck. Ordinary chemical molecules share one characteristic: their electrons (those minute electrical charges swirling around the nucleus of each atom) are paired.[1*] An ordinary chemical bond between two atoms involves two electrons. Each atom ordinarily contributes one. When a chemical reaction takes place and the bond is broken, one fragment ordinarily keeps both electrons.

Not so with free radicals! A bond can break so that each separate fragment keeps one electron. At one time the fundamental laws of modern chemistry (the concepts of valence and molecular weight, if you please) seemed to forbid this. But in the 1930s, oil-industry scientists showed that even though free radicals might have a life span of a mere few thousandths of a second, their activity accounted for some spectacular chemical transformations—the rancification of fats and oils, for example. These discoveries gave birth to the development of the plastics and polymers industry.

In biology it took longer for free radicals to catch on. Enzymes were all the rage then, whereas free radicals looked spooky and forbidding. They are hyperactive. Once generated, they grab on to everything in reach. And once triggered, free-radical reactions tend to be unstoppable, uncontrollable, and irreversible, almost explosive. Blam! Like Sodom and Gomorrah! Turn you into a pillar of rancid fat!

To biologists, conditioned for half a century to the delicate interplay and self-regulating equilibria of enzyme cycles, free-radical reactions seemed irrelevant to life. So it was a feat of considerable insight and perhaps even foolhardy daring for Dr. Denham Harman to propose as early as 1955, and on the basis of preliminary and in retrospect rather unconvincing experiments, that such a major biological process as aging itself might be caused by free-radical attacks against the constituents of the body. He called his proposal the "free radical theory of aging."

Now, while I shall be talking at length about free radicals, I must emphasize that the "free radical theory of aging" is only *one* of at least *six* important theories of aging (See my book *Maximum Life Span* for an explanation of the others), and that some of the others are just as well founded, maybe more so. Indeed, we can explain almost all existing experiments about free radicals and health by supposing that they have much to do with disease (cancer especially) but very little to do with aging.[2]

The reason for all the hoopla in pseudoscientific popular health books and magazines is that the free-radical theory is at least plausible. One can make a reasonable case for it, and having done so, one can promote an almost unending bevy of products (antioxidants) which are supposed to neutralize the damaging free radicals. Some of these products may actually do good, although rarely as much as claimed, but a real danger exists here. Overpromotion of antioxidants, vitamins, and various drugs tends to steer people away from what are far more important for both health and life extension: careful diet, exercise, and stress avoidance. I cannot give a better illustration than to quote from the June 1983 issue of *Whole Life Times* (hardly a medical-establishment magazine, but a part of the health-food industry itself): "It is dangerously deceptive to think that a person who smokes and drinks heavily, eats a high-fat, low-fiber diet, drinks six cups of coffee a day and runs on stress and anxiety with unhealthy social relationships and an oppressive work situation, is going to somehow achieve optimal health and an extended life span simply by consuming the right nutrients and anti-aging substances. Yet this hardly exaggerates the position of [Durk] Pearson and [Sandy] Shaw, who represent one extreme in antiaging thought."

But "I would not knock old fellows in the dust," to quote John Crowe Ransom's fine poem,[3] so let us go on.

The particular free radicals we're concerned with are the products of oxygen metabolism taking place within the energy factories of the cell (the mitochondria). About 2 billion years ago, before oxygen became available in the atmosphere, organisms got energy from breaking down carbohydrates by a process called "glycolysis." This is not very efficient, and life forms, struggling to multiply, evolved the ability to use the new atmospheric constituent oxygen. Free radicals are devilish by-products of this new high-energy metabolism, just as radioactive wastes are by-products of the increased energy we can get from the atom.

Both must be gotten rid of. We're not doing so well with our radioactive wastes, but Nature has had a longer time. Down the ages, she evolved compartmentalization within the cell. The mitochondria, where many free radicals are generated, are separated from the rest of the cell by their own unique membranes. And Nature developed, within each cell, the ability to manufacture protective free-radical neutralizers—"scavengers," or to use the more popular term, "antioxidants."[4*]

Where the Battle Takes Place

Chief sites of attack are against cell membranes, both those inside cells (mitochondrial and nuclear membranes) and those forming the external walls of cells. Major components of these structures are lipids (fats), both saturated and unsaturated. (They are fatty acids really, but I'll use the simpler term.) A greater membrane concentration of unsaturated than saturated fats is essential to the pliability and elasticity the cell needs to move and flex its membranes. But—and here is the big problem—it is precisely these unsaturated fats which are most susceptible to attack by free radicals.

The radicals may also damage DNA, the hereditary blueprint for life within each cell. Indeed, many of the substances that cause or promote cancer may do so by stimulating cells to produce free radicals which then damage or alter the blueprint until the cell becomes cancerous.[5]

Evidence for the Free-Radical Theory of Aging

It's Plausible

The maximum life spans of different species are proportional to the levels of many free-radical scavengers that occur naturally in their blood. Longer-lived species have higher levels of these scavengers in relation to their "lifetime energy potential" (the amount of calories they burn up per pound of animal in a normal life span).[6*]

Some of the damage products from free-radical reactions increase with aging. A yellow-brown age pigment called lipofuscin accumulates in the cells of older animals. It is a breakdown product related to the action of free radicals upon cellular membranes. This waste is taken up by digestive vacuoles in the cells, but it's indigestible; so it piles up with age. In the human heart, for example, the pigment increases at the rate of about 0.06 percent per year. Eventually up to 5 percent of the total heart-muscle volume can be taken up by yellow-brown inert gunk.[7*]

Effects of Antioxidants on Biomarkers of Aging

Can one improve the biomarkers of aging by including antioxidants in the diet? The amount of age pigments in tissues can be substantially reduced by antioxidants such as vitamin E, methionine, BHT, or selenium,[8] or by ingestion of any of a number of brain-reactive chemicals that may have partial antioxidant properties (DMAE and centrophenoxine). However, the joker is that even though these agents retard the buildup of age pigment, the maximum life spans of animals are not increased—at least, not for long-lived strains. So the evidence could be equally interpreted as *against* the free-radical theory of aging, in that you can decrease the production of one of the main adverse products of free-radical reactions without influencing maximum life span. Many other antioxidant experiments present such an equivocal aspect when viewed critically.[9*] But we'll consider the evidence in more detail when we discuss selected individual antioxidants (vitamins C and E, selenium) in the next chapter.

The free-radical approach is a bit like the Bible. Once you are persuaded to believe in the Bible as the literal Word of God, or in this case the free-radical theory as the Word of Nature, you can give a plausible explanation for many phenomena—in this case cell deterioration, a number of diseases, and aging. This ability to explain phenomena is a necessary first step for any scientific theory. But it's only a first step. The second is to use the theory to devise experiments or treatments that will alter the course of a phenomenon in a predictable way: for example, to retard aging, or prevent or cure disease.

Effect of Antioxidants on Life Span

Certain dietary supplements, including antioxidants, will probably extend the average life spans of animals by decreasing disease susceptibility. If one is dealing with a short-lived strain of, say, mice—short-lived because it has a high incidence of disease—then the maximum life span of that strain may be extended if the antioxidant affects the disease. But this does not mean that "aging" has been retarded. Only if we can break the *species* maximum-life-span barrier, not the *strain* barrier, can we say we have retarded aging. No vitamin, antioxidant, or other supplement has been shown to do that in higher animals such as mammals.[10*] If we look at actual survival curves for populations of mice and rats that have received relatively high doses of antioxidants throughout much of their lives, we find the results to be clearly marginal: sometimes a moderate extension is noted, sometimes not. The moderate extension of average life span is often accompanied by a lower average weight, so the effect could be attributed in some (not all) instances as much to a reduced food intake as to free-radical scavenging.[11] And most of the strains used were not particularly long-lived for their species.[12*]

And Now for the Establishment Prejudice

In certain areas (aging and cancer are the best examples), and in reaction against junk advertising and the overenthusiasm of unqualified health nuts and charlatans, of people with inadequate training, poor critical judgment, and no legal responsibility, orthodox medicine strides too far in the opposite direction. With regard to antiaging therapies, it vigorously opposes anything that has not been positively 100-percent proved by experimental evidence. "Orders of probabilty" are not even considered. This widens the gap between huckster and establishment, and the public is caught in the middle.

And not only the public! Three Nobel Prize winners in biology and medicine, Dr. Albert Szent-Györgyi, Dr. Linus Pauling, and Sir Peter Medawar,[13] all take vitamin C far in excess of the RDA quantity. According to a report in the respected journal *Science*,[14] about 50 percent of nurses take multiple vitamin pills. And the National Research Council itself[15] now specifically recommends a diet with "plenty of vitamin C–containing materials." In short, by the back-door route they seem to be recommending more than their own official RDA of a scant 60 mg./day.

The fact is that orthodox medicine has frequently and throughout its history recommended therapies on the basis merely of probable or inferential evidence—on educated guesswork. "Orders of probability" is no new approach; they just won't consider it for aging. Examples: During the period from 1930 to about 1960, medicine adopted a very conservative attitude toward any exercise more vigorous than walking: exercise was thought to cause the body to "wear out" more rapidly, or to undergo "stress." Medicine has now reversed itself: exercise is held to provide a needed stimulus for maintaining structural and functional integrity of a number of systems. For both these views, so firmly held during their times of influence, really hard evidence has been skimpy.[16*]

Vaccination against smallpox and the provision of clean water and drainage at times of cholera and typhus epidemics in 19th-century Europe were instituted without direct "proof" that they would work. Dr. I. P. Semmelweiss in obstetrics and Dr. Joseph Lister in surgery championed use of antiseptic techniques decades before the germ theory of disease was accepted. Many other ancient and modern examples could be cited. Today's official recommendations to decrease sodium and increase calcium intake in the diet are based on high probability rather than absolute evidence. Thus, there is plenty of precedent in medicine for acting on probabilities. But in certain areas,[17*] and antiaging therapy is one of them, establishment medicine tends to insist on absolute proof and to denounce vociferously any departure from a proof-positive policy.

A side effect of this posture is that any reports on toxicity of vitamin or other supplements are apt to be magnified out of proportion to their scientific worth. For example, it is widely believed in the medical fraternity, and often quoted in textbooks and review articles, that large doses of vitamin C may cause kidney stones. A 1984 article in *Nutrition Reviews*,[18] in stating that "vitamin C may be associated with the formation of oxalate stones" in the kidney, lists seven references. Six of these are in fact merely secondary sources, and everything ultimately refers back to a letter appearing in a 1979 issue of the British medical journal *Lancet* which cautions about "theoretically" harmful effects of vitamin C. The letter describes a single patient who excreted large amounts of oxalate in his urine after taking 4 gm. of vitamin C per day. But this patient did *not* actually have kidney stones. Other individuals taking the same amount of vitamin C did not excrete excess oxalate. There are in fact *no* cases reported in the medical literature of actual kidney stones due to oral intake of vitamin C.[19] Yet the idea persists. The same uncritical attitude attaches itself to the idea that vitamin C may decrease the absorption of vitamin B_{12}, that toxicity to B_1 can occur at rather low doses, or that infantile seizures may occur in babies whose mothers took 50–300 mg. of vitamin B_6 during pregnancy.[20] These claims, and many others about possible adverse effects of vitamin C in doses well above the RDA,[21*] do not withstand critical scrutiny. So while the medical profession might be correct in its position that the vitamin-company claims for the health benefits of vitamin C are exaggerated and unproved, its own views about harmful effects are just as prejudiced.

As a second example, let's take a report on the supposed toxicity of vitamin E published in 1981 in the *Journal of the American Medical Association.*[22] The author, a practicing physician, reported that during the previous ten years he had seen many patients with problems that seemed to have been caused by self-medication with large amounts of vitamin E. This article is often cited in medical circles as evidence that vitamin E may be harmful.

Let's look at the evidence in some detail. Among 50 of his patients who had thrombophlebitis (inflammation of the veins of the legs), the author was impressed that 2 had started taking vitamin E several months before the onset of the disease.[23] And the symptoms improved following cessation of vitamin E and the beginning of conventional treatment.

Basically, that's the evidence. As scientific evidence, it's totally unconvincing. Why? Because many other interpretations are possible besides the one that large doses of vitamin E may cause thrombophlebitis: (1) The patients' illness may have prompted many of them to start taking vitamin E, as it is widely (not necessarily correctly) believed to benefit vascular problems in the legs.[24] (2) The report gives no data at all on what proportion of persons who take vitamin E, out of all the large numbers of people who do, develop thrombophlebitis, compared with the percentage of *non*–vitamin E takers who develop the disease. (3) Some of the patients improved when they stopped taking vitamin E, but at the same time they stopped, conventional treatment was started. We cannot know which of these two factors was responsible for the improvement.

The article goes on to discuss a number of other diseases (hypertension, gynecomastia, breast tumors) which the author had encountered in patients who take a lot of vitamin E. He cites published articles implicating excessive vitamin E intake in fifteen additional clinical disorders. And he cites a letter to the *New England Journal of Medicine* which states that 800 units of vitamin E appeared to cause severe fatigue in friends and patients of the author of the letter. He *fails* to cite another letter to the same journal stating that doses of vitamin E from 400 to 1,600 units given daily to hundreds of persons did not lead to a single case of weakness or fatigue.[25*] *Of all the literature cited, only one* could be considered a controlled study; that one involved only 8 subjects, and the results were not statistically significant.

Notice the type of "evidence" the author is giving us—or rather, to his clinical colleagues. It is definitely *not* good scientific evidence. It is "the clinical anecdote," the second-worst form of evidence, as we learned in Chapter 1.

But this report has been widely cited as evidence for potential toxicity of vitamin E at doses which are not all that high.

Orthodox medicine, if it has assumed a particular position (in this case, that whatever the faddists claim must be vigorously combated), tends to treat second- or third-rate evidence as first-rate if it reinforces that assumed position. Although complicated and precise studies are demanded to prove points about any benefits of supplementing the diet with more than RDA amounts, the medical profession hastens to accept merely anecdotal information if it points in a negative direction.[26]

This leaves us between unqualified, uncritical overenthusiastic promotion on the one hand and uncritical reactive prejudice on the other. We must therefore make up our own minds. *You* must make up your own mind. I will take a strong position in advising you about the high/low diet. It will work! Definitely! But as for the health benefits of large amounts of certain supplements, the evidence is merely of a moderate, not high, order of probability.

The Recommended Daily Allowances

Let's talk next about the famous Recommended Daily Allowances, the RDAs. Establishment medicine tends to advise against vitamin and mineral supplements because it is dazzled by the authoritative backup behind these RDAs. More than the RDAs cannot possibly do any additional good! After all, the RDAs were set by the Committee on Dietary Allowances of the National Academy of Sciences. Anything the National Academy of Sciences gets behind becomes rather sacrosanct in science (most of the time for good reason—but not *all* the time).

The Academy decided upon the RDAs for vitamins and other "essential" food substances by sifting together knowledge from a number of sources, then making a very educated and careful but nevertheless subjective guess as to what is needed by the body. The knowledge basis for this estimate involves six criteria: (1) the amount that apparently healthy people consume of the particular nutrient; (2) the amount needed to avoid a particular disease (Example: pellagra was rampant in the Southern United States until its relation to a deficiency in nicotinic acid was recognized; improvement rapidly followed inclusion in the diet of foods rich in this B vitamin); (3) the degree of tissue saturation or the adequacy of physiological function in relation to the nutrient intake (Example: if your vitamin C intake is too low, your capillary blood vessels will be fragile, and you will have bleeding problems; the RDA of vitamin C will correct this); (4) nutrient-balance studies which measure nutritional status in relation to intake (Analyze the amount of the nutrient in all food and all excreta of an individual for 3–5 days, and find the maximum level of intake at which *all* is absorbed and none found in the excreta: that's the minimum requirement, or the point of zero balance[27*]); (5) studies of volunteers experimentally maintained on diets deficient in the nutrient, followed by correction of the clinical signs of deficiency when a certain amount of the nutrient is resupplied; and (6) extrapolation from animal experiments in which deficiencies have been produced by exclusion of a single nutrient from the diet.

All of the above are excellent criteria, but . . . a seventh can be suggested, perhaps the best criterion of all for our purposes but one that the National Academy of Sciences Committee on Dietary Allowances has never considered. To quote the chairman of the Committee, Dr. Henry Kamin:[28] "I must admit that we do not have much information about the intake of specific nutrients and *remote* [my italics] rather than short-term effects."

The Seventh Criterion

Suppose that separate groups of animals (and by implication humans) were fed the same basic, well-balanced diet but with increasing amounts of a particular supplement from small to megadose quantities. Keep this up throughout their whole lives. Keep records on survival, cancer types and frequencies, and other diseases for all the animal groups. Now let's set the RDA at that dosage of the nutrient which is associated with the longest average or maximum survival, the lowest overall disease frequency, and evidence of improved function. This new RDA may be quite different and larger, indeed much larger, than the RDA established by the six standard criteria outlined above, the only ones actually used.[29*]

In considering the Seventh Criterion, we are pretty much restricted, in terms of longevity and disease information, to extrapolating from animal experiments in the literature of gerontology, supported by studies of the effects of supplements on functional parameters in humans. The immune-response capacity in humans, presumably important in resistance to disease, can be enhanced by administration of more than RDA amounts of, for example, vitamins C[30] and E.[31] In addition, vitamins C and E plus selenium and the sulfur-containing amino acids may display antioxidant properties quite unrelated to their role in classical nutrition. This additional activity might be beneficial.[32]

In the next chapters I will deal with the various antioxidants, drugs, vitamins, and other chemicals with emphasis on the Seventh Criterion. To what extent have these substances been shown in animal (or human) studies to extend average and/or maximum life span? Do they influence susceptibility to the major killer diseases? Do they improve any of the biomarkers of aging? What precisely is the place of supplementation in the high/low diet program for life extension?

CHAPTER 7

Practical Supplementation

The high/low diet is the only method *proved* to retard the aging process in any mammalian species. But to avoid the possibility of chronic, borderline deficiency in any essential nutrients while you're following this low-calorie regimen, I recommend that you take supplementary RDA amounts of most (not quite all) of the vitamins and minerals. This chapter will specify which ones and how much in each case.

As a second but more controversial measure, I recommend taking considerably larger than RDA amounts of vitamins E and C (plus bioflavonoids) and pantothenic acid, plus modest increases in selenium, B_6, and beta-carotene. These nutrients are all naturally present in the diet anyway. They are innocuous, if the added dose is not too high, and there is some evidence, albeit not conclusive, that they may extend average life span, in part by preventing cancer. They have not extended maximum life span, at least in mammals.

I will also briefly discuss the current status of a number of other agents hailed as having antiaging effects: certain sulfur-containing compounds, BHT and BHA, DMAE, centrophenoxine, thymus hormone, DHEA, Coenzyme Q10, carnitine, and "active lipid." I do not currently recommend any of these, although they are worth discussing briefly because you will hear controversy about them, and some do look promising.

Table 7.1 gives, in the third column, the official RDAs (or, where these are not firmly established, what are referred to as "safe and adequate" dosages) for vitamins minerals, and trace elements. Column four gives my personal recommendations for anyone on the high/low diet, assuming a relatively conservative approach to supplementation. Column five adds a few more agents to make up an approach that is less conservative but still sound. Do not be persuaded by promotional advertising or pseudoexperts to keep adding larger and larger amounts and different products to the list. The high/low diet is the only proved life-extending regimen, and supplements may simply add thereto a modest benefit. Let's review the evidence (And if you want in-depth details, see also the notes to this chapter).

Vitamin E

The best food sources are polyunsaturated vegetable oils like corn, soybean, and safflower oils. A tablespoon of any of these contains over 20 international units of vitamin E, more than the RDA. The vitamin has been lauded as the cure for sterility, old age, menstrual disorders, heart disease, diabetes, skin disease, and muscular dystrophy. None of this is true. But it does have previously unrecognized potential therapeutic benefits, centering around its antioxidant properties.

Once free radicals get going, they can form a self-generating, self-damaging chain reaction. Vitamin E breaks the chain.[1] It is the only significant fat-soluble chain-breaking antioxidant in human blood.[2*]

How about the effect of vitamin E on average and maximum life span? As ever, this is the critical question for us. In lower animals such as worms and flies it has been reported that maximum life span can be extended by addition of vitamin E to the diet;[3] however, the interpretation of these data is not at all clear-cut.[4*]

How about mammals? At least three studies, including one by Dr. Denham Harman, the father and strongest proponent of the free-radical theory of aging, have *failed to show any effect of vitamin E on either average or maximum life span in mice.*[5]

Despite the failure to affect life span in mammals, inclusion of substantial amounts of vitamin E in the diet will greatly slow up the accumulation of yellow-brown age pigment in the cells of the brain, heart, liver, and testes.[6,7*]

Larger-than-RDA doses of vitamin E beef up the immune response in humans, and increase the resistance of

Table 7.1 Supplements for the High/Low Diet.

Nutrient	Units	RDAs and "Safe and Adequate" Values	My Recommendation: Conservative	My Recommendation: Less Conservative	Comments
Vitamin A	I.U.	5,000	0	0	Already in fortified milk, and from carotenes
D	I.U.	200–300	0	0	Already in fortified milk
K	µg.	70–120	0	0	Easily obtained in diet
E	mg. α-TE	8–10	200	200–300	Use the d-alpha (not dl-alpha) product
C	mg.	60	500–1,000	500–2,000	
Riboflavin	mg.	1.2–1.7	RDA	RDA	
Vitamin B_6	mg.	2.0–2.2	RDA	50–100	
B_{12}	µg.	6	RDA	RDA	
Thiamine	mg.	1.0–1.4	RDA	RDA	
Niacin	mg.	13–18	RDA	100	Substitute nicotinamide if niacin causes uncomfortable flushing
Folacin	µg.	400	RDA	RDA	

Pantothenic acid	mg.	4–7	RDA	500	
Biotin	µg.	100–200	RDA	RDA	
Calcium	mg.	800	500–1,000	500–1,000	500 if you take lots of dairy products; otherwise, 1,000
Magnesium	mg.	300–350	500–1,000	500–1,000	
Copper	mg.	2–3	RDA	RDA	Omit supplement if dietary intake is okay
Zinc	mg.	15	RDA	RDA	
Chromium	mg.	0.05–0.2	RDA	RDA	
Iron	mg.	10–18	½ RDA	½ RDA	
Manganese	mg.	2.5–5.0	RDA	RDA	
Selenium	µg.	50–200	100	200	
Molybdenum	mg.	0.15–0.5	RDA	RDA	
β-carotene	I.U.	—	25,000	50,000	
Bioflavonoids	mg.	—	100–200	100–200	
Fish oil (MaxEPA)	gm.	—	—	2	See page 117
Aspirin	gr.	—	—	1¼	One baby aspirin every 2nd day. See page 117
Fiber	gm.	—	20	20	

chickens, turkeys, sheep, and mice to experimental infection.[8] In mice, survival after infection with pneumonia bacteria was increased fourfold by addition of vitamin E in large amounts to the diet. About 300 units per day of vitamin E may be optimal for immunologic stimulation in adult humans.[9,10*]

Will vitamin E influence the frequency of noninfectious diseases? Probably not. The blood's fatty components, including HDL, remained about the same or even slightly higher following 4 weeks of 800 international units of vitamin E daily.[11] Excess vitamin E may increase LDL in the blood, which is certainly not desirable.[12] Vitamin E *may* have some mild ameliorative effects on intermittent leg cramps,[13] fibrocystic disease of the breast in humans,[14] and cataracts in rabbits.[15*] The level of vitamin E in the blood does not correlate with cancer susceptibility in either direction in humans,[16] even though this vitamin is known to exert some cancer-inhibiting effects in experimental mice.[17,18*]

Vitamin E supplementation can partially protect experimental animals from chemical agents such as silver, mercury, lead, carbon tetrachloride, and benzene,[19] and very probably ozone, nitrogen dioxide, and paraquat.[20] Most of these toxicants act by stimulating free-radical reactions. One of them, ozone, is a particularly important component of air pollution (smog). Lung damage begins at air levels of 0.2 to 0.3 parts per million. The Environmental Protection Agency's acceptable daily maximum level is 0.12 parts per million. Many communities in and around Los Angeles were above that level for over 100 days in 1981, and peak values in downtown Los Angeles have exceeded 0.32 parts per million.

How much vitamin E is enough and how much might be too much? Is there any evidence of toxicity? At what dosages?

In one careful human study, giving 600 units of vitamin E daily for a 4-week period decreased the levels of certain thyroid hormones and increased those of blood fats.[21] In another experiment, doses of 5–20 units per kg. per day of injected vitamin E in mice (= 350 to 1,400 units in a normal-sized human) proved optimal in stimulating immune functions, but 80 units were inhibitory, and 400 units caused a fatal degeneration of the liver. The authors of this study concluded that a twofold increase in the *blood level* of vitamin E would give optimal results with regard to immune function. We know that a 10-times increase of vitamin E in the diet is required to double the amount in the blood.[22] This would require supplementing a human diet with about 300 units of vitamin E per day. You could take this as either the alpha-tocopherol or the alpha-tocopheryl acetate or succinate forms. The alpha-tocopherol is less stable chemically but has the advantage of being able to neutralize nitrosamines (cancer-causing agents from certain processed foods) in the stomach and small intestine. Despite this, I would recommend the more stable acetate or succinate forms. While D-alpha-tocopherol has at least 40 percent more biologic activity than an equal weight of dl-alpha-tocopherol,[23] the difference is unimportant since supplements are rated in international units of bioactivity.

Vitamin E is a popular subject and there are many more studies in the scientific literature, both pro and con, than I have troubled you with. But you can see from this sampling that things are not nearly so clear-cut as either the vitamin promoters or establishment medicine pretend. There is no compelling reason for believing that vitamin E will slow down the basic aging process; but amounts quite a bit larger than the RDAs *may* render you less susceptible to several diseases and to chemical pollutants, and may slightly improve your general health for whatever number of years you do have to live.

Vitamin C

Here is a subject that has always been bedeviled by controversy. As early as 1740, James Lind, conducting nutrition experiments on sailors in the British Royal Navy, showed that scurvy could be prevented by a daily ration of fresh lime, lemon, or orange juice. Although his results were published in 1753, it was not until 1795—after 42 years of Royal Navy red tape and the loss of about 100,000 sailormen's lives due to scurvy—that Lind's simple preventive measure became an official regulation for "men-of-war" sailors. Being then the first nation to have warships on long voyages with crews free of scurvy, Britannia began to "rule the waves." In fact, the British Empire was floated on fruit juice. Even so, the news did not get around very fast. In the American Civil War, 30,000 Americans died of scurvy.

In the early 1930s, Dr. Albert Szent-Györgyi isolated in pure form from vegetables and fruits a chemical substance capable of curing scurvy. He called it ascorbic acid or vitamin C, and in 1937 he received the Nobel Prize for his discovery.

Besides being required for the formation of connective tissue, vitamin C both stimulates the immune system and can act as a free-radical scavenger. Giving old people vitamin C by injection for 1 month in amounts of 500 mg. daily led to a substantial improvement in their immune-response capacity.[24] In quantities from 500 mg. to 3 gm. per day, it stimulates the proliferative response of the protective white blood cells known as lymphocytes.[24,25]

As a free-radical scavenger or antioxidant, vitamin C acts both early, tending to inhibit the "initiation phase" of free-radical production, and also later on as a water-soluble chain-breaking antioxidant.[26] But under certain conditions it also has *pro*oxidant properties, acting as a free radical itself (Vitamin E is thought to counteract these prooxidant properties.[27]) Unfortunately, opinions differ as to whether vitamin C is prooxidant at high and antioxidant at low concentrations[28] or the reverse.[29] The bioflavonoids may enhance some activities of vitamin C, and it is my guess that the lack of bioflavonoids in many experiments utilizing pure synthetic vitamin C may have been responsible for the variable results.

Very little work has been done with vitamin C in relation to life extension. In one study,[30] megadoses *decreased* the average life span of guinea pigs; however, there was no significant effect on maximum life span. Large doses also *decreased* the average life span of fruit flies by 5–8 percent when present throughout the lifetimes of the flies.[31] But in some of the fruit-fly experiments, when vitamin C was present only during adulthood, the survival was 5 percent *longer* than that of the controls. And in a recent study, large doses of vitamin C *increased* average life span in mice.[32] Thus the life-span situation is quite unsettled.

The level of intake of vitamin C probably influences susceptibility to cancer-causing agents,[33]* but once you have cancer, taking large amounts may not improve your likelihood of survival. Careful studies at the Mayo Clinic provided evidence contradicting Linus Pauling's view on this important point.[34] Pauling has countered by emphasizing that the Mayo patients, those on vitamin C, all died after their vitamin C was stopped, their deaths possibly accelerated by a "rebound effect."[35] Recent evidence from Pauling's laboratory documents beneficial (preventive) effects of oral vitamin C on development of spontaneous breast cancer in mice.[36]

Again, with vitamin C we are dealing with a scientific and pseudoscientific literature so profuse that you can select and arrange and interpret the reports to support almost any point of view. A lot of judgment is called for. My analysis leads me to recommend 0.5 to 2 gm. of vitamin C per day, along with modest quantities of bioflavonoids (See next section).[37]* The vitamin C should be taken in 2 or 3 divided doses during the day. And if you do take supplemental vitamin C, be consistent about it. Large doses produce high tissue levels, and the body tends to eliminate the excess rapidly. On-again, off-again intake is counterproductive; it may lead to alternating excess and actual relative deficiency of vitamin C, a situation that might account for some of the conflicting results in the literature.[38]

Bioflavonoids

A large group of poorly soluble compounds widely found in plants, the bioflavonoids have antioxidant properties which serve to protect vitamin C and other plant compounds from oxygenation.[39*] They are the pigments present in fruits and vegetables: yellow in citrus fruits, red and blue in berries; present in the skins, peels, and outer layers of lemons, grapes, plums, grapefruit, apricots. The white soft, fleshy part inside lemons and oranges is rich in bioflavonoids (in contrast to the juice, which is not). Onions with colored skins are exceptionally rich. A typical mixed diet might contain up to 1 gram of bioflavonoids, of which probably only half would be absorbable. In a concentrated form (as propolis, the brownish waxy substance collected from tree buds by bees and used by them to caulk their hives), bioflavonoids have been much employed in folk medicine, but not much investigated by orthodox medicine. In the meantime, they are responsible in part for the glorious colors of autumn foliage.

Dr. Albert Szent-Györgyi, of vitamin C fame, discovered bioflavonoids in extracts from red peppers and lemons. He showed that they potentiate the action of vitamin C, and improve the condition of the walls of tiny blood vessels. They may increase the uptake of vitamin C and prevent its conversion to a less active form, although recent evidence is against this claim. Bioflavonoids can be classified as non-essential but "accessory" nutrients. No known diseases are associated with their absence.

Probably the amount of vitamin C you take as a supplement should be matched with ¼ to ½ as much bioflavonoids. There are no reported toxic effects. But commercial forms of bioflavonoids are sometimes processed in such a way as to be almost wholly unabsorbable. Unfortunately, product information on absorbability is usually not available.

Selenium

Named for the moon (*Selene* in Greek), selenium was discovered by a Swedish chemist in 1817 in the lead-chamber deposits in a sulfuric acid–manufacturing plant. He could hardly have foreseen that one day scientists would be investigating Earth's 70th-most-abundant element as a "trace mineral" in preventing disease.

In 1973 selenium was identified as a component of one of the body's major natural antioxidant enzymes, glutathione peroxidase.[40*] Selenium itself (that is, not in the enzyme combination) is also a metabolic antagonist to mercury, lead, cadmium, and arsenic. It combines with and is eliminated along with them.[41]

Still a third way that selenium acts in the body is to influence the so-called "p-450" enzyme systems. In daily contact with simple organic poisons such as gasoline, benzene, naphthol, and naturally occurring organic materials from the environment, the body manufactures the "p-450" enzymes to transform these intruder chemicals into forms that can be readily excreted.[42*]

While selenium is essential for mammals, plants are indifferent to it. If there is none in the soil, plants still grow tall and strong. If the soil is rich, they will soak it up, but generally not to a concentration above 30 parts per million. A few plants, milk vetch, woody aster, and golden weed, known as "selenium accumulators," can acquire concentrations of 1,000 to 10,000 parts per million. These accumulators are no direct threat to humans since we don't eat them, but they can cause the devastating "alkali disease" and "blind staggers" in animals, which wander in circles, stumbling over objects, become emaciated, and finally die. Agricultural runoff water from selenium-rich soil, repeatedly discharged into the 66,000-acre Grasslands Conservation District of California, is building up the selenium there and killing off the wildlife. Dead and deformed birds are being found, and a greatly lowered fertility.

The amount of selenium in our food supply can be small or moderate depending on the soil where the food was grown. Where the soil is selenium-deficient, higher incidences of colonic, rectal, and mammary cancer and (possibly) heart disease occur. On the other hand, we are not apt to eat excessive amounts of selenium, as we do not consume the plant accumulators. Among plants we do eat, potatoes, tomatoes, carrots, cabbage, and especially onions take up the most selenium from the soil.

Half a loaf of bread made from grain grown in the United States could contain from 12 to as much as 200 micrograms of selenium. Examples of the differing selenium levels in plants and dairy and other animal products from high and low areas are shown in Table 7.2. Plants grown in South Dakota, Wyoming, New Mexico, or Utah are good sources. Texas, Oklahoma, Louisiana, Alabama, Nebraska, and Kansas are also selenium-rich states. Connecticut, Illinois, Ohio, Oregon, Massachusetts, Rhode Island, New York, Pennsylvania, Indiana, Delaware, and the District of Columbia tend to be low, as are the states of Washington and Oregon and parts of Montana. Of course in today's market, vegetables may come from afar, so it's hard to tell your local situation exactly.

Will a higher-than-normal selenium intake extend life span? A few studies in which the element was present along with other antioxidants in the diet showed prolongation of average but not of maximum life span. Other studies have shown only a slight effect or none.[43,44*]

While no antiaging effect has been proved, the evidence for selenium's effect on cancer susceptibility is abundant and rather convincing. Substantial selenium increases in the diets of animals decrease the susceptibility to developing both spontaneous cancer, other tumors, and chemically induced cancers.[45]

We do not have direct proof-positive evidence for humans, but the inferential and population evidence is quite strong that high selenium intake leads to lower cancer susceptibility. Figure 7.1 shows that when the populations of

Table 7.2 **(A) Selenium content of various foods from areas where the soil is either poor (Maryland) or rich (South Dakota, Venezuela) in selenium; and (B) average selenium content of different *food groups* in an area where the soil is poor in selenium (Maryland) (adapted from B. Liebman, *Nutrition Action,* December, 1983).**

(A)

Food	Amount	Selenium (in micrograms) Poor Soil	Selenium (in micrograms) Rich Soil
Carrots, raw	1	1.8 to	105.3
Cabbage, shredded	½ cup	1.8 to	316.6
Onion, raw & chopped	½ cup	1.3 to	1513.0
Potato, raw	1 lage	1.0 to	235.0
Tomato, raw	1 large	0.7 to	164.7
American cheese	1.5 oz.	3.8 to	17.9
Swiss cheese	1.5 oz.	4.5 to	16.0
Egg	1 large	4.8 to	86.6
Milk, whole	1 cup (8 oz.)	2.9 to	28.1
Chicken breast	4 oz.	13.1 to	79.3
Pork chop	4 oz.	27.0 to	94.1

(B)

Food	Amount	Selenium (in micrograms)
Vegetables	1 serving	1.6
Fruit	2 servings	0.9
Grains & Cereals	1 serving	12.3
Dairy & Eggs	1 serving	3.6
Sugar	1 tsp.	0.2
Seafood	4 oz.	37.9
Beef, Pork, Lamb, Chicken	4 oz.	22.7
Organ Meats	4 oz.	149.6

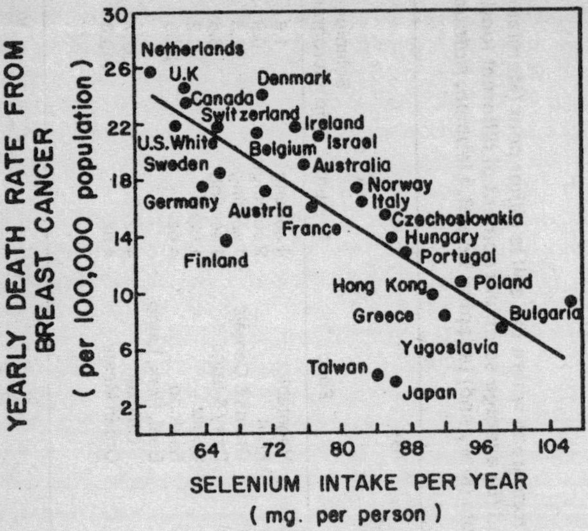

Figure 7.1 Relation between intake of selenium and death rate from cancer of breast.

different countries are compared, high selenium intake correlates with low incidence of breast cancer. And in the United States itself, when the selenium in the blood of people from different regions is compared with the overall cancer death rates in those regions, the death rates are lower when the selenium content is higher.[46]*

What about dosages and possible toxicity at higher-than-average intakes? And which forms of selenium should one use, organic or inorganic?

There is no distinct RDA, but the officially recommended "safe and adequate" range is 50 to 200 micrograms daily. If you are from a high-selenium state, you are probably getting well over 100 micrograms but not 200. If from a low-seleniüm state, you are probably getting less than 100 micrograms daily, which is very likely too low. One way to resolve the issue is to have your doctor test your blood selenium level. The normal value is 15 to 25 micrograms, and you're better off if you're on the high side. Some investigators believe that an intake of about 300 micrograms per day is indicated.[47] That would in most cases require supplementing your diet with either 100 or 200 micrograms per day, depending on where you live.

Toxicity at the above dosage seems very unlikely. Japanese fishermen consume more than 500 micrograms per day without apparent detriment. Though the inhabitants of one county in China developed severe toxic symptoms after consuming 5,000 micrograms a day, the inhabitants of another Chinese county have consumed 750 micrograms a day for many years, and apparently remained healthy.[48]

The organic form of selenium is generally considered both less toxic than at least one of the inorganic forms (selenite), and at the same time to give a greater increase in blood selenium,[49] but there is conflicting evidence. Whereas in one study[50] 2 parts per million of selenite (equivalent to 1,200 micrograms per day in a human) proved extremely toxic to young rats, another study[51] in rodents found anticancer activity and *no* toxicity of selenite (an inorganic form) at a level as high as 6 parts per million. But that much *organic* selenium caused severe liver damage. In view of this controversy, I recommend a 1:1 *mixture* of organic and inorganic selenium, the latter as either selenite or selanate or both.[52*]

The Carotenes

Does a bowl of carrots every day keep cancer away? One raw carrot contains 4,000 to 5,000 micrograms of carotenes, and population studies have suggested that persons with above-average blood levels of carotenes may have a mildly reduced risk of cancer.[53] Since the prinicipal relationship is with lung cancer, it may have been his high consumption of carotene-rich spinach that kept the inveterate pipe-smoking Popeye from developing that terrible malady. The dark yellow–to–red vegetables and fruits (but not citrus fruits or berries) and dark green, leafy vegetables are carotene-rich: carrots, spinach, mustard greens, collard greens, broccoli, squashes, apricots, kale, beets, cantaloupe, and (in Brazil and West Africa) red palm oil. Levels in different foods are shown in Table 7.3.

The most common carotene is beta-carotene. A portion of the ingested beta-carotene may be converted to vitamin A, but only upon demand. Too much vitamin A is known to be toxic, but beta-carotene itself is virtually nontoxic.[54] Only a few milligrams per day are consumed in the average diet, but an average, 160 pound man can handle up to 350 milligrams safely.[55] Of course, beyond one or two dozen milligrams one's skin will turn yellow; but this effect is harmless and will disappear if the carotene intake is re-

Table 7.3 Amounts of carotenes (mostly beta-carotenes) in various carotene-rich foods. Values are in micrograms (adapted from *Nutrition Action*, February, 1982).

Food	Serving	Carotene
Collard greens	1 cup	8,890
Spinach	1 cup	2,670
Squashes:		
Butternut	1 cup	7,870
Hubbard	1 cup	5,900
Acorn	1 cup	1,720
Yellow	1 cup	640
Zucchini	1 cup	430
Cantaloupe	½	5,540
Carrots	1 raw	4,760
Beet greens	1 cup	4,440
Broccoli	1 cup	2,320
Apricots	1	1,730
Papaya	1 cup	1,470
Prunes	1 cup	1,300
Peaches	1 large	1,220
Watermelon	1 cup	560

duced back to normal for some weeks. Just as bioflavonoids are responsible for the color of autumn foliage, beta-carotenes produce the light yellow color of human fat and chicken fat.

Beta-carotene is the strongest available antioxidant for the free radical known as "singlet oxygen,"[56] a very damaging form, being both mutagenic and peroxidizing.[57] In fact, the carotenes are manufactured by plants to protect them against singlet oxygen produced as a by-product of the interactions of light and chlorophyll. And beta-carotene is not a conventional antioxidant like vitamins E and C and selenium. Although it may complement the action of vitamin E,[58] it is in quite another class.

Should we be taking supplemental beta-carotene? Evidence for its alleged anticancerogenic effect is indecisive,[59]* and it has never been tested for life-span effects, although beta-carotene blood levels are higher in the longer-living species.[60] But free radicals are very likely involved in cancer, possibly in aging; beta-carotene fills a unique place among those antioxidants normally present in our food supply and is virtually nontoxic even at high doses. In a relatively few years scientists will know more about its effect on human cancer incidence.[61]*

Other Antioxidants

The Sulfur Compounds

When an atom of sulfur (S) combines with an atom of hydrogen (H), the two form an SH group. Many important chemical reactions in our cells need the SH group. It is one of the major antioxidants and antimutagens in cells,[62] and its concentration diminishes with age,[63] in part because oxidation converts SH groups into SS groups, a less desirable form. At UCLA we have found that these SS groups increase in the proteins wrapped around DNA in older animals, a condition that may diminish gene activity with age.[64]

Gerontologic interest in the sulfur compounds like cysteine, methionine, and glutathione was stimulated in 1965 when Romanian scientists reported that injecting mice and guinea pigs with either cysteine or another sulfur compound (thiazolidin) would increase life span.[65] Animals were treated from 12 to 22 months of age. By 22 months, none of the control mice but 20 percent of the injected ones were still alive; and only 20 percent of the control guinea pigs were alive, compared with 60 percent of the injected ones. Interesting indeed! But we see immediately that if no control mice at all survived to 22 months, the investigators were dealing with short-lived strains, so really very little can be claimed about "aging." Another study[66] reported that giving cysteine produced an increase in average life span in a very short-lived strain of mice, but maximum life span was not influenced. And in two somewhat longer-lived strains of mice, *no* effect on *either* average or maximum life span was found. And one study indicated that methionine supplementation may actually *decrease* life span to a mild degree in mice.

On existing evidence, therefore, I do not recommend any of the naturally occurring sulfur-containing agents for supplementation. In a recent study, the sulfur-containing drug 2-ME gave mildly encouraging results.[67] Newer compounds might be more effective, but we need more animal experimentation at least.[68]*

Nonsulfur Compounds

Many other antioxidant substances have been used in attempts to influence aging, the disease patterns of aging, or the biomarkers. These include BHT and BHA, NDGA,[69] dinitrophenol,[70] and Santoquin,[71] to name most of them. BHT and BHA have been the most studied, sometimes with favorable results. They are fat-soluble antioxidants often added to food in small quantities as preservatives. But at one time considered wholly innocuous, they have recently become too controversial to merit recommending as supplements on existing evidence.[72]*

Overall Comment on Antioxidant Supplementation

The benefits to be gained have been grossly oversold insofar as antiaging effects are concerned. None of the antioxidants and no combination of antioxidants have been shown to meaningfully touch maximum life span. Their occasional extension of average life span may reflect an anticarcinogenic property rather than any true antiaging property. And it is quite possible that any beneficial effects are merely secondary to the fact that antioxidants, when included in large amounts in an animal diet, lead to a 10-to-15-percent weight differential in the test animals—so the mechanism of any benefits might be similar to that of dietary restriction.[73]

If that is the case, you should lose weight directly, on the high/low diet, rather than by daily consumption of a potful of chemicals. I believe that the antioxidants normally present in our food are worth taking in greater-than-RDA amounts,[74*] but we should not burden our diet with every antioxidant that comes along, or we'll be consuming a chemical feast on what is as yet marginal justification. And before considering any new antioxidants or other supplements claimed to influence aging or disease, you should insist on the evidence of survival curves and lifetime disease patterns (in short, the Seventh Criterion, p. 155).

Recommended Nonantioxidant Supplements

Many claims for antiaging, .anticarcinogenic, or pep-up effects of different drugs or vitamins have been made with no real scientific support at all, or even where negative evidence exits. Growth hormone, for instance: people are being encouraged to gobble combinations of amino acids in an attempt to increase growth-hormone output. In adults, growth-hormone excess is associated with a high incidence of heart disease, hypertension, diabetes, arteriosclerosis, and osteoporosis—all these being interpretable as *accelerated* aging.[75] Recent evidence does suggest that a combination of the amino acids lysine and arginine may stimulate thymic hormone secretion in older animals (and humans), and partially reverse the immunodeficiency of aging.[76] The work is well done, but requires a long-term animal follow-up study focused on disease incidence and life span. Indeed the long-term effects of amino acid loading are almost wholly unknown even in animals, much less in humans.

There are a few other nonantioxidant substances which have been claimed to affect either life span itself or major biomarkers of aging. The evidence is inconclusive but not unreasonable. These substances include the B vitamins pantothenic acid and vitamin B_6.

Derived from the Greek word "panthothen," which means "from every side," pantothenic acid is found in many different foods, including whole grains, animal products, and vegetables. It is almost wholly nontoxic in that as much as 10 to 20 grams daily (over a thousand times the ordinary intake) may cause only "occasional diarrhea and water retention."[77]

In the only recorded longevity experiment with pantothenic acid, mice of a long-lived strain were given 0.3 mg. per day in their drinking water (= about 700 mg. for an average human). While the control animals survived an average of 550 days, the pantothenic acid–fed mice, both males and females, lived 653 days—a 19-percent increase in life span.[78] Maximum life spans were unfortunately not recorded. In these experiments the mouse strain was long-lived, but the laboratory conditions were not optimal; in my laboratory at UCLA, the average life span of fully fed mice of the same strain is well over 800 days.[79] Nevertheless, I would attach at least some significance to this early life-span study, although it ought to be repeated under modern conditions.

Large doses of pantothenic acid may augment the ability

to withstand stress, as shown by seeing how long rats can swim in cold water (39 degrees Fahrenheit) before sinking. In one such experiment, rats on pantothenic acid lasted 62 minutes; those on a normal intake, 29 minutes.[80] Correspondingly, when men were immersed in cold water and their blood tested for certain chemical agents, those given large doses of pantothenic acid (10 grams daily) for 6 weeks prior to exposure showed improved adaptation to stress.[81] On the other hand, 1 gm. of pantothenic acid daily for 2 weeks had no effect on highly trained distance runners running to exhaustion on a treadmill.[82]

Vitamin B_6 (pyridoxine) will increase the average life span of fruit flies,[83] and inclusion of vitamin B_6 in the amount of 100 mg./kg./day, beginning at 18 months of age, in the drinking water of a long-lived strain of mice increased average life span by 11 percent. But this would be quite a toxic dose level for humans. Twenty-month-old B_6-treated mice performed better than untreated mice of the same age in a test situation perceived by them as dangerous and requiring quick action.

The concentration of vitamin B_6 in the human body declines with age, and more than 20 percent of persons over 65 years of age appear to be vitamin B_6–deficient.[84] Senescent mice, it is indicated by chemical studies of their brains, are generally vitamin B_6–deficient.[85]

But don't go overboard on B_6. A recent report in the prestigious *New England Journal of Medicine*[86] described toxic manifestations in seven young adults after daily ingestion of 2 to 6 *grams* of vitamin B_6 for 2 to 40 months: difficulty in walking, tingling sensations in the extremities, and other manifestations of central-nervous-system effects. While these cases indeed establish toxicity, the doses were massive—at least 10 times what even the vitamin overpromoters might recommend. Little or no toxic effects have been observed at doses up to 200 *milligrams* daily over periods of many months.[87] Fifty to 100 mg. should be the upper supplementation limit.

I am no more than lukewarm in recommending pantothenic acid and vitamin B_6 as antiaging or health-enhancement agents. But they are naturally present in our foods, are nontoxic at doses considerably larger than the RDAs, and may have some positive effects.

Other Potential Supplements

Many have been suggested. Some theorists believe that the "clock" which regulates how fast we age resides in the brain.[88] Drugs are known that may influence brain aging, including transmission of signals between cells, cell-membrane integrity, levels of brain hormones, and perhaps even some of the psychometric tests which serve as biomarkers for aging. These drugs include centrophenoxine and the related DMAE, L-dopa, piracetum, choline, lecithin and phosphatidylcholine, hydergine, and vasopressin. I do not recommend supplementation with any of these at present, although current evidence suggests that centrophenoxine (available only in Europe, however) may substantially and definitely influence at least one major biomarker of aging, the accumulation of age pigment.[89]*

Thymus hormone

The capacity of our immune system to protect us from foreign invaders and internal killers such as cancer cells declines greatly with age. At the same time, our immune system begins turning against us in the autoimmune reaction which is an important part of aging. These undesired changes could be in part due to a decreased output of the hormones secreted by the thymus gland, which sustain the immune system.[90] Getting the hormones by injection or an appropriate pill might delay aging.[91]*

Thymosin, one of the best-known thymic hormones, is likely to be the first "antiaging drug" to be marketed in the United States with the support of orthodox medicine. It is an effective immunostimulant in old animals. Nevertheless, it has not yet been shown to extend maximum life span in long-lived strains of animals.

DHEA

This adrenal-gland hormone reaches high concentrations in human serum at about the time of puberty, then declines substantially with age (see page 54) so that by the 7th decade the levels are barely detectable. Given to mice, it exerts significant preventive activity against both breast cancer and chemically induced tumors.[92] It may extend the life span of short-lived strains of mice.[93*] However, in its present form DHEA should definitely *not* be taken by humans. Dr. Arthur Schwarz, the main investigator in this area, has found that on very long-term administration of DHEA to mice, the incidence of tumors of the pituitary gland is increased. Chemical analogs of DHEA are being investigated which do not have this effect, and the results so far look quite promising, but it's too soon to judge. In the meantime, the Food and Drug Administration had banned the sale of DHEA in health-food stores, where it was being promoted as an antiobesity agent.

Coenzyme Q10

Coenzyme Q10, or CoQ10, acts like a vitamin, although it can be manufactured by the body and does not have to be obtained from the diet. Essential in certain large enzyme complexes, it is itself a small molecule which carries electrons from the inside of membranes to the outside, where it releases them to another complex. This process is called "electron transport"—a sort of Flying Tigers airline in the cell.

CoQ10 is an essential part of the membranes of the energy factories of the cell. Thus it plays a critical role in the respiratory chain providing energy for life. It may also have an antioxidant function.[94]

A single injection of CoQ10 into old mice partially restored their age-related decline in immune response.[95] In the only antiaging study reported with CoQ10,[96] 17-month-old mice (equivalent to a 50-to-60-year-old human) were injected weekly with 50 micrograms of CoQ10. Average survival of the uninjected controls was another 5 months, and of the injected mice, another 11 months. This amounts to an 18-percent extension of average survival figured from time of birth, or 56 percent *if figured from the time when the injections began*. Maximum life span for the control mice was 26 months; for the injected mice, 36 months—an extension of 40 percent if considered from time of birth, or of 210 percent if considered from time of injection. But we note again that a short-lived strain was involved. The maximum life span of the mouse species was not exceeded.

Carnitine

Carnitine is another transport material. It is absolutely required for the transport of fatty acids across the membranes of the cells' energy factories, the mitochondria.[97] Mammals can generally synthesize their own carnitine, using the amino acids lysine and methionine. Also, it is present in a normal diet. Meat and dairy products are major sources. The redder the meat, the higher the carnitine content. Cereals, fruits, and vegetables contain very little.

A variety of beneficial effects have been claimed for carnitine in both animals and man—for example, an improved stress tolerance in damaged heart muscle in man[98] —and antifatigue effects have been described in healthy individuals who suffer oxygen lack during a prolonged muscle effort.[99] And in one study the oral administration of 900 mg./day of D,L-carnitine for 8 weeks was said to reduce serum triglycerides, one of the blood's fatty components, from 840 down to 186 mg.[100]

In rats given 50 mg. of carnitine per kg. per day beginning at 25 months of age,[101] 70 percent of the treated rats but only 43 percent of the controls were still alive by 28 months. In addition, the treated rats showed distinct improvement in a mental test and a significant increase in cardiac work ability. A dosage of 10 to 30 mg. L-carnitine per kg. of body weight per day (= about 3 gm. for an average-size man) has been suggested for possible human use. Carnitine looks mildly interesting as a possible antiaging drug, but the experimental results are still skimpy.

Active Lipid

With aging the membranes of brain cells and white blood cells show an increased amount of cholesterol, which makes the cell membranes stiff and interferes with function. Israeli scientists have developed a compound called "active lipid" which seems to extract the cholesterol and raise membrane fluidity[102] in cells from old animals and also old humans.[103] This refluidization is accompanied by partial reversal in a number of age-related phenomena.[104] "Active lipid" looks promising as a potential antiaging supplement, but the results need confirmation by independent investigators. We are studying "active lipid" in my laboratory at UCLA.

Conclusion

Table 7.1 shows the supplements I recommend to accompany the high/low diet. They are mainly at RDA levels to avoid the possibility of malnutrition on a low-calorie intake, but a few are in greater-than-RDA amounts. As for the other supplements, many look promising. But when you apply the Seventh Criterion, subjecting the claim to the test of the survival curve(s) and using long-lived strains of experimental animals, the results are often disappointing —or there are no results at all, because the experiments have not been done. Let those who claim miraculous antiaging benefits from their product(s) show us survival curves comparable to those of Figure 3.1 (page 59). When that has been accomplished, you may believe the claims. Until then, be skeptical and selective.

CHAPTER 8

The Size of Exercise: How Much Is Too Little and Too Much

Joggers, 20 million strong, an army of the fit, fanatically striving for perpetual youth and good health, along with hordes of tennis players, cross-country skiers, Nautilus pumpers, aerobic dancers, long-distance walkers, swimmers: millions of Americans are pursuing the great lay religion of today—physical fitness. A whole generation of fitness fanatics has risen out of easy chairs in late youth or middle age and started exercising because they believe the gospel preached by Dr. Kenneth Cooper of Dallas (author of five books on the subject—12.5 million copies in 29 languages) and other fitness gurus that by so doing they will live longer, more enjoyable lives.

There is good evidence to back up part of this faith. But like much else in the lay health field, the value of exercise and fitness has ballooned into a sky-high, free-for-all, no-questions-asked ride. Exercise makes you healthy and sexy, and the more you exercise, the healthier and sexier you get. In the movie *Pumping Iron*, champion bodybuilder Arnold Schwarzenegger declares, "I'm *coming* all the time."

The value of exercise depends on what you want to optimize. Regular sports competition has nothing *necessarily* to do with health as a primary aim.[1]* But exercise can be fun; it generally makes you feel good; it helps relieve stress and depression, improves blood-sugar metabolism, and increases cardiovascular fitness.[2]

The goals of my program are to optimize longevity, health, and freedom from disease. Does exercise actually promote these? What kinds of exercise? Is a certain amount helpful and too much not helpful in relation to longevity? How do diet and exercise compare in importance?

Let's look at the evidence. It derives from animal studies; from human-population studies; from studies of the effects of exercise on the biomarkers of aging in humans, on "risk factors for disease" in humans, on actual disease incidence, and on human longevity; and from studies of the interplay between diet and exercise.

Animal Studies

Used constantly in breathing, the diaphragm muscle of old rats shows little or no change with age in the number and diameter of its muscle fibers. But in contrast to the active diaphragm, the leg muscles of inactive (caged) rats deteriorate as they grow old. It's a "use it or lose it" physiology. In rodents, exercise begun in youth or middle age (12 months) and continued throughout life gives a 10-to-15-percent increase in *average* life span, but if it is not started until 24 months, an actual decrease occurs.[3] Lifelong exercise benefits cardiac function in rats as judged by enzyme patterns (they stay at a younger level).[4] However, at a certain point in life (over 24 to 27 months in the rat, equivalent to perhaps a 70-year-old human), a "threshold of age" appears. When previously sedentary 24–27-month-old rats were put on a vigorous exercise program, cardiac function was damaged.[5*]

Aerobic exercise in mice and rats does *not* decrease the accumulation of age pigment in their hearts. In mice started on a running schedule at 14 and 24 months of age, there was no difference in the amount of age pigment in their hearts compared with that of sedentary mice.[6] And in a rat study, a *greater* accumulation of age pigment occurred in the hearts of old exercised rats than in sedentary controls. By this particular biomarker exercise does not do so well.[7]

The animal data suggest that exercise may protect against certain diseases, such as arteriosclerosis,[8*] thereby increasing average life span, but may fail to retard the basic process of aging. It might even accelerate that process. The data also suggest that starting exercise in youth or middle age and keeping it up throughout life is productive, but beginning *vigorous* exercise *too late* in life may be counterproductive.

Human-Population Studies

In a variety of occupational groups (indoor versus outdoor workers, skilled versus unskilled laborers, active compared with inactive post-office workers), a greater incidence of heart disease has been found among the more sedentary. These population studies suggest that the frequency of coronary disease is roughly 50 percent lower in physically active than in sedentary individuals.

That sounds straightforward, but in fact there are problems with such data. People in different occupational groups have different habits. Businessmen generally have more sedentary jobs than manual laborers, for example, but they also eat differently. They eat more caviar, hollandaise sauce, and marbled red meat. And people of different physical types (genetically obese vs. genetically slender) tend to enter different occupations in the first place, and maybe it's the physical type rather than the occupation itself that influences the disease susceptibility. So we cannot conclude much of anything from such human-population studies. There are just too many variables.

Effect of Exercise in Humans on Biomarkers and "Risk Factors for Disease"

Biomarkers and risk factors relating to heart function and susceptibility to arteriosclerosis are favorably influenced by exercise.[9] Exercise promotes a higher level of the beneficial HDL in the blood and lowers LDL as well as the total cholesterol/HDL ratio—the best predictor among all blood-fat factors of cardiovascular disease.[10] Increased blood HDL has been demonstrated in middle-aged male and female runners, young elite distance runners, Norwegian skiers, middle-aged Finnish runners and skiers, joggers, and male marathon runners.[11,12]* In both sexes, the beneficial effect on HDL levels is reached only when a person exercises until his pulse reaches 70 to 85 percent of its theoretical maximum rate (estimated very roughly by subtraction of his or her age from 220) for at least 20 minutes 3 times a week.

Exercise increases the insulin sensitivity of the tissues and improves carbohydrate metabolism.[13] And the physically fit person has only about 60 percent as much chance of developing high blood pressure as a sedentary person.[14]

Exercise can work against the slowdown in reaction time that occurs with age. Men in their 60s who have exercised vigorously for 20 or more years display reaction times equal to or better than those of inactive men in ther 20s.[15] And at both young and older ages the more fit individuals display a higher level of "fluid intelligence"—a term that refers to the ability to reason, to think things out, as opposed simply to memory.[16] Thus very possibly the aging organism can postpone, by chronic exercise, the decline in oxidative capacity of the brain that usually occurs with aging.[17]

These results were derived mainly from studies of aerobic exercise, like running or swimming. What about resistance training, such as weight lifting or bodybuilding? The evidence is that this does not affect cardiovascular fitness (unless it is also done aerobically, in what is referred to as "circuit training"), but it does favorably affect some of the other biomarkers of aging—those concerned with carbohydrate metabolism, for example.

Everything seems rosy, but to these encouraging data we must add a qualifier. We learned in Chapter 2 that the maximum oxygen consumption, known as the VO_2 max, declines rather steadily with age. This measurement of your "aerobic capacity" is one of the very best measurements of "physical fitness."[18,19*] The lowered VO_2 max with age is due in part to diminished capacity of the tissues to extract oxygen quickly from the blood and partly to a lower maximal heart rate with age. Aerobic exercise will boost the VO_2 max of a sedentary person to a substantially higher level. Some men in their 60s and 70s are able, for example, to increase their VO_2 max levels above those of healthy but untrained younger men. However, we saw in Figure 2.2 (p. 47) that the *rate of decline* of the VO_2 max with age may be steeper for trained than for untrained persons. One can thus argue that while exercise training increases physical fitness and therefore resistance to certain types of disease (cardiac disease especially), it may actually slightly accelerate the rate of aging. The boosted VO_2 max declines from a higher point, but does so more rapidly, and eventually reaches the same level as for an old, sedentary person.[20*]

Effect of Exercise on Actual Disease Incidence and Longevity

It must be admitted that while the risk factors are certainly altered, conclusive long-term follow-up studies confirming the positive effects of exercise training on susceptibility to coronary-artery disease and heart attacks have been slow to materialize.[21] In the National Exercise and Heart Disease Project, a supervised exercise program displayed only a marginal effect on 3-year mortality and 3-year frequency of repeat heart attacks in patients who had already suffered one.[22] But a recent large follow-up study of 16,936 Harvard alumni from 1962 to 1978 did indicate that habitual postcollege exercise—rather than amount of athletic participation as students—coincided with a low death rate from heart disease. Sedentary alumni, *even former varsity athletes*, were at higher risk.[23] But while the death rates declined as the amount of exercise increased from less than 500 to more than 3,500 kilocalories per week, beyond 3,500 the death rate increased slightly.

The Pritikin group[24] have presented evidence that their program of diet and exercise inhibits the progression of peripheral vascular disease, coronary arteriosclerosis, and adult-onset diabetes. But their studies do not differentiate between the benefits of diet and those of exercise.

A common fallacy about exercise and heart disease is

that exercise is more effective than diet in preventing an attack. That's not true. The idea that diet is rather irrelevant as long as you exercise strenuously is a myth. Jim Fixx, author of the 1977 best-seller *The Complete Book of Running*, who transformed himself from a chubby 214-pound, two-pack-a-day smoker into a sleek 160-pound marathon runner, died at the age of 52 from a heart attack while pounding the road in Vermont. He paid dearly for his expressed belief that running all by itself would suffice to prevent heart disease.

Do not fall so deeply into the myth of exercise that you neglect other preventive health measures. Diet is the most important, even for heart disease, although exercise provides additional benefit. But there is absolutely no evidence in either animals or humans that exercise influences the rate of cancer, the second major cause of death after cardiovascular disease, and we know that cancer is very heavily influenced by diet.

The Interplay Between Diet and Exercise

Let us consult a study made by scientists at the National Institute on Aging. They allowed one population of mice to eat as much as they wanted, but gave them no access to exercise wheels; a second population ate as much as they wanted but also exercised daily; a third population was calorie-restricted and not allowed to exercise; and a fourth, calorie-restricted population was allowed to exercise. What were the life spans of these populations? Figure 8.1 shows the results. Exercise increased the life spans of animals allowed to eat as much as they desired, but *decreased* the otherwise very extended life spans of the calorie-restricted animals.

This means that the relationship between diet and exercise is complex. They are not simply additive. Exercise does not automatically increase life span, as everyone seems to think. A fine-tuning between exercise and diet is necessary

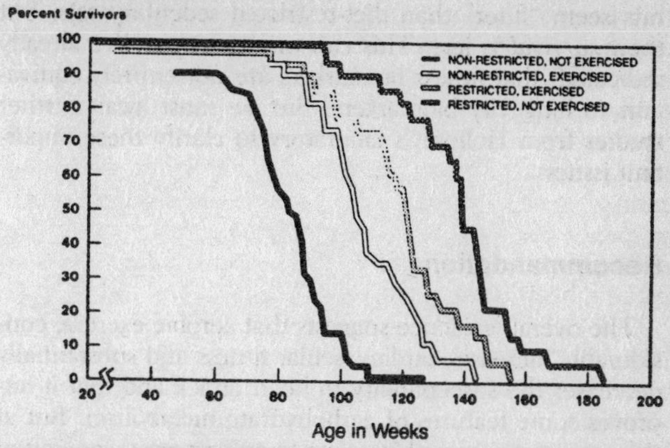

Fig. 8.1 The effect of exercise on survival of food-restricted and non-restricted mice (adapted from C. Goodrick, cited by *Science News*, Dec. 1, 1979, p. 375).

for the optimal effects. And people who do crash dieting, or nutritionally unsound dieting, and couple it with vigorous exercise to "burn off" even more calories are doubling the harm of their bad dieting technique.

Detailed diet/exercise experiments are being performed by scientists at Washington University in St. Louis, in the laboratory of Dr. John Holloszy, whom I consider one of the best exercise physiologists in the world. The studies compare fully fed sedentary rats, fully fed and exercising rats, and calorie-restricted sedentary rats. At time of writing, 50 percent of the fully fed exercising rats were alive at 34 months of age compared with only 25 percent of the fully fed sedentary rats. But again the calorie-restricted non-exercising rats were surviving the longest. The fat cells of fully fed sedentary rats were resistant to insulin, those of diet-restricted animals sensitive to insulin, and those of exercisers still more sensitive ("sensitive" is good, in terms of health and fitness). Blood cholesterol levels followed the same patterns. So in this important study the exercising rats seem "fitter" than diet-restricted sedentary rats, but their *survival* is less. This can ony mean, as I've already indicated, that fitness biomarkers are not entirely equivalent to longevity biomarkers. But we must await further studies from Holloszy's laboratory to clarify these important issues.

Recommendations

The overall evidence suggests that aerobic exercise considerably increases cardiovascular fitness and substantially decreases the susceptibility to heart attack and that it improves some features of carbohydrate metabolism. But at the same time—possibly owing to an increased generation of free radicals or a temporary increase in metabolic rate—it may slightly accelerate the basic rate of aging. Exercise definitely has a good effect and possibly a mild bad effect.

The fitness effect increases rapidly up to a certain point as you exercise more and more, but beyond that point the benefit may level off. According to Dr. Kenneth Cooper of Dallas, running tops out its aerobic benefits at 15 miles a week. He says, "If you run more than that, it's for something other than fitness." Others agree with this assessment.[25]

My own view is that the optimal combination for health and longevity is the high/low diet plus the equivalent in aerobic exercise of about 15 miles of jogging per week, coupled with a modest amount of weight-resistance training (bodybuilding).

CHAPTER 9

The Whole Program

Introduction

On the basis of the evidence I've given you throughout this book, the present chapter will outline my specific program designed (1) to increase your resistance to the "diseases of aging" by 50 percent or better and (2) to extend not only your average, but your maximum life span.

The degree of extension of maximum life span will depend upon how old you are when you start the program and how well you stick to it. If you start in your early or mid 20s and adhere well to the plan, your maximum life-span potential could be 140 to 160 years. That would put you on a new survival curve, one terminating at 140–160 years instead of the present one that crosses zero at 110. Of course, I cannot foretell when you might fall off the new curve. Even though the normal curve today ends at 110 years, very few people actually live that long. In fact, only 3 to 5 persons out of every 100,000 reach even 100 years of age. But quite a few do live to be 80–90.

On an extended life-span curve ending at, say, 140–160 years, only a few people will live to the end of the curve, but a large number will reach 120. So on the present plan, and starting as a young adult, you should be able to add 20 to 40 years to your life. And these are not just old years tacked onto the decrepit end of a normal span, but largely an extension of youth and middle age.

If you start later in life, the degree of extension would of course be less; but even as late as between the ages of 50 and 60, you should be able to enjoy an extension of 10 to 15 years, assuming that you do not already have cancer, moderately advanced heart disease, diabetes, or other such maladies. The program is preventive. I cannot claim it to be curative.

In addition to the prospect of a longer life, and as more immediately recognizable benefits, you should feel a much greater sense of physical well-being, more vitality, and an enhanced "younger" intellectual performance, whatever your chronologic age.

How do I know this is true? You realize by now that I don't know absolutely. My prediction is based on translating from animal to man an enormous body of well-controlled and many-times-repeated experiments, plus a modest amount of direct evidence from human populations and experiments. Look at the evidence presented in the previous chapters and decide whether it's worth the gamble. The stakes are high and it's a fair amount of trouble, but you are holding something like four aces or a straight flush in the poker game with Death. If those odds are not good enough, have another pork chop, jelly roll, Twinkie, soda pop and see how soon he wins the hand.

If you opt for the program, carefully reread the evidence I've presented. You must have the firm conviction that the human body can maintain its vigor and productivity to well over the age of 110 or 120. And you must have the desire to make your life worthwhile—enjoyable and purposeful—for all those added healthy years; otherwise, you won't stick to the regimen long enough to convince yourself of its benefits.

A major stumbling block to changing one's lifestyle enough to ensure that life lasts longer is the unfortunate acceptance of what we may call the "normal" goals for health, fitness, and life span. "Normal" means average or mediocre, and this is far from the best achievable. "Normal" means acceptance of premature disability and death, at age 75 or earlier, rather than freedom from degenerative diseases and an active life to well past the century mark.

You should also recognize that many of the reports and opinions coming from governmental agencies, accredited scientists, and august nongovernmental bodies such as committees of the National Academy of Sciences are prejudiced in several peculiar ways. They resist recommending anything in the way of nutritional change that in their judgment would not be "acceptable" to a large public, or that would constitute a fairly radical departure from what people are already doing or eating. There are three reasons for this. First: before recommending radical change, officials want the evidence to be absolutely 100 percent secure and overwhelming. Such an ultrahigh scientific posture is usually expressed by assertion that the data are inadequate, the conclusions premature, or there's need for more research. "Highly probable" will not do. In terms of *curative* medicine, that attitude is fine, but in terms of *prevention* it means that many people will not benefit from what we know today to have a high order of probability of being true.

It is highly probable that a drastic reduction in total fat intake will markedly decrease the frequency of heart disease and cancer; nevertheless, you will not find such a recommendation in any governmental or official report. Thirty percent of calories derived from fat is as far as they will go. And you will find such overtly asinine statements as the following from President Reagan's former Secretary of Agriculture, John R. Block, the hog farmer from Illinois: "Hogs are just like people. You can provide protein and grain to a hog and he will balance his ration. People are surely as smart as hogs . . . I am not so sure that Government needs to get so deeply into telling people what they should or should not eat."[1]

The second reason for the ultraconservative position is that the whole subject is highly political. In 1977, nearly half of the bills brought to the attention of Congress were related to food and nutrition. In 1979, 14 congressional committees and 20 subcommittees were looking into national nutritional needs,, each group with a slightly different ax to grind.[2] In 1983, nine physicians, scientists, and nutritionists on a federal advisory panel appointed by Agriculture Secretary Block engaged in a politically charged controversy about changing the dietary guidelines previously published by the Carter Administration in 1980.[3] The most hotly contested of these "radical" guidelines advised Americans to "avoid too much fat, saturated fat, and cholesterol." This hardly immoderate language was interpreted as anti-egg, anti-red-meat, and anti-dairy-product. The Midwest Egg Producers Association sent Secretary Block a letter of complaint containing the following language: "Midwest Egg Producers endorsed Ronald Reagan's campaign for the presidency primarily in response to the Carter Administration's promotion of [these] dietary guidelines."

It's the same overseas. In 1983 a government-appointed group of British nutritionists cooked up a dish of recommendations that also proved too hot for their nation's food industry. They recommended a reduction of fat from its existing level of 38 percent of total calories down to 30 percent; that sugar and salt intakes be cut in half; and that total energy intake should remain unchanged, the compensatory calories coming from an increase in starches. In 1984 the ninth and most sanitized version of this report was still having trouble being published. Striking against publication, the British Nutrition Foundation—a food-industry spokesbody—drew attention to "worldwide economic implications" that would follow substantial reduction of sugar or butter consumption. This posture of public concern over financial losses involved in directing the population toward more healthful habits seems morally corrupt.

Still a third reason behind ultra-slow-foot dietary advice from accredited sources stems from the existence of two opposing schools of thought. One school, including the American Medical Association, brings a wholly clinical perspective to the issue. These people, whose bandwagon has been jumped on by livestock and egg and dairy organizations, believe that dietary advice is best dispensed by physicians on an individual-patient basis and cannot be prescribed effectively for the general population. The opposing school, represented by the American Heart Association and many nutritionists, believes that statistical and epidemiological surveys and laboratory evidence show that a large group of people can follow certain dietary practices without health risk, and in fact with great benefits.

With all these forces at work, and even if the scientific view were totally clear-cut, an official consensus opinion on dietary guidelines would be unlikely. You must, therefore, make up your own mind. You must know the evidence, and you must accept the responsibility of knowing how to evaluate the evidence.

General Health Measures

Smoking, Drinking, Stress, Accidents

Naturally anyone who wants a long life should not smoke. If you are smoker, there are already plenty of books, schools, and methods to help you stop. I won't attempt to add to these. If you smoke one pack of cigarettes a day, in addition to a 700-percent increase in your chance to develop lung cancer, your chance of cancer of the mouth increases by 900 percent, cancer of the larynx, 700 percent, of the esophagus, 300 percent, of the pancreas, 170 percent. Heavy smoking increases your risk of heart disease 2 to 3 times. Smoking actually causes more deaths from heart disease than from cancer, although lung cancer is the major danger perceived by the public.

Mild to moderate alcohol intake is not necessarily unhealthful, and in fact may be a slight positive factor in preventing heart disease. However, alcohol does mean empty calories, with no accompanying nutritive value in terms of the RDAs, so the less booze the better. Table 9.1 gives the caloric content of common alcoholic beverages. Be moderate!

The combination of alcohol and tobacco is particularly bad. Cancers of the mouth and throat are twice to 6 times as common among heavy drinkers as among nondrinkers, and the combination of heavy drinking and heavy smoking raises the risk to 15 times. Among moderate smokers, those who drink heavily face 25 times the risk of cancer of the esophagus as nondrinkers.

There is no convincing evidence that stress in and of itself accelerates the basic aging process, although it may potentiate the development of arteriosclerosis, heart dis-

Table 9.1 Caloric content of alcoholic beverages.

Beverage	Approximate Measure	Calorie Content
Beer	8-oz. glass	114
Brandy	1 brandy glass (30 cc.)	73
Crème de menthe	1 cordial glass (20 cc.)	67
Daiquiri	1 cocktail glass (90 cc.)	122
Gin, dry	1 jigger (1½ oz.)	105
Highball	8-oz. glass	166
Martini	1 cocktail glass (4 oz.)	160
Rum	1 jigger (1½ oz.)	105
Whiskey, Scotch	1 jigger (1½ oz.)	105
Wine		
California, table wine	1 wineglass (4 oz.)	84
Champagne, domestic	1 wineglass (4 oz.)	84
Sherry, dry, domestic	1 sherry glass (2 oz.)	84
Port or Muscatel	1 wineglass (4 oz.)	180
Vermouth, dry	1 wineglass (4 oz.)	120
Vermouth, sweet	1 wineglass (4 oz.)	190

ease, and possibly even cancer (by its effect on the otherwise protective immune system). Stress experiments in mice performed years ago at Brookhaven National Laboratories did not show any effect on survival curves. Stories that sudden fright may turn the hair white overnight are all merely testimonial evidence. Animal studies involving the "general adaptation syndrome" suggested at one time that certain forms of stress—those which put the animal into a "fight-or-flight" frame of mind—cause a sudden outpouring of adrenal hormones, and that too much of these hormones may accelerate some features of aging. But this "general adaptation syndrome" has not in fact been accepted as a good model of aging. The relation of stress to "aging" is unsettled.

But in terms of disease susceptibility, you must try to avoid certain forms of stress: not so much that of hard work, which is probably beneficial, but the stress of anxiety and/or frustration.[4] For some time it was thought that so-called "Type A behavior," characterized by ambitiousness, competitiveness, and a sense of time urgency, predisposes to increased risk of heart disease, but this idea is now being questioned. The study of how socioeconomic and behavioral factors, like stress in the workplace and loneliness at home, influence the risk of heart and other diseases is almost a new medical specialty. For a while at least we shall hear conflicting views. A recent study of 2,320 men who had suffered a first heart attack undertook to evaluate risks for a second. The men were classified according to the amount of stress in their daily lives and the degree to which they were socially isolated. Second-attack rates in stressed, isolated persons were 4 times as frequent as in others, but there seemed to be little or no correlation with "Type A behavior" or with the "intensity" of the personality.[5]

Fast cars and dangerous pastimes may shorten your life expectancy, but not by accelerating aging. Five percent of deaths are due to accidents, and it can be shown mathematically that if *all* diseases were eliminated and aging itself completely halted but the accident rate remained at today's level, maximum life span would extend to about 600 years.[6] That's not too bad, and in any case your personal perils are your personal business, your own pleasure. Having hitchhiked and riverboated across Central Africa for my 58th birthday,[7] I won't tell you to sit carefully at home and avoid danger. But that's the third factor on our survival curve: aging, disease, then accidents.

Finding a Longevity Doctor

It's easy for me to find a well-qualified medical doctor. Being a doctor myself, I know where to look, whom to ask, and what to ask for. But if I need a good lawyer or accountant, I feel a bit helpless. I may ask my friends. Probably they had asked their friends. The quest becomes a daisy chain, in which none of the participants really knows how to tell a good professional from a mediocre or even an inadequate one. They judge mainly on whether the practitioner has a pleasing and persuasive manner, whether he seems to know what he's talking about. Clearly that's not good enough.

Finding a well-qualified physician requires a little insight, but it's easier than you think. Most physicians are members of the county medical society, although some doctors who are full time in medical schools may not bother to join. Call up the medical society in your vicinity. In Los Angeles, for example, you would find it listed as "Los Angeles County Medical Association." Say you want to inquire about the availability and qualifications of physicians in your area of the city—Hollywood, for example. The receptionist will connect you to the person who has that information. Say you are interested in finding a doctor in Hollywood who is a general practitioner, a specialist, or whatever it is you think you need. If you want an all-around doctor to give you an initial examination, to supervise you in a preventive health program such as mine, you probably want either a general practitioner or a physician certified by the Board of Internal Medicine. Ask for recommendations in that category.

The county medical society will not recommend a specific person. Nor will it supply information on fees and such matters. But it will gladly give you a list of 4 or 5 practitioners located in your area and in good standing with the society. It will tell you where these physicians went to school, where they served their internships and residencies, how long they have been a member of the county society, and their hospital or medical-school affiliations. If they are on the attending staff of a well-known hospital—Cedars-Sinai Hospital in Los Angeles, for example—that's a plus. Being a member of the recently formed American College of Gerontology would also be a plus.

Or if you do start by asking your friends, ask more than one. Compile a short list of physicians whom your friends recommend as attentive individuals. Then call the county society and ask for the credentials of these physicians: what medical schools they graduated from, and so on.

Several orgaizations now publish lists of longevity doctors for different regions of the United States. None that I've seen has been very discriminating. The lists include a mishmash of M.D.s, some good, some borderline, plus chiropractors, nutritionists, acupuncturists, and so on. There are some good people in each of these categories, but you ought at least to know what type of basic credentials you are getting. For example, "Dr." Robert Haas, author of the best-selling book *Eat to Win: The Sports Nutrition Bible*, is not a medical doctor at all. His "Dr." is a Ph.D. from an unaccredited "university."[8] If that's okay with you, it's okay with me, but *know* what you are getting. The county medical society is apt to have information on M.D. and non-M.D. alike. Seek out this information.

Having selected a short list of possible practitioners by one of these methods, call them up. Ask what their fees are, and (if you want to follow my program) whether they are interested in preventive medicine, nutrition, and antiaging remedies. Don't be bashful! If they don't want to talk frankly, go elsewhere. Don't tolerate the authoritarian mystique that has grown up around organized medicine.

Ideally, you want somebody with satisfactory credentials and an open mind on the subject of antiaging remedies. If he does not take the present book seriously—because it is a popular book for the lay public—see if he has read or will read the book by Dr. Richard Weindruch and me, *The Retardation of Aging by Dietary Restriction*. Our book does not exactly parallel this one, but it's close enough, and it is a fully documented, high-tech science book. A biologist-physician may in part disagree with it, but he or she cannot avoid taking it seriously. And now you have your physician!

Checkups and Biomarkers: What Exactly to Do or Have Done

The General-Status Examination

Start the program with a general medical checkup. The precise nature of this will be up to your physician. It's interesting that a task force of the Canadian Medical Association, reporting on a "cost-effective" basis what the "periodic health examination" should consist of (in terms of how much hidden disease per dollar spent might be found in a population)[9] recommended the following for symptom-free individuals: a blood-pressure determination, examination of the mouth, evaluation of hearing, a test for possible hypothyroidism, and after age 45 a test for traces of blood in the stool. The task force specifically did *not* recommend a routine history and physical examination, *any* X-rays, *any* blood chemistries, urinalysis, or electrocardiograms.

Since you want personalized service and are not part of a large-scale "cost-effective" screen, your physician will be correct in doing a history and physical examination, a urinalysis, and a test for anemia. I would not personally recommend any X-rays, blood chemistries, or electrocardiograms, except those included under your "biomarker for aging" tests, unless something shows up on the history and physical examination.

Body Fat

Before or soon after going on the high/low diet, you will want to know your initial percentage of body fat. The simplest way of doing this (although not the most accurate) is by determining skin-fold thickness in certain parts of the body. Much of your fat lies right beneath the skin, and the thickness of this layer is a good indicator of your overall percentage of body fat. Many people whose actual weights are within normal limits are in fact carrying excess body fat. By correlating body weight with subscapular (shoulder-blade) skin-fold thickness in men, or with thigh and triceps (back-of-upper-arm) skin-fold thickness in women, one can make a good estimate of body fat. The measurement requires special calipers, which your doctor should have (see Readings and Resources, p. 418). Body fat (in kilograms) can be calculated from the following formulas:

For men: body fat (in kg.) = 0.28 × body weight (in kg) + 0.51 × subscapular skin fold (in mm.) − 16.3.

For women: body fat (in kg.) = $0.49 \times$ body weight (in kg.) + $0.16 \times$ thigh skin fold (in mm.) − $0.39 \times$ triceps skin fold (in mm.) − 13.6.

You can then estimate your percentage of body fat by dividing your body fat (in kg.) by your total body weight (in kg.) and multiplying by 100. A thin man might have only 6 percent body fat; an average man, 12 percent; a plump man, 15 percent; a fat man, 20 percent or over. A thin woman might have 15 percent body fat; an average woman, 19 percent; a plump woman, 25 percent; a fat woman, 30 percent or over.

A more accurate way to estimate body fat is by the density method, whereby you are weighed while submerged in water (Chapter 5, p. 106). Your doctor can arrange this. It is also available at many of the sports and fitness clubs that have become popular around the country (at The Sports Connection in Los Angeles, for example, where part of the John Travolta/Jamie Lee Curtis film *Perfect* was made).

What percentage of body fat should you aim for on the high/low diet? The "set point" approach (pp. 69–71) applies here just as it does to how much you should weigh. If you neither overeat nor diet, you will drift toward a set-point characteristic for both body weight and percentage of body fat. Ultimately, on the high/low diet, your percentage of body fat should be about half that initial set point. But this may not apply if you are pregnant or are trying to become pregnant.[10*]

Your Personal Biomarker Program

The different biomarkers were discussed in detail in Chapter 2. Here I shall simply summarize what you should have done early in your program and again every one or two years. Evaluating human biomarkers for usefulness is a high-priority undertaking for the National Institute on Aging. As much as possible you should follow the progress of this work and adjust your own program accordingly.

The tests you can do by yourself or with a friend (Chapter 2: skin elasticity, the falling-ruler test, static balance, and visual accommodation) are more toys than serious or definitive tests except for static balance, which is in fact quite a reliable marker.

Two very important tests your doctor can do are the Vital Capacity and the test for autoantibodies in your blood. Both have predictive value for how much longer you may expect to live. A low Vital Capacity and/or the presence of autoantibodies (antibodies to "self" reactive with DNA, with thyroid-gland tissue, with the rheumatoid factor, or any others) are unfavorable signs for a long life. Fortunately, there is an excellent chance, on the basis of studies in my laboratory, that the high/low diet will diminish or entirely eliminate the autoantibodies.[11] And that it will slow down the rate of loss in Vital Capacity with age, although it probably will not rejuvenate Vital Capacity to that of a younger age.

Other tests to be run early in the game include creatinine clearance (a test for kidney function), the Glucose Tolerance Test, measurement of serum cholesterol, and determination of blood levels of HDL and LDL.

After being on the high/low diet for about 2 months, but before starting a new exercise program, you should have your maximum oxygen consumption determined by means of the treadmill or stationary-bicycle test. An electrocardiogram is done concurrently with this—an added advantage because physical stress will tend to unmask slight or hidden cardiac abnormalities. Determining your maximum oxygen consumption, as you recall from Chapter 2, is more a test of cardiovascular fitness than of aging itself, but if yours is not high you will want to increase it by your life-style changes.

The remaining biomarker tests I recommend are listed in Table 2.2 (p. 54). Have these done at your convenience any time during the first six months of your new life.

The Dietary Program

Specific menu suggestions will come in the next and last chapter. Here I'll sumarize some of what we have learned in prior chapters and point that knowledge toward my particular program.

How Much Should You Weigh?

Having selected an appropriate doctor and undergone the initial biomarker tests, you must gradually adopt a change in dietary lifestyle that allows you, on a very-high-quality diet, to lose weight gradually, over a period no shorter than 4 to 6 years, until you are 10 to 25 percent below whatever your set point is for body weight (10 percent if your set point places you as already slender, 25 percent if obese) and/or about 50 percent below whatever it is for body fat. Set point, you recall, is what you weigh when for a considerable period of time you neither overeat or undereat. It is probably about what you weighed for most of your life, but in particular during your young-adult years. For example, I weighed about 155 pounds in high school, college, and thereafter. When captain of the wrestling team at the University of Chicago, I trained down to 145 to 147, to make my weight class. And from ages 40 to about 55 I weighed around 150. So my set point is clearly in the range of 150 to 155 pounds. To translate the animal experiments to my own lifestyle, I should lose from 15 to 37 pounds over 4–6 years. At the moment, 3 years into the program, I weigh about 140 pounds.

If you are an average-size person, neither thin nor thick, 10 to 25 percent below the weights given by insurance-company tables for body weight for a person of your height and build will amount to about the same degree of loss. But to go by set point is best, although a little more difficult to define in terms of actual poundage.

Suppose that to be 20 percent below your set point you need to lose 30 pounds. Buy yourself a scale like one of those in a doctor's office, a scale that is accurate and will remain so. (If you are going to embark upon a long-term project, it makes no sense to settle for a cheap, inaccurate bathroom-type scale.) Now suppose you started at 150 pounds. Losing 30 pounds over 6 years amounts to 5 pounds per year, or a little less than one-half pound per month. Of course you cannot do this perfectly smoothly; you do it in little jumps. Start with a goal of, say, 148 pounds. Reduce to that and stay there for a few months. Weigh yourself when you get up in the morning. One morning it will be 147; another, 149 or even back to 150; another morning, 148. But hover around the 148 average point for 4 months, always on a high-quality diet, then drop your hover point another 1 or 2 pounds.

What Calorie Level to Settle On?

The answer to this frequent question is *There is no particular level.* The daily food combinations of the next chapter are pitched at less than 1,500 calories. That's a basal level. You must probably eat more or you'll lose weight too fast. But using the basal level as a guide, simply decrease your average caloric intake to whatever level allows you to lose weight very gradually.

If you change from the typical American high-fat diet to the diet described in this book (Chapter 10), you are apt to lose weight faster than planned. That's all right for the first 3 to 6 months; it will encourage you; but then you must slow down. Remember that animal studies show that crash diets leading to rapid weight loss are counterproductive: they *shorten* life span.

If you want to lose weight—for cosmetic reasons—more rapidly than I've prescribed, that's a personal choice. But at least do it on the high/low diet. That will injure you the least, and once you level off at the new cosmetic weight you want, you'll be more apt to stay there, because you'll feel better and will not be going through the loss/gain/loss/gain swings of malnourishing fad diets.

There is no great need to fast one or two days a week, as

I often do. But some people find it advantageous. It cuts your weekly calorie intake, and if you grow accustomed to a one-day-weekly fast, you won't experience difficulty if one morning your scale indicates that you should eat very lightly indeed that day, because you have zoomed above your new weight goal.

As you adapt to the high/low diet over a period of months, or after the first year, you will find that you tend to gain weight a bit more easily and on less intake than before. That's a good sign. It means that your metabolic efficiency has increased. Instead of burning off 70 percent of the ingested calories without benefit, and producing excess free radicals and other damaging by-products, your body is headed for the 50-percent mark of maximum metabolic efficiency.

Amounts of Protein, Fat, Cholesterol, Carbohydrate, and Fiber

The high/low diet calls for 60 to 90 gm. of protein per day. This would correspond to deriving 16 to 24 percent of your calories from protein if you consume 1,500 calories per day, or 12 to 18 percent at a 2,000-calorie level. No more than 20 percent of calories should come from fat, including all kinds of fat. Cholesterol intake should not exceed 300 mg. on any one day: for example, don't save up your allotment and eat seven eggs on Sundays! The rest of your calories should come from carbohydrates, preferably complex ones. Your daily diet should include 40 grams or more of fiber—preferably up to about 60 gm. depending on your size.

The Dietary Allowances Committee of the National Academy of Sciences estimated that the daily protein quantity of the U.S. diet should be 0.8 gm./kg. of body weight. This amounts to 56 grams for an average man and 46 for an average woman. However, the actual needs are known to be highly variable and individualistic.[12] With advancing age the protein intake should be somewhat lower than in younger age groups. A diet too high in protein over a long time may damage the filtration appratus of the kidneys. In addition, the specific dynamic effect of excess protein (the need to produce energy to metabolize the excess) requires unnecessary energy expenditure, a kind of metabolic stress in itself. And diets too high in protein exert a negative effect on calcium balance, with excessive excretion of calcium in the urine. I advise you to say "No, thanks" to those "high protein" drinks you see so heavily advertised.

A protein is "complete" if it contains the essential amino acids in the same proportions as given by the RDAs for those amino acids. If one or another amino acid is in short supply in the protein, that amino acid is said to be "limiting," which means that the other amino acids cannot be fully used for building the structures of the body. What cannot be used gets burned off in so-called "futile cycles" (See p. 72).

The completeness of a protein can be expressed as a score.[13] A perfectly balanced protein, as found in human milk or in whole eggs, merits a score of 100. Rice protein scores as 75, soy flour as 70, wheat flour as 50. Two different protein sources may mutually supplement what each lacks, so the two together yield a high score. Beans and brown rice make a good twosome.

On a daily basis your food selections should include material from four of the five food categories: from vegetables, legumes, and nuts as the first; from cereals and grains as the second; dairy and egg products as the third; and fruits as the fourth. The fifth category, meats and fish, may be omitted if you are a vegetarian. But it's a bit difficult to concoct fully adequate 1,500–2,000-calorie food combinations with no meat at all. Fish foremost and chicken or turkey next are preferable to red meats, in part because of the lower fat content. It's high/low time the cattle industry began breeding for leanness rather than marbling of the flesh it peddles. Even the fat content of commercial chickens is substantially greater than it once was.

Food Types to Favor

Among meats, fish is best, containing both fairly complete proteins and the so-called "omega-3" fatty acids (EPA, or eicosapentaenoic acid, and DHA, or docosahexaenoic acid), which appear largely responsible for the low incidence of arteriosclerosis in Eskimos, despite their high-fat diet. The fattier fishes contain more of these omega-3 compounds (herring, mullet, anchovies, mackerel, freshwater trout, catfish, smelt, sardines, and salmon) as opposed to fishes of medium fat content (rockfish, sea trout, flounder, ocean perch, halibut, and swordfish) or low-fat fishes (cod, haddock, lake perch, sole, whiting, red snapper, and pike). White-meat albacore tuna is of medium fat content and contains omega-3s, but in other kinds of canned tuna the fatty acids are apt to have been removed in processing. Shellfish are low in fat but relatively higher in omega-3 fatty acids than other low-fat "fishes." While for years shellfish were regarded as a forbidden food for people with high blood cholesterol, their cholesterol content is now known to be far lower than previous studies indicated; the early studies were picking up noncholesterol compounds along with cholesterol.[14] Table 9.2 displays the percent of calories from fat and the amount of omega-3 fatty acids in various fishes.

Among vegetables and legumes the only fairly "complete" protein is soybean. You can achieve protein completeness in a meal by combining legumes (low in the amino acids tryptophan and methionine, but high in lysine and isoleucine) with one of the grains or cereals (high in tryptophan and methionine, but low in lysine and isoleucine).

The cruciferous vegetables are a favored food. These include cabbage, broccoli, brussels sprouts, cauliflower, and turnips. They contain unidentified substances that seem to stimulate your immune system and p-450 enzyme system, which help protect against cancer-causing agents.

Carbohydrates should be complex, not simple ones like

Table 9.2 Percentage of calories from fat and amount of omega-3 fatty acids in different fishes.

Species	% cals from fat	omega-3 gm./4 oz.
Low-fat Fishes		
Haddock	7	0.2
Cod	8	0.3
Pike	9	0.2
Sole	9	0.3
Tuna, light, in water	10	0.2
Red snapper	11	0.4

Species	% cals from fat	omega-3 gm./4 oz.
Medium-fat Fishes		
Flounder	13	0.3
Rockfish	14	0.6
Tuna, white meat, albacore	14	0.5
Halibut	17	0.4
Ocean perch	23	0.3

Species	% cals from fat	omega-3 gm./4 oz.
High-fat Fishes		
Catfish	30	0.7
Salmon, Atlantic	35	0.4
Salmon, pink	36	2.2
Salmon, sockeye, canned	36	1.8
Herring	43	1.3
Mackerel	52	2.5
Salmon, chinook	58	3.0

plain sugar, molasses, or honey, which contain largely empty calories. The complex carbohydrates—potatoes, whole-wheat bread and cereals, and grains—also contain other nutrients such as protein, vitamins, minerals, and fibers. For many years it was assumed (without actual testing of the assumption) that complex carbohydrates or starches such as rice and potatoes were slowly digested and absorbed, causing only a small rise in blood sugar, whereas simple carbohydrates like table sugar were readily digested and rapidly absorbed, producing large and rapid increases in blood sugar and insulin levels. Upon experimentation, however, investigators found the situation to be quite variable.[15] The so-called "glycemic index"[16] was devised to express the true situation for individual foods. The index expresses the blood-glucose response for any particular food as a percentage of the response after the same weight of carbohydrate is taken in the form of pure sugar (glucose). The index of glucose would thus be 100 percent and the indices of other foods less. Surprisingly, the response does not closely correspond to whether a carbohydrate is simple or complex.[17]* The response of blood glucose (and blood insulin) to some starches (white potatoes, for example) is nearly as great as to refined sugars, whereas other starches (most grains, for example) give a low response. Pasta is lower than cereals. Milk is low, but cheese and bread give a high response.

The glycemic indices for a number of foods are shown in Table 9.3. We see that carrots are rather high on the list and sweet potatoes low. The reasons for all these seemingly haphazard differences are not entirely known. Fiber content does not seem to be a factor in cereals, but fibers such as the guar and pectin found in fresh fruits and vegetables greatly influence the rate of carbohydrate absorption and subsequent blood-sugar responses. Legumes are digested less rapidly than other foods, so produce lower, flatter glucose responses.

Other things being equal, for your high/low diet choices select foods with the lower glycemic index. The list given in Table 9.3 is accurate and usable. One should not be led astray by listings which show that such items as potato chips and ice cream have low glycemic indices. They do indeed, but in these cases it's because the foods are high in fat, and fat delays emptying time of the stomach. A low glycemic index at the expense of a high-fat meal is a poor trade-off.

Fiber is also a favored substance in the high/low diet. As we recall from an earlier chapter, the term "fiber" refers to the indigestible portions of plants, the chemical substances usually present in the cell walls that give plants their struc-

Table 9.3 Glycemic Indices
The "glucose tolerance" response for each food is expressed as a percentage of the response to the same amount of carbohydrate given as pure glucose.

100%
Glucose

80–90%
Carrots
Cornflakes
Parsnips
Honey

70–79%
Whole-meal bread
White rice
Millet
Broad beans
White potatoes

60–69%
White bread
Brown rice
Shredded Wheat
Bananas
Raisins
Muesli

50–59%
Corn
Buckwheat
White spaghetti
All-Bran
Yams

40–49%
Whole-meal spaghetti
Porridge oats
Sweet potatoes
Navy beans
Oranges
Dried peas

30–39%
Butter beans
Green beans
Black-eyed peas
Chick-peas
Apples
Nonfat milk
Whole milk
Yogurt

20–29%
Kidney beans
Lentils
Fructose

10–19%
Soybeans
Peanuts

ture and form.[18*] And different kinds of fiber have different effects on the body. For an average-size person, fiber intake should reach 40 grams per day.[19*] Depending on your present intake, you may have to work up to 40 grams gradually to avoid temporary flatulence and bloating. But 40 grams is a minimal amount, and most vegetarians consume a lot more. Sixty grams may be a quite reasonable amount. A word of caution: consuming very large amounts of fiber between meals in the form of processed material like guar gum can cause sigmoid volvulus, a twisting and impaction of the colon.

The amount of fiber should be split more or less equally between cereal fibers, such as bran, and the gums and pectins, found especially in apples, pears, peaches, oranges, rolled oats, and dried beans. Bran fiber does not influence cholesterol, but adds build and softness to the stool. Miller's bran can be added to your breakfast cereal; two tablespoonfuls weigh about 3 grams. The pectins and gums can reduce cholesterol levels. Fruits, vegetables, and beans will supply these fiber types. Oat and rice bran will also reduce cholesterol.

A high-fiber diet will also help you control your weight. Fiber is filling but adds virtually no calories. Three apples contain about 24 grams of fiber, but their carbohydrates content equals that of only one fiberless candy bar.

Many cereal manufacturers and some bread makers include fiber information in their nutrition rundown on the back of the package. Look for the words "dietary fiber," not just "crude fiber." You want the former. "Crude fiber" dates back to 1887, and the test on which it is based doesn't pick up a number of materials now recognized as being "fiber." In Table 5.4 (pp. 122–23) I listed the fiber contents of representative portions of a number of common foods. Others are given in the appendix to this volume.

How to Put Together Daily Menus

The goal is to devise each day's food intake so as to optimize nutrition and minimize calories. You want to approximate or exceed the RDA amounts of each essential nutrient, with protein, fat, cholesterol, carbohydrate, and fiber within the conditions outlined above. Figure in a sufficient caloric restriction to enable you to very slowly lose weight. To fulfill all these requirements takes a lot of doing.

This "diet problem" is an example of a special "linear programming problem," to give the mathematical term. It is usually expressed in economic terms applicable to the situation of Third World countries. A Third World inhabitant has dietary requirements like everyone else's: so much vitamin A, so much vitamin C, and so on. But he has less money. He must select his foods so that all nutrient requirements are met but the food *costs* as little as possible.

In the larger sense, what is the minimum cost per person to feed a Third World population adequately? The first thorough consideration of this "diet problem" was undertaken in 1944 by the economist George Stigler, who considered nine nutritive requirements: calories, protein, calcium, iron, and vitamins A, B_1, B_2, niacin, and C. A diet was constructed that satisfied these basic but limited requirements and cost only $39.93 a year (less than 11 cents a day) at 1939 prices. The diet consisted solely of wheat flour, cabbage, and dried navy beans. Of course, with the 31 items of the high/low diet, rather than merely 9, the problem becomes much more difficult.

Our high/low "diet problem," of course, is to minimize calories rather than cost. But we are still dealing with what is more popularly known in mathematics as a "bin-packing" problem: how to get all the essential nutrients into a bin that will not hold more than a certain number of calories, a certain number of grams of protein, with less than 20 percent of calories from fat, and so forth. There is no general mathematical solution, but the problem can be solved for a number of special cases. For my book *Maximum Life Span*, I arranged for a mainframe computer to look randomly at an enormous number of combinations of food substances, eliminate those combinations which did not measure up, and print out the others. In computerese, this is called solving the problem by "brute force." Many bin-packing problems can be solved only by brute force. Some of the food combinations and menus in the last section of this book were also arrived at by this technique. But there are other methods.

For those of you who own computers, I am putting out a software package allowing an easy solution to the food-selection problem. Called *Dr. Walford's Interactive Diet Planner*, it will permit the user to devise daily food combinations which, at any desired calorie level and with other of the above restrictions, will approach or exceed RDA amounts of the essential nutrients (See Readings and Resources, page 416, for details).

Appendix A of this book gives you representative complete food combinations for 20 days, with a number of specific menus. The 20-day menu combination is quite enough to live on with rather full variety, but if you wish you can begin to vary it, using the complete nutrient listings for 150 foods given in Appendix B. If you do not own a computer, the easiest way to devise new daily combinations is to take any good popular diet book, such as any of Pritikin's books, or the Weight Watchers books, or *Jane Brody's Nutrition Book*, see what their menus are deficient in by reference to my Appendix B, and do mild rearranging. The combinations in all these popular diet books were put together without reference to the complete RDA list, and with fewer restrictions than we require. They almost never measure up to our needs, but they are often excellent starts. And with that start, your rearrangement will almost inevitably be nutritionally better than anything else in the literature of cuisine.

If a 1,500–2,000-calorie complete daily diet leads to weight loss more rapid than our 4–6-year rate, fill up with enough calories of just about any type (except fat and certain obvious no-no's) to hold you to the gradual weight-loss rate.

Eating Out

For the high/low dieter, eating out is not a major problem. It's the total weekly or monthly caloric intake that is important, as long as the quality is high. If you eat out often, you must be somewhat restrictive. But *concentrate mainly on the quality* of the diet, rather than on simply its caloric content. Don't eat the white bread and butter most restaurants put on the table for you to nibble while you are waiting for the main course. Either don't choose a high-fat meal (roast duck, pork, or the like) or, with your doctor's permission (a prescription is necessary), 15 minutes before the meal take one packet of cholestyramine (brand name, Questran) in a glass of water. Cholestyramine largely prevents the absorption of fats (Table 5.3). It appears completely safe: it was used in the 7-year National Heart, Lung and Blood Institute study of the effect of lowering cholesterol on heart disease (see page 113), and was taken by several thousand men at the rate of 6 packages per day without evident harm. Pectin has a similar but less powerful effect in hindering fat absorption.[20]

A number of good books contain suggestions about how to dine out without being too unhealthful. Pritikin's is one of the best, and again, *Jane Brody's Nutrition Book* has excellent suggestions. But if you are careful to stay on the high/low diet at home, you can be more liberal outside, provided that you insist on *quality*. In addition, look on the menu for items cooked without added fat: steamed, cooked in own juice, broiled, roasted, or poached would be okay. Avoid items sautéed, fried, braised, creamed, escalloped, pickled, or smoked.

You may also take advantage of the fact that some restaurants are now offering low-calorie, low-fat meals, which in some instances are of gourmet quality. Marriott Hotels calls this its "Good for You Program." It follows the guidelines set by the American Heart Association. The meals are on its regular menu but are marked with the American Heart Association seal. The seal is also on special meals served at Sheraton Hotel restaurants, and on American Airlines. Fairmont Hotels have a similar "Fairmont Fitness Menu." The entire chain of eighteen Four Seasons Hotels presents its low-calorie "Four Seasons Alternative" in which a three-course dinner totals no more than 650 calories. Hyatt Hotels has 600-calorie "Perfect Balance" meals on its menus. Holiday Inns is introducing a "Gourmet Health Menu" into its Asian chain. Sumptuous diet food is now the aim of many a resort from coast to coast: Gurney's Inn in Montauk, New York; Palm Aire in Pompano Beach, Florida; Sonoma Mission Inn in Sonoma, California. The trend was started some years ago with the "spa cuisine" of New York's Four Seasons restaurant. ("Spa cuisine" accounts for about 25 percent of the meals served there. It's excellent.)

In adopting the high/low diet for health and longevity, first concentrate on switching toward the highest possible quality of food. You will find it far easier to limit your calories if the quality is high. And as you become accustomed to a perfectly balanced, high-quality intake, you will very likely begin spontaneously to lose weight, and it will be easy to keep this up by a gradual reduction in total calories.

Supplementation

But why not just eat tasty fast foods daily to the tune of 1,500–2,000 calories and take care of your deficiencies by ingesting RDA amounts of all the essential nutrients? That way you'd be losing weight, not have to be very careful about quality of food, and still get adequate nutrition! Right? Wrong.

There are a number of reasons why that won't work. First, there is still much we don't know about nutritional needs. Guinea pigs placed on a totally synthetic diet that contains ample amounts of *all the known essential nutrients* will not thrive at all. Not all essential nutrients have been identified. A high/low diet will probably include these unknowns; a fast-food/quick-pill or processed-food diet very likely will not.[21*] The nature of the problem is dramatically illustrated in Table 9.4, which shows the susceptibility of rats fed two different diets to the cancer-causing effects of three different chemical agents. Those on the semisynthetic diet were far more susceptible to the carcinogens than those on a natural whole-food diet. Now, this semisynthetic diet is analogous to a fast-food diet with vitamin supplements. Clearly that's not the best choice.

Second, the form in which nutriments are taken is also important. While one can absorb essential amino acids either as pure amino acids or as complex peptides (amino

Table 9.4 Effect of type of diet fed to rats on their susceptibility to cancers induced by different chemicals (adapted from P. M. Newberne and V. Suphakarn, *Nutrition and Cancer* 5: 107, 1983).

Chemical	Location of Cancer	% of Rats with Tumors: Semisynthetic Diet	% of Rats with Tumors: Natural Whole-Food Diet
AAF	breast	91	33
	liver	67	29
DMH	colon	67	42
ethinyl estradiol	liver	96	48
	ovary and uterus	67	11

acids strung together into one compound) or as protein in food, retention in the body of nitrogen derived from the peptides or proteins may be as much as 16 times that from amino acid mixtures. You cannot wholly depend on supplementation, even for *known* essentials.

A third reason for not settling for a poor but supplemented diet is that poor diets are bad for you not just because of what they lack, but because of what they contain: large amounts of saturated fat, for example.

While supplements cannot compensate for a poor diet, they can add to the quality of a good one, and I do recommend them as part of the high/low program. But you do want top-quality supplements. Unfortunately, in the vitamin/mineral business there are no reliable industry standards for protecting the consumer, no national monitoring service with any power to inspect and enforce, and no governmental protection except for general laws on food purity, cleanliness, and false or misleading advertising. Because vitamins and minerals are defined legally as foods, legal standards are much more lenient than for drugs. In fact the industry is rife with rip-offs for the consumer. You must take care not to be hoodwinked into buying second- or third-rate products.

Because the processing equipment needed to extract or

synthesize vitamins from raw materials costs millions of dollars, only a few big companies like Hoffmann–La Roche or Eastman Kodak actually *produce* the vitamins. These are then sold to either a vitamin company or a vitamin broker. The vitamin company puts together a final product (pill, powder, capsule, or liquid), packages it, and markets it either directly to retail stores or to distributors. But if the vitamin made by the original big-company producer is bought by a vitamin broker, quite a different route takes place. He sells either to another vitamin broker (There may be a string of these) or to a contract manufacturer. The contract manufacturer then puts together a product designed for any marketing company that gives him an order. The marketing company then sells to a distributor, to a retail store, or by mail order directly to the public. Thus, the route the product takes through a marketing company may be quite roundabout. More people are involved, more time, more add-ons, less control. Exceptions there may be, but in most instances, products that come by this circuitous route are much less reliable. Look on the label. If it says "manufactured by," you are dealing probably with the shorter route through a vitamin company (Thompson, Solgar, or Plus, for example). If it says "manufactured *for*" or "produced *for*" or "distributed *by*," you are probably dealing with the longer route. The most hazardous procedure is to deal with a mail-order company. Such vitamins have taken the longest route of all, and while there are exceptions, these companies have the worst record for quality.

Carefully inspect the label on the bottle. Do not be influenced by any promotional literature not part of the actual bottle or package. The label itself must conform to certain legal requirements that restrict false claims or misinformation, but accompanying literature can promise nearly anything the ad department decides is catchy. And even the label can be misleading. If you intend taking 500 mg. magnesium as a supplement and you buy a product whose label reads "100 mg. magnesium gluconate," you would have to take 56 *tablets*, because there are only 9 mg. of magnesium in 100 mg. of magnesium gluconate. The other 91 mg. are the gluconate.

The word "natural" on any food product has no legal definition. It is so abused you should totally disregard it. Synthetic vitamins are neither worse nor better than those derived by direct isolation from foods, possibly excepting vitamin E. The food-derived vitamin E molecule, D-alpha-tocopherol, differes in structure from the synthesized mixture of molecules dl-alpha-tocopherol (a mixture of 8 isomers). The d-alpha form is the more potent on a weight basis. On the other hand, the synthetic acetate or succinate form of vitamin E is effective and is not susceptible to becoming rancid, so might be preferred by some.

Look for the product that gives the most precise and specific wording on the label. Ideally, all labels should give batch number, date of production (the most important date), and date of expiration. Not a single company provides all three of these. If you have the batch number, you can call the company and learn when the product was made and by whom.

Buy the freshest substances possible. Vitamin E should be no older than 6 months from date of production, and no other supplement should be older than 18 months.

It would be a great boon for the consumer if some of the larger, better vitamin companies banded together to finance a separate agency to set up standards for and certification of products. Something like the Good Housekeeping Seal of Approval, only better. In my opinion the Linus Pauling Institute or the Orthomolecular Society would be a good candidate to serve in this role.

Don't believe what the retailer in the store tells you about vitamin products. Most retailers know pathetically little about nutrition, and also they have big financial axes to grind. Don't go for "good deals" on vitamins. You will just get inferior quality. Expect to pay more for well-labeled, top-quality material. The "good deal" will be the length and quality of your life.

Glass bottles are better containers than most plastic. The

polyethylene and polystyrene bottles used to package many supplements are not impervious to air. Their "oxygen barriers" are too low and the vitamins inside are subject to oxidation. The *worst* supplements you can buy are those packaged in little plastic, cellophane, or foil envelopes. Plastic bottles with the required properties can be made, but they require very costly equipment. Glass jars with nitrogen flushing would yield adequate protection, but no vitamin company offers this because of the expense.

Unfortunately, heavy advertising and promotion are greater keys to success in the vitamin/mineral business than quality of product. And because of intense competition there is pressure all along the line to minimize costs, which translates into inferior products. You must educate and protect yourself, and insist on more responsibility from this industry.

As a particularly bad example of what goes on, I may mention that one company has chosen to call itself "MLS (Maximum Life Span)," adopting the name of my own earlier book, and has implied in its advertising that I am somehow associated with it. I do not in fact have any association whatsoever with this company, and I definitely do not recommend its products. I have no association of any nature with any commercial health-food or vitamin company.

Exercise

My exercise program is aimed at balancing the positive effects of physical fitness on disease susceptibility against the potentially negative effects of exercise and increased energy turnover on the generation of free radicals.

The best exercise program is one that fits readily into your daily life, is varied and perceived as fun, emphasizes endurance and flexibility, does not depend too much on other people, and can be followed throughout your life. The multimethod type of training is recognized as superior for middle-level athletes, which is about the level we seek. Sticking to only one type of exercise, like swimming or jogging, is not best for your health. Deep adaptive shifts are undergone by the body for specialized performances. Heavy specialization is one of the reasons for the high performance records of Soviet athletes.[22] The elite athlete is thus quite different from the average athlete. But he is not necessarily healthier.

Studies performed at the Washington University School of Medicine give us a target range for exercise. Fourteen persons 65 years of age were followed through a 12-month, two-part exercise program. All started from a sedentary status. They first completed 6 months of low-intensity training, including moderately vigorous walking 3 times per week for a half-hour each time. During the second 6 months, they did high-intensity training, consisting of 30 to 45 minutes of endurance activity (cycling or jogging) at least 3 times per week. Maximum oxygen uptake, the best indicator of fitness, increased 12 percent during the low-intensity phase and 18 percent more during the high-intensity program. There was definite improvement in the blood fat and cholesterol levels and in the ability to metabolize glucose.

After you have had a cardiovascular-fitness examination by your doctor, I recommend spending three or four 15-to-20-minute sessions each week at an aerobic exercise during which your heart rate is at 70 to 85 percent of its maximum. Your maximum heart rate can be determined as part of your initial fitness examination. Subtract your age from 220 and multiply that figure by 0.70 and 0.85 to obtain an estimate of the lower and upper limits of your target cardiac range.

For aerobic exercise to be beneficial, it must be continuous and steady. The most convenient method I have found is to use a stationary bicycle upon rising in the morning. An excellent model (unfortunately expensive) is the Schwinn XR-7. You may have to work up from 5-minute intervals to the 15–20-minute ride. This morning program will not interfere witih your daily activities at all but will gradually bring you to a substantial degree of physical fitness.

I believe it is important for top health to vary the exercise pattern. After a time, substitute a 2-mile morning jog for the stationary-bicycle ride. As a third alternative, you may walk briskly for 30 minutes. Walk to work, perhaps, or park far enough from your job to necessitate a 30-minute walk.

Other forms of aerobic exercise may of course be substituted, although they usually require special effort, such as going to a jazz exercise class, or swimming. But the exercise has to be continuous. Tennis, gymnastics, and other stop-and-go sports, although acceptable, are not quite as good as continuous aerobics.

I also recommend one or two days per week of resistance weight training, for about 30–45 minutes each period. Bone will increase its content of calcium in response to short hard pulls more readily than to long sustained pulls. This means using Nautilus or Universal gym equipment or a regular weight lifters' gymnasium. Previously sedentary persons who do weight training 3 times a week for 45–60 minutes can expect a small drop in blood cholesterol within 12 weeks, and an increase in HDL.[23]

Resistance weight training, or bodybuilding exercises, exerts a favorable influence on the blood-fat profiles, altering them in a way that reduces cardiovascular risk.[24] Blood-sugar metabolism also improves. There is a good chance that aerobic and resistance exercises in combination are additive in their benefits.

You now have an excellent all-around physical-fitness routine, and except for the weight training, you will hardly notice any interference with your regular life. Tailor your own program, depending upon your interest in sports. But remember that beyond the equivalent of about 15 to 20 miles of jogging per week, you won't gain proportionately in terms of increased cardiovascular fitness, and you may well lose something by the increase in metabolism and generation of free radicals induced by exercise. Don't overexercise unless you are doing it not primarily for health, but for enjoyment.

One final point. Once you are on an exercise program, you must stay on it or the cardiovascular benefits quickly disappear. The level of HDL in the blood, for example, drops rapidly (within about 3 weeks) if exercise is discontinued.

CHAPTER 10

Foods and Tips for a High/Low Cuisine

Although neglected by historians, food has played a fascinating part in American history. Hunting and fishing, gathering nuts, wild seeds, berries, and herbs, and raising corn, squash, and beans, the Indians enjoyed a richer and more varied diet than anyone except the wealthiest Europeans. The Pilgrim settlers nearly starved their first winter, and had to kill and boil the great mastiffs they had brought with them from England for protection; but they planted seeds of cabbage, turnips, onions, and peas, and after their first harvest survived without mastiff stew. Thomas Jefferson served elaborate White House dinners prepared by an imported French chef. He considered food important in the art of diplomacy, and introduced macaroni to American cuisine—an innovation foreshadowed in the song "Yankee Doodle." Tom Jefferson stands as our Yankee Doodle par excellence.

Our more recent forebears, male and female, were not gourmets but gourmands of gargantuan capacity. Full-fleshed women, like the 200-pound Lillian Russell, were much admired in the early 1900s. A large belly was the sign of affluence in a man. William Howard Taft, "Diamond Jim" Brady, and Teddy Roosevelt exemplify the globular silhouette that was the period's popular look. These heroic trenchermen wore vests and watch chains and sat down to multicourse meals, starting off with a dozen oysters to "open the appetite." Indigestion and gout were widespread.

This same astonishing epoch and its aftermath saw the invention and development of modern food technology, another mixed-blessing American gift to the world. Hot dogs hit the market in 1904, processed cheese in 1915, Wonder Bread in 1921, potato chips in 1925, Hostess Twinkies in 1930, Spam in 1937. The first McDonald's hamburger was sold in 1948, the first TV dinner in 1954.

We are now, I hope, passing into a new era from gourmet to gourmand to good sense. The influence of the environment, particularly diet, upon health, disease susceptibility, and longevity is being fully realized. People are beginning to refuse to eat themselves into mental deterioration, disease, accelerated aging, and early death.

In this chapter combined with Appendix A I will give you menus, food combinations, and general advice on how to set up a high/low nutrient-dense diet that involves all the principles we have learned up to now. The diet will be limited in calories, approaching or exceeding the RDAs for all important nutrients, with calories derived from fat not less than 8 percent and rarely more than 20 percent, with an unsaturated-to-saturated-fat ratio of about 1 to 1, high in fiber, with a total protein content generally between 60 and 90 gm. per day. Nor will the dishes be complicated to prepare—you certainly don't want to spend your 120+ years in the kitchen.

I'll outline a 20-day menu program (Appendix A). Eat your way through it three times, which will take about 2 months. This may take some effort, but the high/low diet is clearly the most important part of my program and you should give it your personal experimental test. Two months will suffice to change your food habits, enhance your sense of physical well-being, and fill you with energy. When you feel that good, you'll want to go for the 120+ years. During these 2 test months, take no supplements beyond what you may now be taking. Don't change your habitual exercise pattern, whatever it is. I want you to experience the beneficial effects of the diet without wondering whether *part* of the good feelings might be due to a new exercise program, or to extra vitamins. One trick of vitamin/protein-drink weight-loss faddists is to put people on a diet and *also* sell them pills. The people feel better because they lose weight, but the faddist sells them on the idea that it's because of the miraculous pills. Let's not play that huckster game. For the first 2 months just stay on the high/low diet. Don't change anything else in your lifestyle.

All the food combinations we'll be using were derived by computer techniques applied to extensive tables of food values (Appendix B). You can check out the nutrient values of other published diets, or devise your own combinations, by means of the software program I am making available independently (*Dr. Walford's Interactive Diet Planner*—see Readings and Resources), or by plugging in the information given in the tables in Appendix B. For a long-term low-calorie diet, it's not enough just to pick good-looking items from the five food groups, as many nutritionists seem content to do.

Before starting the high/low diet, stock your larder with all the staple items to be used in the three 20-day cycles. The herbs, spices, grains, cereals, and dry legumes should last the whole 2 months. The produce should be bought fresh once a week, or more often if possible. Inquire where you shop on what day of the week its produce is delivered. With supermarkets it's usually only once a week. Shop there on that or the following day to be sure of fresh produce.

Stocking the Larder

Reserve a place on your shelves and in your refrigerator for the following foods. Buy 1-quart canning jars with stick-on labels for the grains, cereals, legumes, nuts, seeds, and fresh herbs. Keep the fresh herbs in the refrigerator in canning jars with ½ inch of water in the bottom (except for ginger, which should be stored dry). Oils, nuts, seeds, and of course vegetables, meats, and dairy products should also be refrigerated.

Grains and Cereals
- Brown rice
- Wild rice
- Barley
- Buckwheat
- Oat flakes, raw
- Rye flakes, raw
- Bran, wheat
- Bran, oat

Herbs, Fresh
- Basil
- Chives
- Cilantro
- Dill
- Ginger
- Marjoram
- Parsley

Herbs, Dried
- Basil
- Bay leaves
- Dill
- Marjoram
- Oregano
- Rosemary
- Sage
- Tarragon
- Thyme

Flour and Pasta
- Cornmeal
- Whole-wheat flour
- Whole-wheat pasta (various shapes)

Vegetables
- Beets
- Beet greens
- Broccoli
- Brussels sprouts
- Cabbage (red)
- Carrots
- Cauliflower
- Chard
- Corn
- Kale
- Lettuce, Romaine
- Onions
- Peppers, red
  green
- Potatoes, new
  sweet
- Radishes
- Spinach
- Squash, zucchini
  yellow
- Tomatoes
- Turnip greens

Miscellaneous
- Raisins
- Seaweeds: nori
  kombu
  wakami
- Vegetable bouillon cubes (low-fat)
- Vinegar (Aceto balsamico, top-grade (Reading and Resources); cider and red and white vinegar
- Worcestershire Sauce
- Dry white wine
- Dry sherry
- Tofu

Legumes (Beans)
- Black beans
- Black-eyed peas (cowpeas)
- Garbanzo beans
- Kidney beans
- Lentils
- Lima beans
- Navy (white) beans
- Pinto beans
- Soybeans

Nuts and Seeds
- Almonds
- Peanuts (actually, they are legumes)
- Pumpkin seeds

Spices, Dried
- Allspice
- Cardamom
- Chili powder
- Cinnamon
- Cumin
- Cloves, ground
- Coriander seeds
- Curry powder
- Cayenne (red) pepper
- Red pepper flakes
- Saffron

Oils
- Corn oil
- Olive oil (extra-virgin)
- Safflower oil

Fruit
- Apples
- Bananas
- Berries
- Figs
- Grapefruit
- Melons
- Oranges
- Papaya
- Peaches

Meats
- Liver (1 or no portions per week)
- Red meat other than liver (1 or no portions per week)
- Seafood (1 to 2 portions per week)
- Poultry (1 or no portions per week)

Dairy Products
- Nonfat yogurt
- Skim milk (nonfat)
- Buttermilk
- Low-fat cottage cheese
- Eggs
- Low-fat cheese (St. Otho's)

Equipment

Besides the standard equipment like knives, long-handled cooking spoons, saucepans (2- and 4-quart), plastic food containers and freezer bags, oven cooking bags, a wooden cutting board and salad bowl, and measuring spoons and cups, you should have the following:

- Blender and/or food processor
- Double boiler

Frying pan, nonstick: I highly recommend the new T-FAL ware.

Kitchen weighing scale: None of the scales in the usual stores are very good, as they are very inaccurate in the low weight range. Go to a biological- or chemical-supply house, where you will find a large selection. I recommend the Ohaus #720, which is a balance scale with a large removable scoop.[1*] It is hard to break, easy to use, and accurate to 1 gm. or less over the entire range of 1 to 500 gm. Price about $90. Contrast this with the food-store top-of-the-line Soehnle Computer Kitchen Scale, accurate only to within about 8 gm. and costing close to $85.

Labels and a marking pen: to label foods on your shelves or in your freezer.

Soup pot, 8-quart

Vegetable steamer

Microwave oven: While not necessary and not integrated into the menu instructions for this book, a microwave oven will save you a lot of time. Microwave cooking is also less destructive of the nutritive values of foods than fire cooking. However, microwaved foods do not crisp or brown, and do not always cook evenly. They may require stirring or turning during the heating process, and tough cuts of meat may not become as tender as with slow-fire cooking. Microwave cooking is really an art in itself. Taking a short instructional course is better than just bumbling into it.

Nutrient-Dense Menus

For our menu data bases we require daily food combinations approaching full RDAs of 31 major nutrients, but with less than 1,500 calories. The list of 31 includes the essential amino acids, vitamins, minerals, and trace elements plus biotin, which is not established as "essential." It does not include essential fatty acids, sodium, and phosphorus, as it is almost impossible not to get enough of these except on the most artificial type of diet.

If you are of average size, limiting yourself to less than 1,500 calories will induce a considerable weight loss over a 6-month period—perhaps 25 percent of your body weight. That's 5 to 10 times too rapid. So for a slow weight-loss program, you can eat more, and within limits (not too much fat) you can eat whatever you want, since you're already over the RDAs.

Full food values for 150 of the highest-quality foods are given in Appendix B. Selected foods that contain substantial amounts of 2 *or* 3 *or more* essential nutrients were featured in Table 4.3 (pp. 82–87). Table 10.1 shows the foods highest in each individual category. By using these tables, you can build the basic nutrient-dense, low-calorie daily food combinations. Start with what you like, and then add what you need to bring the combination up to par for the day. It can be done simply with my computer software (See Readings and Resources), and with some effort by hand, using Tables 4.3 and 10.1 and the nutrient values given in Appendix B.

Table 10.1 Best food sources for vitamins and minerals according to food categories; (1) meat, (2) fish, (3) dairy, cheese, eggs, (4) bread, cereals, grains, (5) vegetables, (6) legumes, (7) fruit, (8) nuts and seeds, (9) oils, (10) seaweed, (11) miscellaneous.

+ Top quality, sometimes approaching 100% of RDA *per ordinary portion*

○ 2nd best, but still good, *per ordinary portion*

Vitamins		
Vitamin A	+	(1) liver, (2) shark, (5) sweet potato, kale, turnip greens, chard, carrots, beet greens, (10) nori
	○	(2) Swordfish, crab, (5) broccoli, spinach, Romaine lettuce
Vitamin D	+	(2) sardines, mackerel, (10) kombu, nori, wakami

	O	(1) veal, (2) salmon, oysters, herring, tuna, shrimp
Vitamin K	+	(1) liver, (4) wheat germ, (5) Romaine lettuce, tomatoes, cabbage, brussels sprouts, broccoli, turnip greens, cauliflower, carrots, asparagus, (6) soybeans
	O	(1) ham, pork, (3) Ricotta cheese, cottage cheese, (4) wheat bran, (5) celeriac, spinach, (7) strawberries
Vitamin C	+	(5) kale, broccoli, brussels sprouts, turnip greens, red peppers, (7) cantaloupe, papaya, oranges, strawberries
	O	(1) liver, (5) cauliflower, chard, cabbage, asparagus . . . , (7) grapefruit, persimmon, lemon, watermelon, banana
Vitamin E	+	(5) kale, sweet potato, (4) buckwheat, (6) soybeans, (8) sunflower seeds, almonds, (9) safflower oil
	O	(2) shrimp, (5) turnip greens, asparagus, celeriac, (7) avocado, apple, (8) peanuts, (9) corn oil, olive oil
B-1 (Thiamine)	+	(1) pork, (2) catfish, (6) soybeans, cowpeas, (11) yeast
	O	(1) ham, lamb, veal, (2) snapper, salmon, (4) brown rice, bulgur wheat, (6) lima beans, lentils, split peas, garbanzos
B-2 (Riboflavin)	+	(1) liver
	O	(2) mackerel, catfish, (3) yogurt, milk, (4) wild rice, millet, (5) turnip greens, mushrooms, kale, broccoli, (6) soybeans, (7) banana, (11) yeast
B-6	+	(10) kombu, nori
	O	(1) liver, chicken (light meat), turkey, rabbit, pork, beef, (2) salmon, mackerel, halibut, catfish, (4) millet, brown rice, (5) kale, turnip greens, cabbage, (6) soybeans, lima beans, lentils, garbanzos, (10) yeast
B-12	+	(2) oysters, salmon, mackerel, herring, sardines, crab, clams, catfish, etc., (10) seaweeds

	O	(1) liver, turkey, rabbit, pork, beef, (3) yogurt, eggs
Niacin	+	(1) rabbit, liver, chicken, (10) wakami
	O	(1) turkey, capon, veal, lamb, etc. (2) halibut, mackerel, swordfish, salmon, shark, tuna, catfish, (4) brown rice, wild rice, bulgur wheat, whole wheat pasta, (5) mushrooms, (8) peanuts, (11) yeast
Folic Acid	+	(1) liver, (11) yeast
	O	(5) Romaine lettuce, turnip greens, beet greens, brussels sprouts, (6) garbanzos, soybeans, pinto beans, lima beans
Pantothenic Acid	+	(1) liver, (5) mushrooms
	O	(1) turkey (dark), chicken (dark), veal, pork, (2) salmon, (3) yogurt, eggs, (5) broccoli, kale, sweet potato, (6) soybeans, lentils, garbanzos, lima beans, (7) avocado, (11) yeast
Biotin	+	(1) liver, (6) soybeans
	O	(1) chicken, (2) mackerel, salmon, sardines, (3) eggs, (4) barley, (6) cowpeas, garbanzos, (7) cantaloupe, banana, watermelon, (8) peanuts, (11) yeast
Minerals		
Calcium	+	(3) milk, yogurt, cheese, (5) turnip greens, (10) kombu, nori, wakami
	O	(2) salmon, (5) kale, chard, broccoli, (6) soybeans, garbanzos
Magnesium	+	(6) soybeans, lima beans, cowpeas, (10) kombu, nori, wakami
	O	(4) buckwheat, wild rice, brown rice, millet, whole wheat pasta, (5) beet greens, chard, turnip greens, corn, (6) garbanzos, lentils, split peas, (8) cashews, almonds
Copper	+	(1) liver, (2) squid, oysters
	O	(1) rabbit, (2) cod, lobster, (4) wheat bran, millet, brown rice, barley, (6) garbanzos, lentils, split peas, (8) sunflower seeds, cashews, (11) yeast

Zinc	+	(2) oysters, cod
	O	(1) beef, liver, hamburger, turkey (dark), veal, lamb, (4) wild rice, (5) turnip greens, (6) soybeans, split peas, lentils, garbanzos, lima beans, cowpeas, (8) sunflower seeds, (11) yeast
Chromium	+	(1) liver, (3) American cheese, (6) lima beans, green beans
	O	(1) beef, chicken, turkey, lamb, veal, pork, (2) sole, salmon, haddock, shrimp, tuna, crab, oysters, (3) skim milk, buttermilk, Swiss cheese, eggs, (4) rye and whole wheat bread, (5) white and sweet potatoes, broccoli, corn, brussels sprouts, lettuce, (8) peanuts, (11) yeast
Potassium	+	(1) liver, (10) kombu, nori, wakami
	O	(1) beef, veal, hamburger, ham, pork, (2) clams, oysters, scallops, (5) chard, kale, turnip greens, mushrooms, (6) soybeans, lima beans, split peas, garbanzos, lentils, (8) pumpkin seeds
Iron	+	(1) liver, (2) clams, oysters, (5) soybeans, lima beans, split peas, (10) hijiki, nori, wakami, (11) yeast
	O	(1) beef, veal, ham, pork, turkey, rabbit, lamb, chicken, (2) tuna, scallops, (4) millet, (5) chard, beet greens, (6) garbanzos, lentils, cowpeas, (8) pumpkin seeds
Manganese	+	(5) beet greens, turnip greens, (6) soybeans, (8) chestnuts, (10) nori
	O	(4) wheat bran, wheat germ, millet, brown rice, barley, rolled oats, buckwheat, (5) beets, chard, kale, sweet potatoes, (6) garbanzos, lima beans, (7) pineapple, grapes, raspberries, (8) peanuts
Selenium	+	(1) liver, beef, (2) tuna, herring, ocean perch, mackerel, cod, sardines, (4) barley, whole wheat bread and pasta, (6) soybeans
	O	(1) pork, lamb, chicken, (2) oysters, lobster, shrimp, (4) brown rice, (5) brussels sprouts, (6) lentils, (7) lemon, (8) sunflower seeds, (11) yeast

Appendix A provides 20 days of combinations and menus at less than 1,500 calories per day. You will be surprised at how much you can actually eat if you select nutrient-dense foods. To these daily menus you may add black coffee or tea or whatever is calorie-free or -low, as you prefer. After laying in your supplies, skip a couple of days. Eat out! Then start on the first day of your first 20-day cycle. After three 20-day periods, your eating patterns will have changed. If you must eat dinner out during the 60 days, 10–15 minutes before the meal take 1 pack of cholestyramine (Questran) to inhibit absorption of fat. Questran is a prescription drug and you will have to ask your doctor for it. Also, carry your own small packet of low-fat salad dressing (Dieters' Gourmet Low-Cal Dressing, for example, comes in small individual-serving packets; or make your own, p. 237). Remember, the high/low diet is not intended as a 20-day quick-weight-loss program, although you can easily misuse it to that end. It's a reprogramming. After the 60 days, you must choose your own direction, following the precepts I've laid down, and depending on how healthy and long-lived you want to be and how much gluttony you want to sacrifice for enhanced physical well-being. Habit and social pressure will be more of a problem than hunger.

Dressings, Sauces, and Broths

A few commercial dressings are low in calories, but most are quite high in sodium. Among 60 commercial dressings tested by *Consumer Reports* (August, 1979, issue), the *lowest* sodium content was 210 mg. per 3 tbsp. (Wish-Bone Deluxe) and the highest 1,080 (Ann Page Chef Style). The average was 600. One average tablespoon contains more sodium than Paleolithic man got in his whole daily diet. So all these commercial dressings were too high in sodium. A more recent comparison is shown in Table 10.2. Most commercial salad dressings also contain sugar. Wish-Bone

Table 10.2 Calorie, fat, and sodium content of some leading commercial Italian dressings (values are per tablespoon) (adapted from *Nutrition Action*, October, 1981).

	Calories	% calories from fat	Fat (gm.)	Polyunsaturated fat (gm.)	Saturated fat (gm.)	Sodium (mg.)
Regular						
Kraft	80	97	8	5	1	240
Wish-Bone	80	94	8	5	1	284
Seven Seas	70	96	7	3	1	400
Reduced-calorie						
Kraft	6	0	0	0	0	220
Wish-Bone	30	90+	3	2	0	192
Walden Farms	9	90+	1	1	0	300
No-oil						
Kraft	4	0	0	0	0	220
Herb Magic	4	0	0	0	0	NA
Aristocrat	6	0	0	0	0	2

"Russian" dressing, for example, contains about 2 teaspoons of sugar per tablespoon of dressing.

A number of recipes follow for low-fat, low-calorie dressings (including mayonnaise and "cream cheese"), sauces, and broths. Most of these (including "the four sauces" for vegetables) can be thickened by addition of a solution of gums. Guar gum, gum arabic, and gum tragacanth are the most common (See pages 120–21). You may wish to substitute Worcestershire sauce for soy sauce or tamari in your cooking. Worcestershire has 55 to 95 mg. sodium per tsp. (depending on brand), whereas soy sauce characteristically contains 330 mg.

Dressings

Low-Calorie Mayonnaise

Blend the following until smooth: 1 raw egg, whites of 2 hard-boiled eggs, 2 shallots, ½ clove pressed garlic, 1 tsp.

lemon juice, 1 tsp. dry mustard. Pour into dish and fold in ½ cup nonfat yogurt. Store in covered jar or plastic container. Yields 21 calories per tbsp.

Tofu Mayonnaise

Blend the following until smooth: ½ cup nonfat yogurt, 200 gm. (7 oz) tofu, ½ clove pressed garlic, 2 tbsp. cider vinegar, 1 tbsp. lemon juice, 2 tsp. safflower oil, 3 tsp. Worcestershire sauce.

Tofu Cream Cheese

Blend the following until smooth: 1 cup (200 gm.) tofu, 1 tsp. umeboshi paste (Japanese salted plum paste), ¼ tsp. tahini (sesame-seed paste). Add 1 tbsp. finely chopped scallions, ¼ stalk finely chopped celery, 1 tsp. finely chopped parsley, and ¼ grated medium carrot, and stir into mixture.

Low Calorie, Low-Fat Vinaigrette

Add ½ cube vegetable bouillon and 1 tbsp. Worcestershire sauce to ½ cup boiling water and stir until bouillon is dissolved. Allow to cool, then add 2 tbsp. lemon juice, 4 tbsp. vinegar, 1 clove of pressed garlic, ½ tsp. dry mustard, ¼ tsp. each of dried marjoram and tarragon, 3 tsp. chopped fresh herbs (either dill or basil), and 2 tbsp. safflower oil. Mix in blender and store in glass jar in refrigerator. For a still lower-fat vinaigrette, substitute ½ cup low-fat or nonfat yogurt for the safflower oil.

Buttermilk Dressing

Stir or blend together 1 cup buttermilk, 1 tbsp. prepared mustard, 2 tbsp. finely chopped scallions, ¼ cup grated cucumber, ¼ tsp. dillweed, 2 tsp. lemon juice, and ¼ tsp. black pepper.

Yogurt-Balsamic Dressing (my favorite!)

Stir or blend together 1 cup low-fat or nonfat yogurt, ½ cup top-grade balsamic vinegar, ½ cup buttermilk, 2 tsp. extra-virgin olive oil (The oil can be omitted), and ½ of a peeled, finely chopped lemon.

Cottage Cheese Dressing

Process the following in a blender until smooth: ½ cup buttermilk, ½ cup low-fat cottage cheese, ¼ cup balsamic or other vinegar, 1 tsp. Worcestershire sauce, 4 small red radishes, 2 to 3 chopped green onions.

Yogurt Middle Eastern Dressing

Blend 1 cup yogurt, 1 tbsp. olive oil, 1 tbsp. fresh lemon juice, 1 small clove pressed garlic, 1 tbsp. fresh chopped mint.

Yogurt Green Goddess Dressing

Blend the following until smooth and very green (about 2–3 minutes): ¾ cup yogurt, ¼ cup Low-Calorie Mayonnaise (see above), 2 tsp. vinegar, 1 tsp. dried or 1 tbsp. fresh tarragon, 2 tbsp. chopped green onions or chives.

Sauces

Mock Sour Cream

Blend until smooth: 2 tbsp. low-fat or skim milk, 1 tbsp. lemon juice, 1 cup low-fat cottage cheese.

Mock Cream Cheese

Blend powdered milk into the above to thicken to the desired consistency.

Tofu Cream Sauce

Blend until completely smooth: ½ lb. tofu, ½ cup nonfat yogurt, 1 tbsp. each of sesame tahini, miso, and lemon juice. Will keep up to a week in refrigerator.

Creole Sauce

Cook 2 tbsp. chopped onion, 2 tbsp. chopped green pepper, and ¼ cup sliced mushrooms in nonstick skillet over low heat for 5 minutes. Add 2 cups stewed tomatoes with juice, ¼ tsp. pepper, and ½ tsp. basil. Simmer until sauce is thick, about 30 minutes.

Bean Sauce

Blend 1 cup low-fat or nonfat yogurt, ½ cup mashed, cooked beans, ¼ cup chopped chives, 2 tbsp. green chili salsa. Cover and store in refrigerator.

Salsa

Chop the drained tomatoes from a small can of salt-free peeled tomatoes. Add ½ stalk of finely chopped celery, ½ of a finely chopped green pepper, 1 jalapeña or yellow pepper seeded and finely chopped, ⅓ cup of lemon juice or apple-cider vinegar, 1 tsp. cumin, ½ tsp. chili powder, 2 tbsp. chopped cilantro (optional), and some freshly ground pepper. Mix well.

The Four Sauces

Tofu White Sauce

Blend the following until completely smooth: ½ package (7 oz. = 200 gm.) tofu, ½ cup low-fat or nonfat yogurt, ¼ cup water, 2 tsp. miso, 2 tsp. tamari, 1½ tsp. grated ginger, 2 tbsp. sherry, ¼ of a peeled lemon, and ½ of a freshly grated nutmeg. (Makes about 1 cup.)

Fruit Sauce

Finely dice 1 apple, 1 pear, 4–5 plums, 1 peach (Can leave out any one of these but not the plums). Place in a saucepan; add 1 cup water, ¼ cup good-quality cider vinegar, 1 tsp. sugar, 2 tsp. tamari (or Worchestershire sauce), 1 clove of pressed garlic. Bring to boil and simmer on low flame for ½ hour. (Makes 1½ cups.)

Garlic Potato Sauce (another favorite)

Boil two average-size white potatoes, skin them, and place in a blender. Add 6 cloves pressed or minced garlic, 1 tsp. tamari, ¼ cup cider or ½ cup wine vinegar (whichever you like), and ½ cup low-fat or nonfat yogurt. Blend until smooth.

Tomato Vegetable (TV) Sauce

Finely chop 1 bunch of scallions, 2 garlic cloves, and ¼ cup of parsley. Poach in water to cover the bottom of a large frypan, while stirring, until the onions are golden or very wilted (about 10 minutes). Add water if necessary during this time. Meanwhile chop 6 ripe fresh tomatoes (or use a 28-oz. can of tomatoes, drained). Add the tomatoes to the onion mixture and mix until the tomatoes are heated through. Add 1 tbsp. oregano, 1 tbsp. fresh, crushed mint (or a dash of dried mint), 2 bay leaves, and ½ cup of sherry, and simmer for 15 to 20 minutes only.

Broths

Chicken Broth

Place 3–4 lb. chicken, mostly bony parts like backs and necks, with most of the skin removed in large pot with 1 large quartered onion, 1 sliced stalk of celery, 2 small or 1 large sliced carrots, 4 parsley sprigs, 1 leek divided into 2-inch slices, 1 bay leaf, 2 cloves of sliced garlic, 8 peppercorns, and 4 quarts of water. Bring to boil and simmer for 2–3 hours. Remove chicken bones. Strain and chill broth. Allow fat to rise to top and remove. Boil down further to concentrate the broth. Freeze in ice-cube trays, then store the cubes in a plastic bag. Each cube may be used like a bouillon cube and diluted with water.

Bouillon Broth

Place 4 cups of water, 3 vegetable-bouillon cubes, 2 cloves pressed garlic, and ¼ cup Worcestershire sauce in a pot, bring to boil, and simmer until bouillon dissolves. Freeze in ice-cube trays and store cubes in a plastic bag.

Bytes and Tidbits

These are alphabetically arranged notes on healthful foods (or unhealthful foods), including how to make a healthful cuisine more fun. For example, an apple a day *can help* keep the doctor away, but eating a Red Delicious every day could get boring. Did you know, however, that almost 100 varieties of apples are still in cultivation, ranging from dark red to pale yellow, from sweet to tart, with all consistencies of firmness? Many varieties do not travel well in bulk, so only three or four types appear in the supermarkets. But in the proper season, you can have any of the others, or a selection of them, mail-ordered to your home.

Apples: For variety in apples, write to Applesource, Tom Vorbeck, Route 1, Chapin, Illinois 62628.

Bioavailability: The term "bioavailability" refers to how much of the nutriment in a food can actually be absorbed, and also to the materials present in this or other foods that may interfere with its absorption. The bioavailability of zinc, for example, varies widely. Meat and seafood zinc is more readily available than that from vegetables. Indeed, one can develop actual clinical zinc deficiency on a completely vegetarian diet when the theoretical amount of zinc in the diet is far in excess of the RDAs. Iron can be a problem too. The body absorbs twice to four times as much of the iron present in meat, fish, and poultry as it does of the iron in plant foods. Vitamin C facilitates iron absorption. When drunk with or within an hour *after* a meal, tea may interfere with iron absorption by as much as 85 percent, and coffee by 40 percent. If it is drunk an hour *before* the meal, this does not occur. In multivitamin preparations, the presence of calcium carbonate and/or magnesium oxide may interfere with the absorption of iron in the same preparation. Too much bran in a meal, or a large amount of calcium, may bind certain elements like iron, copper, and zinc into insoluble complexes and prevent their full assimilation.

The phytic acid present in cereals and nuts (in the bran and germ) seriously intereferes with absorption of dietary calcium. In the presence of calcium it will inhibit absorption of zinc and iron. When the cereal is soaked for 15 to 30 minutes before it's brought to a boil, the enzyme phytase renders the phytic acid less active. Spinach is high in calcium but contains substances that interfere with calcium absorption.

Absorption of iron from mineral supplements may be much less if the supplements are taken with meals. My advice: take major calcium and magnesium supplements *separate* from trace elements (iron, zinc, copper, chromium, selenium) and take both between meals.

Bread: Pita, sometimes called pocket or Bible bread, is made of whole-wheat flour, water, yeast, and salt. Avoid the white-flour version in supermarkets. A basic loaf of good bread might contain only whole-wheat flour, water, and yeast, but other materials are usually added: oils, molasses, honey, and salt, and/or other grains. Avoid any kind of white flour, enriched or not. Avoid anything labeled merely "wheat flour," as that could just mean ordinary white flour. Tortillas and chapattis are simply whole-wheat flour and water. Or you may get corn tortillas, in which case they should be made from whole-grain cornmeal (Most store-bought varieties are *not* so made). These and sprout bread (sprouted wheat berries put through a coarse grinder and baked), having no oil, are low in calories. If you must eat crackers, be guided by the data in Table 10.3 to select those low in both fat and sodium. I was surprised to learn how much fat Wheat Thins contain, and how loaded with sodium they are. Stoned Wheat Thins, even though manufactured by a company with the reassuring name of "Health Valley," are hardly better.

Caffeine: Sir T. H. Herbert wrote about coffee in 1626, "It is said to be healthy when drunk hot. It destroys melancholy, dries the tears, softens anger and produces joyful feelings. Tradition has it that it was invented by Gabriel to restore the sinking Mohammed." That's the positive report. Each year Americans brew 2½ billion pounds of coffee, and 8 out of 10 persons drink an average of 3–5 cups per day. A typical cup of coffee contains 100 mg. of caffeine; of tea, 20–50; the colas, 30–45; and Dr Pepper has 60 mg. per 12-oz. can.

Whether caffeine is bad for you, and if so, how bad, remains debatable. A study from Finland reported that 1–4 cups of coffee per day would increase blood cholesterol by 5 percent, and 9 cups by 14 percent; but 3 of 5 other studies did not confirm this one. It might be important how the coffee is prepared, or what it is drunk with. The Framingham study found no association between coffee consumption and the risk of heart disease. In laboratory tests, caffeine appears somewhat mutagenic (potential cancer-causing), but there is no evidence of such an effect in human coffee-drinking populations. Coffee may contain

Table 10.3 Comparison of selected crackers for content of calories, fat, and sodium per ounce of cracker (adapted from *Nutrition Action*, April, 1983).

Cracker	Calories	Fat (g.)	Sodium (mg.)
Whole Wheat Matzo (Manischewitz)	110	0	3
Whole Grain No Salt Flatbread (Ideal)	72	0	188
Ry-Krisp, Natural (Ralston)	100	0	220
Golden Rye Krisp Bread (Wasa)	98	0	312
Dark Caraway Rye Wafers (Finn Crisp)	100	0	—
Wheat Melba Toast, Unsalted (Devonsheer)	112	0	7
Bran Wafers, No Salt (Venus)	100	2	4
Stoned Wheat Thins (Interbake)	128	2	111
Ry-Krisp, Sesame (Ralston)	120	3	302
Wheat Wafers (Sunshine)	119	3	—
Harvest Wheats (Keebler)	140	4	—
Herb Wheat Crackers, No Salt (Health Valley)	134	5	101
Triscuits (Nabisco)	140	5	210
Stoned Wheat Crackers (Health Valley)	134	6	189
Wheat Thins (Nabisco)	140	6	240
Toasted Wheat Crackers (Keebler)	144	7	—
Wheat Goldfish Thins (Pepperidge Farm)	140	8	260
Ritz Crackers (Nabisco)	150	8	270
Sesame Wheats (Nabisco)	150	9	281

residues of toxic insecticides banned in the United States but sold to coffee-producing countries.

Cereals (See also Grains): "Shredded" cereals are probably the closest to "wholeness" in a mildly processed cereal. Many of the highly processed mainstays of Kellogg, Post, General Mills, and General Foods are high in sugar content, up to 30 percent. Those low in sugar include Kellogg's Special K, Nutri-Grain Corn, Nutri-Grain Shredded

Wheat, Puffed Rice, Puffed Wheat, corn flakes, Corn Chex, Rice Chex, and Grape-Nuts.[2] Processed cereals both low in sugar and best in nutritional quality include Cheerios, Grape-Nuts, Shredded Wheat, Instant Cream of Wheat, Instant Quaker Oatmeal, and Maypo 30-Second Oatmeal.[3]

Grape-Nuts is among the most nutritious of the processed cereals. Like many of the others, it is "fortified." According to studies by *Consumer Reports*, however, a serious question exists about the actual bioavailability of the added materials in "fortified" cereals.[4]

Whole cereals and grains, with as little processing as possible, are best. Flakes are next best and retain a fair amount of their original nutritive values—as examples, wheat flakes, rye flakes, barley flakes, triticale flakes, and soy and oat flakes, which are also referred to as rolled oats, rolled rye, and so on. Creams vary widely in nutritive value. They are good if made from freshly ground 100-percent-whole-grain flour, but poor if made from processed flour. In puffed cereals, nutritional losses are substantial, so in general avoid them. "Hulled" millet, which cooks up in 15 to 20 minutes, is as close to a whole grain as you can get, only the outer hull having been removed. One of the most nourishing of grains, it makes an excellent breakfast porridge. As much a grain as a cereal, amaranth seed can be eaten in pancakes and porridge. It was a basic food in America before Columbus arrived, and is just becoming popular again. Amaranth protein is closer to a complete protein than that of any other cereal or grain, having more lysine, in which the others tend to be poor. The leaves of amaranth are also highly nutritious.

To cook most whole cereals, simmer 1 part of cereal with 2 parts of water for about 15 minutes, until the water is absorbed. If you need to save time in the morning, soak the cereal in cold water overnight and it'll cook in just 3 to 4 minutes. Wheat germ has been overpublicized as a health food. It *is* a concentrated source of protein and contains a lot of vitamin E, but its major component is oil, and it becomes rancid easily. The best form is that delivered to health-food stores from local mills on the same day each week, the day it is made. Buy it that day, refrigerate it, and use it up in the next few days.

Complementarity: There are eight amino acids essential for adult humans. When these are present in the ratios represented in the RDA amounts, *all* of the protein can be used in making the building blocks of the body. If the supply of one is deficient, a proportionate amount of the others is merely converted into energy—burned off. If a single one is in great excess, the excess also is simply burned off. Achieving complementarity has been in and out of favor among nutritionists. The position now is that as long as you are above the RDAs in all eight, an excess amount of one, two, or three is irrelevant. But that's probably not true for antiaging regimens. "Burning off" an excess intake of any kind may create additional free radicals, and/or use up your lifetime caloric allotment (the so-called "lifetime energy potential").[5] So complementarity is in fact important, at least for us. Eggs and milk afford the most complete protein followed by red meat, then fish. Soy products are fairly complete. Rice is deficient in isoleucine and lysine, but can be complemented with broccoli, cauliflower, spinach, or beans. Millet and corn are deficient in lysine: add tofu, pumpkin seeds, nuts, soy products, brussels sprouts, broccoli, spinach, or mustard greens. Beans tend to be low in methionine and tryptophan. Most nutritionists take the position that rice, millet, and the cereals, for example, can be "complemented" by addition of a small quantity of dairy products or meats. That does indeed bring everything above the RDAs, but still leaves an imbalance, and the excess will have to be burned off. For antiaging purposes, we want as close to a real *balance* as can be achieved. This can be done best by computer techniques.

Dairy products and eggs: Milk, cheese, yogurt, and eggs are all sources of complete protein, vitamin A, calcium, and essential fatty acids. Unfortunately, some supply saturated fats and cholesterol. Whole eggs contain a considerable amount of cholesterol, although in the Framingham study there was no close relation between egg intake and either blood cholesterol or coronary-artery disease. If eggs are eaten along with a source of vitamin C—for example, with a glass of orange juice—one may get an increase in HDL without an increase in LDL.[6] Total fat intake may be more important than cholesterol intake in controlling blood cholesterol levels.[7] And oxidized cholesterol may be much worse than plain cholesterol in causing arteriosclerosis. The oxidized form may be found in dehydrated or powdered eggs (as found in many noodles) and in cooked meats that are stored unfrozen for an appreciable time before eating.[8]

Regular cheese like cheddar, Swiss, and other "natural" cheeses derives about 65 percent of its calories from fat, and some cheeses much more (cream cheese, 90 percent; blue cheese, 74 percent). Even so-called low-fat or part-skim cheese still derives 50 percent of its calories from fat. Thus, with a few exceptions, low-fat cheese is not really low in fat. The one exception among regular natural cheese may be St. Otho's, which is reputed to be only 5 percent fat. Unfortunately, St. Otho's is hard to find. Regular cottage cheese and part-skim mozzarella (Kraft) derive about 35 percent of their calories from fat. Dorman's makes a low-fat skim Edam cheese which derives about 25 percent of its calories from fat. On the other hand, "low sodium" chese is truly low in sodium. Unless you buy the no-salt-added kind, cottage cheese may be quite high in sodium; also, unlike other dairy products, it is not a good source of calcium. Low-fat cottage cheese derives only 10–25 percent of its calories from fat. At 180 calories a cup, it can be used in recipes to replace ricotta cheese (430 calories per cup). Pot or farmer cheese is low in fat and can replace cream cheese at ¼ the calorie count.

Whole milk is 3.3 percent fat by total weight, which doesn't sound bad, but 50 percent of the calories in whole milk are derived from fat; 36 percent of the calories in 2-percent, or "low-fat," milk in fact comes from fat; skim milk, or "nonfat" milk, derives 10 percent of its calories from fat. Use skim, or "nonfat," milk when possible, with added vitamins A and D, in which case take no supplemental vitamin D. And of course sunlight is a major source of vitamin D.

Many non-Caucasian adults and even a few Caucasians are troubled by cramps, gas, and diarrhea when they drink milk. These problems develop because of genetically determined low levels of the intestinal enzyme lactase in many adults. Present in all children of every race, lactase is low or absent in the intestines of 30 percent of adult non-Caucasians and 10 percent of adult Caucasians. Lactase is necessary to digest lactose, the sugar in milk. If milk disagrees with you in this fashion, try Lact-Aid, which can be added to milk to predigest the lactose. Sweet acidophilus may also be tolerated, and mild evidence exists that it has a beneficial effect on colon cancer and blood cholesterol levels.[9] Since there are few dietary sources of vitamin D besides milk, people who consume no milk might want to consider a vitamin D supplement, but care should be taken that vitamin D in the diet not be excessive.

Through the ages, a good deal of folklore has grown up about yogurt. According to a Persian tale, an angel taught Abraham how to make it. Well tolerated by lactase-deficient people, it has all the nutritional content of milk, except that low-fat and nonfat yogurt are usually not fortified with vitamins A and D. Regular yogurt contains 150 to 210 calories per 8-oz. serving; low-fat yogurt, 140 to 160 calories; nonfat yogurt, 90 to 110. Most flavored yogurts contain about 6 tsp. of sugar per cup (or enough to make up 25 to 50 percent of the total calories in Dannon fruit yogurt, for example). Avoid these.

Fiber: Water-soluble fibers such as pectin and the various gums will lower cholesterol. These "soluble fibers" are found in dried beans and peas, fresh peas, corn, sweet potatoes, pears, prunes, and oat bran. Fibers in Chinese vegetables such as pea pods, bamboo shoots, and Chinese lettuce are especially good cholesterol binders. Water-*in*soluble fibers such as those in wheat bran help normalize bowel function and prevent bowel cancer and diverticulosis. Large quantities may inhibit absorption of iron, calcium, zinc, and other minerals because the phytates in them tend to combine with the minerals, rendering them insoluble (See Cereals, p. 243). In ways not well understood, fiber contributes to satiety and prolongs the time before you are hungry again.[10] Diets should contain 30 or more grams of dietary fiber for every 1,000 calories. The average American consumes, in his 3,000+-calorie diet, only about 20 grams total—much too little. If you want to increase your fiber intake with wheat or oat bran or other additives, do it slowly, as a rapid increase may cause intestinal discomfort. Fiber contents of a number of foods were given in Table 5.4 (pp. 122–23). Wheat bran, incidentally, is not merely inert roughage, as many assume. It contains substantial amounts of manganese, magnesium, niacin, and vitamin K per 15-gm. portion.

Fish: Most fishes afford complete protein and either are low in fat (cod, haddock, halibut, lake perch, whitefish) or contain the kind of fat that inhibits the development of arteriosclerosis. White-meat albacore tuna, mackerel, and pink salmon, followed by freshwater trout, herring, anchovies, and catfish, all contain eicosapentaenoic acid (EPA) and docosahexaenoic acid (DHA) (See p. 208). Whitefish and bass are both low in fat and fairly high in EPA and DHA. Unfortunately, some seafoods from some locations are contaminated: mercury in tuna and swordfish, and insecticides and other chemical residues in other fishes, especially the fatty ones. Residues such as the PCBs tend to accumulate in fatty tissues, and may be high in fish that live all or part of their lives in shallow estuaries (bluefish, striped bass, Atlantic sturgeon, white perch, and white catfish, depending on where they come from, and Chinook salmon from the Great Lakes). Santa Monica Bay off Los Angeles, San Francisco Bay, New York Bay, and Chesapeake Bay are hot spots of contamination, as well as the whole East Coast from Chesapeake Bay to Boston. Eighty to 90 percent of the tomcod population over 2 years old from the Hudson River have liver tumors due to pollutants. The contaminant danger is not great enough that it should scare you off fish, but be wary. The safest fishes are small white-fleshed ocean varieties plus a few others including snapper, sea bass, sole, cod, flounder, mackerel, perch, herring, and sardines. Two fish dishes per week will help prevent heart disease (See p. 117).

Stick to fresh fish or to frozen plain varieties. To freeze a fillet, drop it into cold water, place on foil, and freeze 20 minutes, then transfer to a plastic bag and seal. Such a fillet can be cooked directly from the frozen state; simply add 50 percent to the usual cooking time. Avoid supermarket prepared fish. For example, Van de Kamp's "Light and Crispy" fish fillets contain 68 percent of calories derived from fat. Fast-food fish are no better; Carl's Jr.'s Fillet of Fish Sandwich contains 43 percent of calories from fat, and McDonald's Fillet-O-Fish, 52 percent.

Garlic and Onions: A few years ago at a hearing of the House Committee on Aging, Representative Claude Pepper asked a number of octogenarians to what they attributed their longevity. The commonest claim among the oldsters was that they ate a lot of onions. Of course, that's only testimonial evidence—the very worst kind.

Onions and garlic (especially garlic) do have a long folkloric history. Egyptian pharaohs were entombed with carvings of garlic and onions to ensure that the meals in their afterlife would be well seasoned. Roman nobles fed garlic to their soldiers to make them brave, and to their women to make them strong. Elizabethans hailed garlic as an aphrodisiac. It was used against the plague in the 18th century and was the main ingredient of the "Vinegar of Four Thieves," a concoction invented by four thieves and supposedly enabling them to burglarize the houses of the dead and dying in plague-ridden Marseille without catching the plague themselves.

The oils of onions and garlic appear to inhibit tumor promotion by certain cancer-causing agents,[11] although how many onions and garlic cloves one would have to eat to produce a measurable effect is not certain. Onion oil contains at least 55 components. Which are the tumor inhibitors is not known at present. Gangshan County in China has the lowest gastric-cancer death rate of all of Shandong Province, and Quixia the highest. Gangshanites regularly eat up to 20 gm. of garlic daily (about 5 cloves), Quixiites little or none.

A number of animal and human studies have indicated that garlic and garlic oils may lower blood cholesterol and fat levels.[12] In one study in humans, the consumption of 0.5 ml. of fresh garlic juice per kg. of body weight per day over a two-month period led to an average fall in serum cholesterol of about 28 percent. Well-controlled studies of the Jain sect in India indicate that populations eating more garlic and onions have lower blood cholesterol levels.[13*]

There are several types of garlic. The small red-skinned variety is the strongest, and keeps the longest. Purple or violet garlic is medium in strength, and the familiar white variety the mildest. Elephant garlic has very large white-skinned cloves and is quite mild in flavor. It and other varieties can be obtained (seasonally) from Willacrik Farm, P.O. Box 599, Templeton, Calif. 93465.

To peel garlic, squeeze the ends of a clove so that the skin cracks and then proceed. In preparing onions and/or garlic for sauces and dressings, one usually sautés them in a small amount of oil. As an alternative, one can poach them by covering with water which is brought to a boil and allowed to simmer for 4–5 minutes, draining the water, and using cold water to cool them. Elephant garlic is good steamed. Commercially produced garlic powders and salts are in general not recommended. "Garlic salt" is usually 90 percent plain salt.

Grains (See also Cereals): We are here concerned with barley, buckwheat, corn, millet, rice, wild rice, rye, and wheat. Wash thoroughly before cooking. Generally a dry grain expands to 2½ times its volume when cooked. Cooked grains will keep up to 3–4 days in the refrigerator, so make enough for two meals if you wish. Cooking times and amounts of water to be added per cup of different grains are shown in Table 10.4.

A few minutes before the grain is wholly cooked, you can add cinnamon or cloves for a sweet flavor, basil or oregano for an Italian flavor, finely chopped fresh ginger, coriander, or cumin for an Indonesian flavor, or curry power for an Indian. Of all the grains, rye (and amaranth—see Cereals) has the highest percentage of the essential amino acid lysine. Rice, wheat, and bulgur are deficient in isoleucine and lysine. Rice is also low in riboflavin, although wheat is not. Use hulled or, even better, unhulled barley, not pearl barley. Pearl barley is too far along the big-food-company chain; it's a polished product lacking in insoleucine and lysine. Nutritionally one of the best grains, millet is the staple of the Hunzas of India, an allegedly long-lived population. Millet has one of the most complete proteins of all the grains. Although listed here, buckwheat

Table 10.4 Cooking times and amounts of water to be added per cup of different grains.

Grain	Amount	Water	Cooking Time	Equivalent
Buckwheat	1 cup	5 cups	20 minutes	Makes 3 cups
Bulgur	1 cup	2 cups	15 minutes	Makes 2½ cups
Brown rice				
short-grain	1 cup	2 cups	35–40 minutes	Makes 2½ cups
long-grain	1 cup	2½ cups	35–40 minutes	Makes 2½ cups
Rye	1 cup	4 cups	60 minutes	Makes 2⅔ cups
Triticale	1 cup	4 cups	60 minutes	Makes 2½ cups
Wheat berries	1 cup	4 cups	60 minutes	Makes 2½ cups

is not a grain at all; it is related to rhubarb. "Groats" are buckwheat with the hull removed, and when these are roasted, constitutes "kasha." Buckwheat has 2½ times as much of the B vitamins as whole wheat, and lots of potassium, phosphorus, and biotin.

Heat, effect on nutrients: Cooking has positive and negative effects on the nutrients in foods. It decreases some nutrients, but it also destroys some contaminants. The pesticide EDB, which causes cancer and genetic mutations, is about 80 percent destroyed by cooking. The B vitamin folacin is easily destroyed by heat, so when using dark green leafy vegetables, eat them only slightly cooked (steamed).

Labels: "Organic," "natural," "raw," "uncooked," "unfiltered," "low-calorie," "sugarless," "sugar-free," "enriched," "fortified": don't fall for these prohealth buzzwords! Some of them are meaningful, others not. "Organic" is understood to mean grown without artificial chemical fertilizers, herbicides, or pesticides, but in fact the word implies no legal requirement. It means nothing unless the grower has been certified by an organic growers' association, and you may have trouble confirming this. However, true "organic" food is better if you can get it, to avoid pesticide residues. During the past 30 years pesticide use has increased by 1,100 percent. In setting acceptable residue limits, the U.S. Department of Agriculture assumes a person eats no more than ½ pound *per year* of avocados, artichokes, brussels sprouts, cantaloupe, eggplant, melons, mushrooms, radishes, and summer and winter squash.[14] That ½ pound may be the yearly American average, but it's not the level in a good diet; hence the allowable residue limits are simply too high.

Food products that are claimed to be "natural" often contain lots of sugar as well as unbleached wheat flour. In fact, when I see the word "natural" on a product, I regard it as a phony label, an attempt to fool the customer, and I'm apt not to buy that product. For example, "Ragu' Home-style" spaghetti sauce contains, for each 74 calories, 2 gm. of fat, 470 mg. of sodium, and no added sweeteners, whereas "Ragu' 100% Natural" spaghetti sauce has 3 gm. fat, 770 mg. sodium, plus added sweeteners. So the "home-style" is better than the "natural." But does either of these terms make any nutritional sense? None whatever.

The terms "raw," "uncooked," and "unfiltered" also have no legal definition, so they mean very little on a label. Legally, "enriched" means that thiamine, riboflavin, niacin, and iron have been put back into refined cereals or breads to the level they had before processing. "Fortified" is used interchangeably with "enriched." Neither of these terms means you are getting any more nutrients than in the simple unprocessed food. "Sugar-free" and "sugarless" just mean no *sucrose* (table sugar); the material may still have large amounts of fructose, glucose, sorbitol, mannitol —all just variants of table sugar. "Reduced calorie" legally means ⅓ or more fewer calories than the regular product, but if there were a lot to start with, ⅓ fewer are still a lot. "Low calorie" is the only meaningful term in all this misleading verbiage. Legally, foods whose label says "low calorie" must contain no more than 40 calories per normal serving.

Whatever you are buying should bear a complete list of ingredients on the label, in descending order of quantity. Read this and pay no attention at all to terms like "natural." *The most important thing a health-conscious public can demand is full and proper labeling.* We are certainly not getting it.

Legumes (Beans and Peas): Legumes are plants in which the seeds develop in pods. Besides what we usually think of as "beans," alfalfa, clover, and peanuts fall into this category. Except for lentils, split peas, and adzukis, beans need to be soaked for several hours or overnight before cooking. The soak water should be discarded. A small amount of nutrients will be lost, but well-soaked beans cause much less flatulence. Two of the carbohydrates in beans, stachyrose and raffinose, which can be partially removed by soaking, are indigestible by the enzymes of the small intestine and are passed along to be digested by bacteria in the colon, with the formation of gas. Cook lentils, split peas, fresh black-eyed peas, and adzuki beans for 1 hour, the other beans for 1½ to 3 hours. Beans are fiber-rich, contain no cholesterol, and are low in fat (except for soybeans, which derive 40 percent of their calories from fat). Adzuki beans have an exceptionally low fat content, for a bean, and do not need to be presoaked. Legumes have a significant iron content, but its bioavailability is low. We must seek our iron elsewhere.

Mushrooms: They come in many varieties. For a good sampler of chanterelles, French morels, Italian porcini, and French cèpes, with recipes, write to Key Gourmet, Box 3691, Beverly Hills, Calif. 90212.

Nuts: Nutritious but tending to be murderously high-fat, nuts have lots of calories. One cup of peanuts contains as many calories as 4½ cups of brown rice or 8 baked potatoes. You could hardly eat that much rice or potatoes, but could easily munch away a cup of peanuts. Brazil nuts, macadamias, filberts, and pecans are especially high in fat (93 percent of calories); pecan pie is perhaps the world's highest-calorie desert! Pistachios derive 88 percent of their calories from fat, and walnuts, 81 percent. "Low-fat" nuts include cashews (45 percent fat), almonds, and peanuts. But hail to the chestnut! Quite unlike any other of the common nuts, it is high in carbohydrates, low in fat, and low in calories. You can obtain vacuum-packed chestnuts from Williams-Sonoma, Mail Order Dept., P.O. Box 7456, San Francisco, Calif. 94120-7456.

Because of their high largely unsaturated oil content, nuts tend to become rancid. If you want them to keep longer, buy only unshelled nuts, and shell them yourself before use; or at least buy unbroken nuts, and store them in a closed jar in the refrigerator, not on a shelf.

Oil: Oil and fat are really equivalent, since fats are simply oils that are naturally solid at room temperature. The structure of fats and oils consists of a glycerol backbone to which three fatty acids are attached. The differences between various oils reflect which among many different fatty acids are actually present. Some of the carbon atoms in these fatty acids are joined by what are called "double bonds" and some by "single bonds." The double bonds designate "unsaturated" and the single bonds, "saturated" sites. The unsaturated sites or bonds tend to protect against arteriosclerosis, but they are subject to oxidation and the generation of free radicals.

In general, the lower the fat content of your diet the better, whether the bonds be unsaturated or saturated, although a minimum essential amount is required (equivalent to 4 to 6 percent of calories from fat per 2,500 calories, depending on the type of fat or oil). It's almost impossible not to consume enough essential fatty acids (unless you stick to highly processed oils), and dangerously easy to get too much. The average American takes in over 21 pounds of salad and cooking oil per year, whereas for a tablespoon's worth of corn oil from the natural source, you would have to eat 14 ears of corn. Furthermore, regular commercial corn oil has probably been heated to about 400 degrees C., and in animal experiments heated corn oil is more prone than unheated oil to cause arteriosclerosis. It is possible that margarine, which is apt to be highly processed and hydrogenated, is in fact worse for your arteries than butter. High-quality corn oil does happen to be one of the better polyunsaturated oils. High in vitamin E, it is less apt to go rancid than, say, safflower oil, which is highly polyunsaturated and not especially high in vitamin E.

Processed or highly refined oils are not recommended. These categories include both "hydrogenated" and "partially hydrogenated" oils or fats. Natural fatty acid is the so-called "cis" form, whereas in processed oils as much as 60 percent may have been converted to the "trans" form. Crisco and Spry are partially hydrogenated. Avoid them.

Avoid anything that is simply labeled "vegetable" oil. It is apt to be highly processed.

You may be surprised to learn that pork fat is probably better for you (or less harmful) than beef fat, since the former contains mainly oleic and linoleic fatty acids (Linoleic is an "essential," unsaturated fatty acid), whereas beef fat contains mainly palmitic and stearic fatty acids, both fully saturated. Furthermore, the pork industry is now breeding hogs that are 50 percent leaner than 30 years ago, and lean cuts of pork have the same cholesterol content as beef (60–80 mg. per ¼-lb. serving). Recall (page 31) that wild animals and free-roaming grass-eating beef have far lower fat contents than the fatted calves and steers most of the cattle industry is serving up to us.

Italian olive oil is government-regulated, the better qualities being by law designated "virgin," "superfine virgin," and "extra virgin." Obtained by manual pressing of the olives between cold stone wheels, "extra virgin" is the best. It may then be filtered through cheesecloth to be clarified. If unfiltered, it is cloudy, dense, and called "mosto." While of the highest quality, "extra virgin" is subject to oxidation, so should be used over a period of weeks to months, not years. Highest-quality Italian brands are Badic, Coltibuono, and Colavita from Tuscany, and Il Castelluzza from Umbria. Olive oil and peanut oil are monounsaturated, and chemically stand between saturated and polyunsaturated oils, but biologically they may be just as antiarteriosclerotic as the polyunsaturated oils or even more so.[15] They all lower LDL and cholesterol, but the polyunsaturated oils may also lower HDL, while the monounsaturated oils do not. (Remember that you want low cholesterol, low LDL, and high HDL.) Olive oil is the best oil to use on a low-fat diet, if you use any at all. The term "pure" olive oil means oil extracted from the second pressing, at a higher temperature and pressure, followed by the use of hot-water treatment or solvent extraction. Not at all of the quality of "extra virgin"! Olive oil, as well as any other oils, should be refrigerated once opened, to avoid oxidation or rancidity. Put a drop on your wrist, rub it in, and smell it: if it smells good, it's probably okay. A few oils are packaged with nitrogen flushing, which cuts down on the oxidation. The label should tell you this.

The term "cold pressed" on many domestic oils means little—another health-food buzzword. There may be no such thing as a truly cold-pressed large-scale commercial American oil; any that you buy has been mechanically pressed, involving temperatures up to 150 degrees. The term "100 percent virgin" on an American oil is the top designation, and indicates the first pressing of the olives, no additives, and that it is unrefined. The Marsala and Sciabica oils may carry this designation, and are among the best domestic oils. The term "prepressed," while somewhat misleading, indicates a better product than "cold pressed." "Unrefined" as applied to oils means no refining, bleaching, or deodorizing, but it does not exclude extraction with hexane (instead of pressing) followed by distillation to get rid of water. "Unrefined" oils smoke more when cooked, become rancid faster, and tend to be darker with sediment, which should be shaken into the oil before using.

Pasta: At the Chamber of Commerce in Bologna there is a solid-gold noodle, 1mm. thick, and 6 mm. wide—the standard dimension of the perfect raw tagliatelle noodle. Pasta is made from the flour of durum wheat, whose starch is too hard for making bread but ideal for pasta, which must stay together while being boiled, baked, or steamed. Good pasta is nutritious, but you should use only pasta made from "whole durum wheat flour," *not* from *semolina*, which is refined for the sake of color and variety. Other grain and vegetable powders are sometimes added to the basic durum wheat flour: spinach, artichoke, soy, buckwheat. Take advantage also of pasta's endless shapes and textures. Shells or fusilli catch the sauce better than long slim shapes.

To cook pasta, add a teaspoon of olive oil to boiling water

to prevent sticking, and drop in the pasta. Cook until firm and slightly chewy but not starchy. If you can easily bite all the way through a noodle, it is done. Drain in a colander and toss with sauce in a bowl to coat and separate the noodles. Do not rinse with cold water, as it renders pasta soft and gummy. If you use cheese, the best Parmesan is Reggiano; the best Romano, Pecorino. Use only freshly grated cheese.

Poultry: The fat content of commercial chickens has tripled in the last 25 years. In 1960 it was 5 gm. per 100 gm.; now it is 15 gm. This increase has been due to selection for larger size and more rapid growth rate and use of less expensive feeds. It's the same unhealthful commercial pattern we have already seen in the cattle industry. (As fish farming becomes big business, here also we shall probably see the lean turned into fat.) In chickens, the skin and the fat pad between the skin and the meat contain about 85 percent of the fat. To a considerable extent these can be separated off and discarded. Chicken breast without skin derives 19 percent of its calories from fat; chicken thigh without skin, 47 percent.

Seasonings: Important as they are nutritionally, many foods such as grains and legumes are rather bland. Vegit and Jensen's Broth & Seasoning are excellent general-purpose seasonings for rice or beans. It's more interesting to use pure seasonings, bought fresh weekly when possible. Among liquid seasoning, beware of the sodium content. Examples: regular soy sauce and tamari contain about 1,200 mg. sodium per tablespoon—much too much. Worcestershire sauce is similar in flavor and much lower in sodium. Miso has excellent food value but is high in sodium. Sugarless ketchup, to be preferred on a high/low diet, must by law be labeled as "imitation ketchup." By quirks of the law like this one, some things which must be labeled "imitation" are in fact more healthful than the real thing. Mayonnaise is another example.

To clue into the different seasonings, to find out what tastes best to you, divide the dish into two or three equal portions and flavor each differently. Suggested combinations might be as follows:

Cabbage:	oregano, savory, tarragon
Carrots:	mint, thyme
Eggplant:	basil, marjoram, sage
Green beans:	dillweed, marjoram, savory
Lentils:	oregano, sage
Lima beans:	oregano, sage
White potatoes:	dillweed, mint, oregano, rosemary, thyme
Rice:	cumin, coriander, thyme
Spinach:	marjoram, mint, rosemary

Having tested these separately, mix them together for the combined effect.

Seaweeds: These plants are becoming popular in the United States, and with good reason. They are highly nutritious, being particularly rich (for a nonmeat source) in iron, as well as calcium, vitamin B_6, probably vitamins B_{12} and D (There is some dispute about these), and other nutrients. To North American tastes, dulce is the most palatable of the seaweeds. But unlike other seaweeds, it contains a fair amount of fat. It requires only gentle boiling. Become familiar also with nori (which is used to wrap sushi, but can be cut up and added directly to salads), with sweet kombu, wakame (Needs moderate boiling), and single-bladed and finger kombu (Both require rather long boiling). Kombu will reduce the starchiness of beans, shorten the cooking time, and eliminate the flatulence. It's one of the highest nonmeat sources of iron. Best (freshest) kombu brands are Erewhon and Westbrae. High in calcium, iron, and possibly vitamin B_{12}, the seaweed wakame (Alaria) contains lot of alginic acid, which precipitates heavy metals such as mercury, lead, and cadmium if these contaminate the food source.

Seeds: Like nuts, seeds are nutritious but high in fat, mostly unsaturated. However, they are more nutrient-dense than nuts and so are the wiser choice. Pumpkin seeds (pepitas) are quite high in iron and zinc. Iron is often too low or at best borderline on a low-meat diet, and zinc is the element most often deficient in the American diet. If possible, buy only mechanically hulled sesame seeds, as the common variety has had the hulls removed by chemical solvents (usually lye), which may diminish the nutrient value. Seeds, like nuts, can go rancid as a result of their high fat content. Store them in the refrigerator.

Sprouts: These have the nutritive value of greens, rather than that of the seeds they emerged from. For example, soybean sprouts are nutritionally more like broccoli than like soybeans. A sprout from a grain would be nutritionally similar to lettuce. Sprouts are delicious and good for you, but don't use them to replace grains in your diet.

Tofu: A fairly recent addition to the American diet but long a mainstay in Asian cooking, tofu is a good replacement for meat and dairy products, thanks to a somewhat lower percentage of fat (40 percent calories from fat), mostly unsaturated (15 percent saturated, 52 percent polyunsaturated). Soybean curd, tofu, is low in calories (72 calories for 3½ oz. serving). It goes well in recipes calling for cheese—as examples, in sauces, pasta, or pizza. It will absorb the flavor of anything you cook with it. Scrambled and with salsa added, it can substitute for scrambled eggs, and it contains no cholesterol. Its protein quality approaches or equals that of meat, although slightly low in methionine.

Tofu comes packed in water. The package should bear a date of production. Use the tofu within about 2 weeks of that date. Once the package has been opened, drain off the liquid, add fresh water, and change the water every 1 or 2 days. To see if you like the taste of tofu relatively neat, try the following: place a block of soft tofu on a plate, top with diced shallots fried in a minimal amount of olive oil, and add soy sauce or Worcestershire sauce and fresh chopped cilantro. Serve this as an appetizer.

Vinegar: Buy only the top quality. Even the most expensive vinegar is comparatively cheap, and top quality will pay handsomely in the excellence of your salads and other dishes. A favorite of mine is the balsamic vinegar available from Williams-Sonoma (address p. 254).

Water: Bottled waters have increased remarkably in popularity in the United States in the past several decades. A great deal of this is due to advertising, which has popularized and internalized the most famous myth in gerontology, the Fountain of Youth. There is also a growing fear of contamination of city water. Whole sections of cities suddenly discover that industrial pollutants have crept into their local aquifer. The underground march of the infamous Stringfellow acid pits in eastern Los Angeles is one gruesome example. Bottled water from carefully controlled springs or other sources should be free of this danger, or so it is hoped.

In fact, only a fourth of the bottled water sold in the United States is truly spring water. Again, labels can be deceiving. If a label carries the word "spring" merely in the company's name, rather than on the product, it's not spring water. If the label says "spring-type," "spring-fresh," or "spring-pure," it is not spring water. Look for a product that is designated specifically as "spring water" or "natural spring water." Anything labeled "natural mineral water" usually comes from a spring. "Mineral water" generally refers more to the total dissolved solids than to the source. In California, whatever is labeled as "mineral water" must contain 500 parts per million or more of total dissolved solids.

Certain areas of the United States are characterized by greater average longevities and lower death rates than other areas. In general, the Southeastern United States (Georgia, the Carolinas, and parts of Alabama, but not Florida) shows decreased longevity in the population. The upper-middle portion of the United States (Nebraska, Colorado, South Dakota, Minnesota, and neighboring states to some extent) plus Alaska generally shows increased longevity. The rest of the country follows a hodgepodge pattern, longevity varying from county to county. Trace elements in the soil or differences in the quality of the drinking water may be of paramount importance in accounting for these differences.

There is a relation between the extent of heart disease in a population and the hardness of water in the area, although it's not easy to pin down just what chemical or chemicals are involved.[16] In the areas of greater longevity the water supplies are characterized by a high density of dissolved solids (over 300 milligrams per liter), very hard water (over 200 mg. of inorganic matter/l.), high calcium content (over 50 mg./l.), high magnesium content (over 30 mg./l), a variable but often high sodium content (10 to 1,000 mg./l.), and a low level of dissolved organic compounds.[17] A high chromium and manganese content might also be important.[18] You can find out about your own water by writing to the Department of Water and Power in your county. In Table 10.5 I have listed some of the characteristics of a number of popular bottled waters and of Los Angeles and New York City tap waters. These data are assembled from various sources, not all of which are in complete agreement, but should be approximately correct. Make your own judgment among the waters. Vichy and Calso are simply too high in sodium to be good choices. Vittel, Deep Rock, Indian Head, Evian, San Pellegrino, and a few others all look good.

We were born in water and we go to dust. The Fountain is the enduring legend. Take a good drink of water and thank your stars you were not born too early in human history to participate in the life-extension revolution.

Table 10.5 Characteristics of selected bottled waters and of Los Angeles and New York City tap waters (milligrams per liter).

	Total dissolved solids	Hardness	Calcium	Magnesium	Sodium
Appolinaris	2,250	1,200	180	240	570
Arrowhead	112	96	16	3	9
Badoit	—	1,550	355	198	205
Calistoga	540	240	80	3	120
Calso	2,910	670	230	3	1,325
Deep Rock	547	320	73	25	55
Deer Park	29	15	3	3	4
Evian	330	295	78	25	7
Fiuggi	120	400	118	25	68
Indian Head	654	367	74	32	33
Los Angeles tap	186	61	21	5	31
Mountain Valley	205	230	79	11	3
New York tap	127	65	18	6	11
Perrier	545	290	88	13	15
Poland Spring	125	50	19	7	4
Ramlosa	—	1	0.2	0.1	3
San Pellegrino	1,100	776	212	60	44
Saratoga	445	—	—	—	64
Silver Springs	150	95	31	7	11
Sparkletts	18	12	1	1	4
Vichy	3,400	105	162	12	1,223
Vittel	465	755	181	41	7

APPENDIX A

FOOD COMBINATIONS AND TASTY MENUS FOR THE HEALTHIEST 20 DAYS OF YOUR LIFE

(An asterisk indicates that a recipe is provided.)

Menus

DAY ONE

BREAKFAST		*% OF RDAs*	
¼ cup cereal, rye		Tryptophan	592
flakes	20 gm.	Isoleucine	663
2½ tbsp. wheat bran	15 gm.	Lysine	881
1 tbsp. yeast	10 gm.	Valine	629
1 glass skim milk	244 gm.	Methionine,	
1 medium peach	100 gm.	cysteine	510

LUNCH

Succotash/Barley Chowder,* 1 bowl
1 slice rye bread with Hummus* or Soy Paste*

DINNER

175-degree steak*	¼ lb.
1 steamed summer squash	130 gm.
1 sweet potato, with 1 tbsp. yogurt topping	180 gm.
1 cup chopped spinach	55 gm.
1 slice rye bread with Hummus or Soy Paste	
almonds, 1¼ tbsp.	10 gm.

NUTRITIONAL INFORMATION

Total calories	1,550
% calories from fat	13
Total protein	90 gm.
Total carbohydrates	256 gm.
Total fat	23 gm.

Threonine	802
Leucine	754
Phenylalanine, tyrosine	782
Vitamin A	532
Vitamin D	69
Vitamin K	134
Vitamin C	218
Vitamin E	145
Riboflavin	146
Vitamin B_6	138
Vitamin B_{12}	98
Thiamine	220
Niacin	127
Folacin	252
Pantothenic acid	209
Biotin	57
Calcium	91
Magnesium	162
Copper	109
Zinc	107
Chromium	215
Phosphorus	165
Potassium	251
Iron	129
Manganese	204
Selenium	120

DAY TWO

BREAKFAST

1 egg	50 gm.
1 slice whole-wheat bread	25 gm.
½ grapefruit	100 gm.

LUNCH

Chicken, light meat	¼ lb.
Cold Green Soup,* 1 bowl	
Yeast, added to soup	5 gm.
1 slice whole-wheat bread	

DINNER

Stuffed Pepper with Beer Sauce*	
1 white potato with yogurt topping	250 gm.
4 brussels sprouts	112 gm.
1 medium tomato with ⅛ wedge romaine lettuce and low-cal dressing	90 gm.

NUTRITIONAL INFORMATION

Total calories	1,288
% calories from fat	17
Total protein	91 gm.
Total carbohydrates	177 gm.
Total fat	24 gm.

% OF RDAs

Tryptophan	658
Isoleucine	650
Lysine	889
Valine	594
Methionine, cysteine	525
Threonine	790
Leucine	722
Phenylalanine, tyrosine	779
Vitamin A	385
Vitamin D	75
Vitamin K	2,427
Vitamin C	919
Vitamin E	144
Riboflavin	128
Vitamin B_6	170
Vitamin B_{12}	196
Thiamine	199
Niacin	151
Folacin	290
Pantothenic acid	210
Biotin	88
Calcium	90
Magnesium	194
Copper	74
Zinc	66
Chromium	326
Phosphorus	130
Potassium	304
Iron	142
Manganese	182
Selenium	258

DAY THREE

BREAKFAST

¼ cup rolled oats	25 gm.
½ cup wheat bran	20 gm.
1 tbsp. yeast	5 gm.
1 banana, sliced	150 gm.
1 glass skim milk	244 gm.

LUNCH

¼ pound marinated halibut	100 gm.
½ cup cabbage (as cole slaw)	50 gm.
1 glass skim milk	244 gm.

DINNER

Oyster cocktail (4 to 8 oysters, depending on size)	100 gm.
Pasta Primavera,* 1 serving	
6–8 leaves kale, steamed, with sauce of choice (see Sauces)	50 gm.
1 slice watermelon, equivalent of 2 cups, diced	320 gm.

NUTRITIONAL INFORMATION

Total calories	1,142
% calories from fat	11
Total protein	76 gm.
Total carbohydrates	178 gm.
Total fat	14 gm.

% OF RDAs

Tryptophan	538
Isoleucine	522
Lysine	742
Valine	506
Methionine, cysteine	455
Threonine	630
Leucine	601
Phenylalanine, tyrosine	599
Vitamin A	256
Vitamin D	150
Vitamin K	674
Vitamin C	511
Vitamin E	73
Riboflavin	116
Vitamin B_6	156
Vitamin B_{12}	698
Thiamine	165
Niacin	146
Folacin	138
Pantothenic acid	169
Biotin	74
Calcium	96
Magnesium	115
Copper	227
Zinc	338
Chromium	177
Phosphorus	144
Potassium	208
Iron	102
Manganese	158
Selenium	283

DAY FOUR

BREAKFAST

½ cantaloupe	400 gm.
½ cup blueberries	70 gm.
1 poached egg	50 gm.
1 slice whole-wheat bread	25 gm.

LUNCH

Sandwich:	
2 slices whole-wheat bread, with Soy Paste*	50 gm.
3½ oz. chicken, white meat	100 gm.
3 leaves romaine lettuce	25 gm.

DINNER

Saffron SLS Soup,* 2 bowls, with 10 gm. yeast added and garnished with ¼ cup chopped parsley	40 gm.
1 glass skim milk	244 gm.

NUTRITIONAL INFORMATION

Total calories	1,311
% calories from fat	16
Total protein	87 gm.
Total carbohydrates	189 gm.
Total fat	23 gm.

% OF RDAs

Tryptophan	601
Isoleucine	608
Lysine	838
Valine	557
Methionine, cysteine	485
Threonine	686
Leucine	672
Phenylalanine, tyrosine	749
Vitamin A	627
Vitamin D	102
Vitamin K	238
Vitamin C	538
Vitamin E	149
Riboflavin	122
Vitamin B_6	148
Vitamin B_{12}	132
Thiamine	246
Niacin	147
Folacin	234
Pantothenic acid	209
Biotin	94
Calcium	94
Magnesium	153
Copper	80
Zinc	70
Chromium	207
Phosphorus	139
Potassium	255
Iron	113
Manganese	168
Selenium	240

DAY FIVE

BREAKFAST

½ cup millet (as porridge)	50 gm.
1 tbsp. yeast	10 gm.
1 glass skim milk	244 gm.
1 banana	150 gm.
1 tbsp. sunflower seeds	9 gm.

LUNCH

Sandwich:	
2 slices whole-wheat bread	50 gm.
¼ can sardines in water or mustard or tomato sauce	50 gm.
4 leaves romaine lettuce	50 gm.

DINNER

Salad #1,* 2 servings	
1 cup skim milk	244 gm.

NUTRITIONAL INFORMATION

Total calories	1,437
% calories from fat	13
Total protein	81 gm.
Total carbohydrates	254 gm.
Total fat	20 gm.

% OF RDAs

Tryptophan	566
Isoleucine	600
Lysine	752
Valine	578
Methionine, cysteine	459
Threonine	660
Leucine	710
Phenylalanine, tyrosine	712
Vitamin A	321
Vitamin D	57
Vitamin K	749
Vitamin C	378
Vitamin E	102
Riboflavin	156
Vitamin B_6	166
Vitamin B_{12}	251
Thiamine	259
Niacin	116
Folacin	249
Pantothenic acid	222
Biotin	65
Calcium	122
Magnesium	148
Copper	130
Zinc	94
Chromium	209
Phosphorus	181
Potassium	255
Iron	116
Manganese	196
Selenium	187

DAY SIX

BREAKFAST

Scrambled Tofu,* 1 serving	
1 slice whole-wheat toast (with Soy Paste*)	
1 citrus fruit	180 gm.

LUNCH

Vegetable Salad #1,* 1 serving	
1 glass skim milk	244 gm.

DINNER

4 oysters (see Oysters with Millet*)	100 gm.
Millet	25 gm.
Yeast, ½ tbsp.	5 gm.
Broccoli (with one of the "4 Sauces")	200 gm.

NUTRITIONAL INFORMATION

Total calories	1,145
% calories from fat	17
Total protein	79 gm.
Total carbohydrates	181 gm.
Total fat	21 gm.

% OF RDAs

Tryptophan	593
Isoleucine	573
Lysine	698
Valine	548
Methionine, cysteine	426
Threonine	642
Leucine	646
Phenylalanine, tyrosine	707
Vitamin A	313
Vitamin D	110
Vitamin K	1,102
Vitamin C	941
Vitamin E	123
Riboflavin	131
Vitamin B_6	112
Vitamin B_{12}	642
Thiamine	206
Niacin	87
Folacin	189
Pantothenic acid	222
Biotin	77
Calcium	107
Magnesium	154
Copper	220
Zinc	333
Chromium	208
Phosphorus	151
Potassium	249
Iron	134
Manganese	167
Selenium	291

DAY SEVEN

BREAKFAST		*% OF RDAs*	
½ papaya	150 gm.	Tryptophan	638
2 glasses skim milk	488 gm.	Isoleucine	641
		Lysine	843
LUNCH		Valine	648
Sandwich:		Methionine, cysteine	437
2 slices whole-wheat or rye bread with Tuna Chutney Spread* and lettuce or sprouts	50 gm.	Threonine	727
		Leucine	723
		Phenylalanine, tyrosine	738
1½ cups Country Cole Slaw*		Vitamin A	360
		Vitamin D	96
		Vitamin K	2,030
DINNER		Vitamin C	670
Baked Stuffed Eggplant,* 1 serving		Vitamin E	87
turnip greens with one of the "4 Sauces"	80 gm.	Riboflavin	135
½ cup lentils with ⅓ cup wild rice, 1 tbsp. sunflower seeds, plus herb seasoning	40 gm.	Vitamin B_6	121
		Vitamin B_{12}	118
		Thiamine	117
		Niacin	119
		Folacin	117
		Pantothenic acid	174
		Biotin	28
		Calcium	117
		Magnesium	129
NUTRITIONAL INFORMATION		Copper	85
		Zinc	79
		Chromium	156
Total calories	1,388	Phosphorus	149
% calories from fat	13	Potassium	230
Total protein	92 gm.	Iron	117
Total carbohydrates	210 gm.	Manganese	110
Total fat	20 gm.	Selenium	330

Note: ½ cup lentils 50 gm.

DAY EIGHT

BREAKFAST

Cereal, rye flakes	20 gm.
1½ glasses skim milk	366 gm.
Banana	75 gm.

LUNCH

Susan's Veggie San,* 1 serving

DINNER

Whole-Wheat Spaghetti with Clam Sauce*	
Asparagus	150 gm.
Mushrooms	70 gm.

NUTRITIONAL INFORMATION

Total calories	1,334
% calories from fat	18
Total protein	89 gm.
Total carbohydrates	208 gm.
Total fat	26 gm.

% OF RDAs

Tryptophan	609
Isoleucine	640
Lysine	724
Valine	614
Methionine	490
Threonine	722
Leucine	700
Phenylalanine, tyrosine	704
Vitamin A	553
Vitamin D	85
Vitamin K	1,079
Vitamin C	962
Vitamin E	185
Riboflavin	179
Vitamin B_6	140
Vitamin B_{12}	937
Thiamine	117
Niacin	110
Folacin	153
Pantothenic acid	289
Biotin	51
Calcium	133
Magnesium	121
Copper	72
Zinc	78
Chromium	265
Phosphorus	142
Potassium	237
Iron	149
Manganese	124
Selenium	238

DAY NINE

BREAKFAST

Porridge of millet and wheat bran	25 gm. / 20 gm.
Yeast	5 gm.
½ cup strawberries	75 gm.
1 glass skim milk	244 gm.

LUNCH

1 orange	180 gm.
3 brussels sprouts	100 gm.
1 banana	150 gm.

DINNER

Cauliflower Soup,* 1 serving	
Chicken with Artichoke,* 1 serving	
1 cup kale, steamed	100 gm.
1 cup turnip greens, steamed	100 gm.
One of the "4 sauces" (on greens)	

NUTRITIONAL INFORMATION

Total calories	1,254
% calories from fat	7
Total protein	88 gm.
Total carbohydrates	203 gm.
Total fat	10 gm.

% OF RDAs

Tryptophan	671
Isoleucine	626
Lysine	859
Valine	574
Methionine, cysteine	525
Threonine	757
Leucine	722
Phenylalanine, tyrosine	728
Vitamin A	380
Vitamin D	93
Vitamin K	2,195
Vitamin C	1,019
Vitamin E	106
Riboflavin	163
Vitamin B_6	199
Vitamin B_{12}	157
Thiamine	234
Niacin	193
Folacin	224
Pantothenic acid	247
Biotin	79
Calcium	120
Magnesium	160
Copper	98
Zinc	67
Chromium	197
Phosphorus	165
Potassium	271
Iron	100
Manganese	221
Selenium	225

DAY TEN

BREAKFAST

Rolled oats	20 gm.
Wheat bran	10 gm.
1½ tbsp. wheat germ	10 gm.
½ cup raspberries, or other berries	70 gm.
1 glass skim milk	244 gm.

LUNCH

California Corn Salad,* 1 serving

DINNER

Broccoli Pasta Casserole,* 1 serving	
½ cup split peas	100 gm.
1 medium carrot	80 gm.
Celeriac	100 gm.

NUTRITIONAL INFORMATION

Total calories	1513
% calories from fat	8
Total protein	89 gm.
Total carbohydrates	260 gm.
Total fat	13 gm.

% OF RDAs

Tryptophan	502
Isoleucine	581
Lysine	721
Valine	568
Methionine, cysteine	425
Threonine	671
Leucine	691
Phenylalanine, tyrosine	743
Vitamin A	371
Vitamin D	28
Vitamin K	1,718
Vitamin C	727
Vitamin E	122
Riboflavin	125
Vitamin B_6	105
Vitamin B_{12}	72
Thiamine	150
Niacin	98
Folacin	151
Pantothenic acid	183
Biotin	40
Calcium	95
Magnesium	135
Copper	79
Zinc	94
Chromium	220
Phosphorus	171
Potassium	262
Iron	116
Manganese	195
Selenium	177

DAY ELEVEN

BREAKFAST

¼ cup millet (as porridge)	25 gm.
2 tbsp. bran	12 gm.
2 tbsp. sunflower seeds	20 gm.
1 banana	150 gm.
1 glass skim milk	244 gm.

LUNCH

Lima Bean Chestnut Salad,* 1 serving	
1 glass skim milk	244 gm.

DINNER

Wild Rice Scallop Casserole,* 1 serving	
1 glass skim milk	244 gm.

NUTRITIONAL INFORMATION

Total calories	1,427
% calories from fat	12
Total protein	79 gm.
Total carbohydrates	235 gm.
Total fat	16 gm.

% OF RDAs

Tryptophan	581
Isoleucine	575
Lysine	527
Valine	586
Methionine, cysteine	460
Threonine	698
Leucine	692
Phenylalanine, tyrosine	673
Vitamin A	53
Vitamin D	146
Vitamin K	470
Vitamin C	101
Vitamin E	159
Riboflavin	132
Vitamin B_6	306
Vitamin B_{12}	282
Thiamine	145
Niacin	75
Folacin	70
Pantothenic acid	160
Biotin	46
Calcium	102
Magnesium	149
Copper	117
Zinc	89
Chromium	116
Phosphorus	163
Potassium	258
Iron	103
Manganese	200
Selenium	137

DAY TWELVE

BREAKFAST		*% OF RDAs*	
½ cup millet	25 gm.	Tryptophan	471
1 medium peach	100 gm.	Isoleucine	488
1 glass skim milk	244 gm.	Lysine	628
2 tbsp. wheat germ	12 gm.	Valine	467
		Methionine, cysteine	394
LUNCH		Threonine	574
Salmon Sandwich:		Leucine	565
3½ oz. canned salmon	100 gm.	Phenylalanine, tyrosine	552
2 slices whole-wheat bread	50 gm.	Vitamin A	180
2 leaves romaine lettuce	25 gm.	Vitamin D	109
1 slice onion	25 gm.	Vitamin K	929
¼ tomato	25 gm.	Vitamin C	541
		Vitamin E	135
		Riboflavin	113
		Vitamin B_6	95
DINNER		Vitamin B_{12}	295
Green Grain Salad with Mustard Dressing,* 1 serving		Thiamine	107
½ pound (1 large stalk) broccoli	225 gm.	Niacin	107
1 glass skim milk	244 gm.	Folacin	150
		Pantothenic acid	192
		Biotin	38
		Calcium	96
		Magnesium	92
NUTRITIONAL INFORMATION		Copper	65
		Zinc	63
		Chromium	132
Total calories	1,152	Phosphorus	143
% calories from fat	16	Potassium	201
Total protein	74 gm.	Iron	73
Total carbohydrates	169 gm.	Manganese	146
Total fat	20 gm.	Selenium	182

DAY THIRTEEN

BREAKFAST

½ cantaloupe	400 gm.
½ cup blueberries	70 gm.
1 poached egg	50 gm.
1 slice whole-wheat bread	25 gm.
1 glass skim milk	244 gm.

LUNCH

Cape Cod Chowder,* 1 bowl

DINNER

Bean/Millet Stuffed Pepper,* 1 serving	
1 glass skim milk	244 gm.

NUTRITIONAL INFORMATION

Total calories	1,296
% calories from fat	16
Total protein	73 gm.
Total carbohydrates	198 gm.
Total fat	23 gm.

% OF RDAs

Tryptophan	556
Isoleucine	577
Lysine	677
Valine	531
Methionine, cysteine	418
Threonine	647
Leucine	653
Phenylalanine, tyrosine	724
Vitamin A	376
Vitamin D	105
Vitamin K	215
Vitamin C	1,023
Vitamin E	149
Riboflavin	145
Vitamin B_6	164
Vitamin B_{12}	176
Thiamine	280
Niacin	91
Folacin	223
Pantothenic acid	208
Biotin	84
Calcium	98
Magnesium	153
Copper	95
Zinc	72
Chromium	249
Phosphorus	155
Potassium	300
Iron	104
Manganese	170
Selenium	204

DAY FOURTEEN

BREAKFAST

⅓ cup rolled oats	30 gm.
4 medium-size figs, fresh	100 gm.
½ apple, diced	75 gm.
Sunflower seeds	10 gm.
1 glass skim milk	244 gm.

LUNCH

1 Baked Sandwich*
2 glasses nonfat milk

DINNER

3½ oz. calf's liver	100 gm.
Beer Slaw,* 1 serving	

NUTRITIONAL INFORMATION

Total calories	1,071
% calories from fat	18
Total protein	76 gm.
Total carbohydrates	156 gm.
Total fat	20 gm.

% OF RDAs

Tryptophan	563
Isoleucine	552
Lysine	722
Valine	550
Methionine, cysteine	436
Threonine	653
Leucine	674
Phenylalanine, tyrosine	702
Vitamin A	531
Vitamin D	85
Vitamin K	496
Vitamin C	436
Vitamin E	116
Riboflavin	267
Vitamin B_6	105
Vitamin B_{12}	2,120
Thiamine	124
Niacin	105
Folacin	140
Pantothenic acid	346
Biotin	142
Calcium	114
Magnesium	81
Copper	313
Zinc	88
Chromium	184
Phosphorus	167
Potassium	181
Iron	93
Manganese	104
Selenium	240

DAY FIFTEEN

BREAKFAST

⅓ cup buckwheat	35 gm.
Yeast	5 gm.
1 glass skim milk	244 gm.
½ cup strawberries	75 gm.

LUNCH

Vegetable Curry,* 1 serving	
Indian Brown Rice,* 1 serving	
1 glass skim milk	244 gm.

DINNER

3½ oz. black sea bass	100 gm.
Ruth's Italian Zucchini,* 1 serving	
1 cup peas	145 gm.
1 cup beets, cubed	140 gm.
Dessert:	
½ cup low-fat yogurt	122 gm.
½ cup blueberries	70 gm.
1 tbsp. sunflower seeds	10 gm.
1 cup skim milk	244 gm.

NUTRITIONAL INFORMATION

Total calories	1,284
% calories from fat	11
Total protein	88 gm.
Total carbohydrates	220 gm.
Total fat	16 gm.

% OF RDAs

Tryptophan	583
Isoleucine	628
Lysine	923
Valine	641
Methionine, cysteine	477
Threonine	778
Leucine	755
Phenylalanine, tyrosine	769
Vitamin A	309
Vitamin D	112
Vitamin K	1,591
Vitamin C	629
Vitamin E	112
Riboflavin	164
Vitamin B_6	210
Vitamin B_{12}	201
Thiamine	197
Niacin	113
Folacin	185
Pantothenic acid	255
Biotin	67
Calcium	142
Magnesium	139
Copper	105
Zinc	87
Chromium	219
Phosphorus	178
Potassium	290
Iron	88
Manganese	189
Selenium	160

DAY SIXTEEN

BREAKFAST

⅓ cup rolled oats	30 gm.
3 tbsp. wheat bran	20 gm.
1 tbsp. yeast	10 gm.
Breakfast Drink,* 1 cup (on cereal)	

LUNCH

Sandwich:	
Tuna Chutney Spread*	
2 slices whole-wheat bread	
1 glass nonfat milk	244 gm.

DINNER

Eternal Youth Chili,* 1 serving
Lima Bean Chestnut Salad,* 1 serving

NUTRITIONAL INFORMATION

Total calories	1,438
% calories from fat	14
Total protein	90 gm.
Total carbohydrates	218 gm.
Total fat	22 gm.

% OF RDAs

Tryptophan	662
Isoleucine	683
Lysine	956
Valine	683
Methionine, cysteine	534
Threonine	846
Leucine	788
Phenylalanine, tyrosine	817
Vitamin A	91
Vitamin D	149
Vitamin K	781
Vitamin C	448
Vitamin E	79
Riboflavin	134
Vitamin B_6	322
Vitamin B_{12}	283
Thiamine	253
Niacin	150
Folacin	192
Pantothenic acid	186
Biotin	58
Calcium	78
Magnesium	148
Copper	102
Zinc	90
Chromium	209
Phosphorus	177
Potassium	259
Iron	133
Manganese	276
Selenium	369

DAY SEVENTEEN

BREAKFAST

⅓ cup rolled oats	30 gm.
3 tbsp. wheat bran	20 gm.
4 medium-size figs, raw	100 gm.
½ medium apple	75 gm.
½ cup nonfat yogurt	122 gm.
½ tbsp. yeast	5 gm.

LUNCH

Borscht with Greens,* 1 bowl	
Cucumber Fruit Salad,* 1 serving	
Sandwich:	
3½ oz. mackerel	100 gm.
2 slices whole-wheat bread	50 gm.
1 leaf lettuce	

DINNER

Baked Soybeans with Kombu,* 1 serving
Asparagus and Red Pepper Salad,* 1 serving

NUTRITIONAL INFORMATION

Total calories	1,503
% calories from fat	20
Total protein	89 gm.
Total carbohydrates	212 gm.
Total fat	33 gm.

% OF RDAs

Tryptophan	584
Isoleucine	658
Lysine	895
Valine	636
Methionine, cysteine	485
Threonine	772
Leucine	760
Phenylalanine, tyrosine	826
Vitamin A	201
Vitamin D	400
Vitamin K	299
Vitamin C	334
Vitamin E	158
Riboflavin	156
Vitamin B_6	242
Vitamin B_{12}	553
Thiamine	226
Niacin	132
Folacin	237
Pantothenic acid	207
Biotin	110
Calcium	113
Magnesium	210
Copper	93
Zinc	95
Chromium	119
Phosphorus	168
Potassium	299
Iron	136
Manganese	360
Selenium	407

DAY EIGHTEEN

BREAKFAST	
1 grapefruit	217 gm.
2 glasses skim milk	488 gm.

LUNCH	
½ cup brown lentils	100 gm.
½ cup brown rice	100 gm.
2 tbsp. wheat bran	12 gm.
Yeast	5 gm.
Herbs per choice	
1 glass skim milk	244 gm.

DINNER	
Steamed vegetables:	
sweet potato	90 gm.
cauliflower	100 gm.
spinach	60 gm.
eggplant	200 gm.
green beans	100 gm.
carrots	80 gm.
onion	80 gm.
with ⅓ cup Peanut Sauce*	
1 glass skim milk	244 gm.

NUTRITIONAL INFORMATION	
Total calories	1,683
% calories from fat	12
Total protein	86 gm.
Total carbohydrates	283 gm.
Total fat	23 gm.

% OF RDAs	
Tryptophan	609
Isoleucine	631
Lysine	771
Valine	612
Methionine, cysteine	399
Threonine	723
Leucine	729
Phenylalanine, tyrosine	770
Vitamin A	499
Vitamin D	102
Vitamin K	627
Vitamin C	461
Vitamin E	115
Riboflavin	147
Vitamin B_6	147
Vitamin B_{12}	123
Thiamine	182
Niacin	116
Folacin	178
Pantothenic acid	264
Biotin	77
Calcium	132
Magnesium	145
Copper	103
Zinc	87
Chromium	180
Phosphorus	183
Potassium	275
Iron	101
Manganese	201
Selenium	232

DAY NINETEEN

BREAKFAST

1 small pear	75 gm.
2 glasses skim milk	488 gm.

LUNCH

Split Pea Soup,* 1 bowl	
1 glass skim milk	244 gm.

DINNER

Green Grain Salad,* 1 serving	
Mushroom & Spinach Veal Rolls,* 1 serving	
¼ lb. kale	115 gm.

NUTRITIONAL INFORMATION

Total calories	1,303
% calories from fat	10
Total protein	89 gm.
Total carbohydrates	203 gm.
Total fat	15 gm.

% OF RDAs

Tryptophan	620
Isoleucine	721
Lysine	854
Valine	648
Methionine, cysteine	482
Threonine	781
Leucine	766
Phenylalanine, tyrosine	754
Vitamin A	514
Vitamin D	128
Vitamin K	178
Vitamin C	417
Vitamin E	115
Riboflavin	151
Vitamin B_6	108
Vitamin B_{12}	151
Thiamine	111
Niacin	110
Folacin	87
Pantothenic acid	198
Biotin	44
Calcium	104
Magnesium	102
Copper	88
Zinc	86
Chromium	168
Phosphorus	153
Potassium	244
Iron	122
Manganese	91
Selenium	150

DAY TWENTY

BREAKFAST

¼ cup rolled oats	20 gm.
⅛ cup rye flakes	10 gm.
2 tbsp. wheat bran	10 gm.
1 banana	150 gm.
1 glass skim milk	244 gm.

LUNCH

Mackerel, canned	50 gm.
¼ cup brown rice	50 gm.
⅛ cup wild rice	20 gm.
⅓ cup red bell pepper, diced	50 gm.
Nori	10 gm.
2 glasses skim milk	

DINNER

Vegetable Stir Fry with Almonds and Oysters,* 1 serving
1 glass skim milk

NUTRITIONAL INFORMATION

Total calories	1,459
% calories from fat	14
Total protein	84 gm.
Total carbohydrates	229 gm.
Total fat	23 gm.

% OF RDAs

Tryptophan	608
Isoleucine	589
Lysine	742
Valine	600
Methionine, cysteine	461
Threonine	706
Leucine	717
Phenylalanine, tyrosine	691
Vitamin A	217
Vitamin D	421
Vitamin K	546
Vitamin C	745
Vitamin E	81
Riboflavin	189
Vitamin B_6	490
Vitamin B_{12}	840
Thiamine	139
Niacin	122
Folacin	98
Pantothenic acid	236
Biotin	66
Calcium	133
Magnesium	185
Copper	151
Zinc	210
Chromium	180
Phosphorus	182
Potassium	264
Iron	131
Manganese	190
Selenium	333

Average Nutritional Values for the 20-Day Food Combinations of the High/Low Diet

Total calories	1,358
% calories from fat	14
Total protein	85 gm.
Total carbohydrates	212 gm.
Total fat	22 gm.

Amino acids (% of RDAs)

Tryptophan	590
Isoleucine	899
Lysine	782
Valine	590
Methionine, cysteine	464
Threonine	714
Leucine	649
Phenylalanine, tyrosine	725

Vitamins (% of RDAs)

A	353
D	131
K	924
C	606
E	124
Riboflavin	149
B_6	181
B_{12}	417
Thiamine	185
Niacin	126
Folacin	183
Pantothenic acid	219
Biotin *	70

Minerals (% of RDAs)

Calcium	108
Magnesium	143
Copper	121
Zinc	115
Chromium	197
Phosphorus	107
Potassium	254
Iron	115
Manganese	181
Selenium	239

* No data available for many foods, so entered as zero in the data base, giving a falsely low value.

Recipes

(arranged alphabetically)

ASPARAGUS/RED BELL PEPPER SALAD

(4 Servings)

Grated peel from ½ large orange	
1 medium red bell pepper	**100 gm.**
1 lb. asparagus with 2–3 inches of stalks discarded	**400 gm.**
2 tbsp. red wine vinegar	
1 tsp. Dijon mustard	
½ tbsp. olive or safflower oil	
1 tbsp. water	

NUTRITIONAL INFORMATION (per serving)

Total calories	32
% calories from fat	50
Total protein	2 gm.
Total carbohydrates	4 gm.
Total fat	2 gm.

Place orange gratings in boiling water for 3–5 minutes, drain, and set aside. Broil pepper until skin is black all around. Rub off the blackened skin, cut pepper into strips, and set aside. Steam asparagus spears until tender. Allow to cool, then cut into 1-inch lengths. Mix vinegar, mustard, oil, and 1 tbsp. water in a bowl. Add orange gratings, pepper strips, and asparagus. Mix all ingredients thoroughly by hand.

% RDAs (per serving)

Tryptophan	9	Vitamin B_{12}	0
Isoleucine	8	Thiamine	7
Lysine	10	Niacin	5
Valine	8	Folacin	8
Methionine, cysteine	7	Pantothenic acid	9
Threonine	10	Biotin	1
Leucine	7	Calcium	2
Phenylalanine, tyrosine	9	Magnesium	3
		Copper	6
Vitamin A	31	Zinc	3
Vitamin D	0	Chromium	9
Vitamin K	42	Phosphorus	5
Vitamin C	112	Potassium	10
Vitamin E	12	Iron	3
Riboflavin	7	Manganese	5
Vitamin B_6	3	Selenium	0

BAKED SANDWICH
(8 Sandwiches)

½ cup brown lentils	**50 gm.**
¾ cup wheat bran	**40 gm.**
¼ cup oat bran	**15 gm.**
½ cup Soy Paste*	
1 cup skim milk	**224 gm.**
1 tbsp. yeast	**10 gm.**
2 whole eggs	**100 gm.**

2½ cups whole-wheat flour	
1¾ oz. ham	50 gm.
2 tbsp. sugar	
½ cup diced green bell pepper	100 gm.
½ cup chopped onion	100 gm.

NUTRITIONAL INFORMATION (per serving)

Total calories	253
% calories from fat	18
Total protein	14 gm.
Total carbohydrates	38 gm.
Total fat	5 gm.

Wash and simmer lentils for 30 minutes. In a large bowl combine the brans and soy paste, and add slightly warm milk. Add yeast and stir until dissolved. Beat in 1 egg. Gradually add flour and stir and knead until doughy. Cover and let rise until double in volume (about 30 minutes). Hard-boil remaining egg. Dice ham into small pieces. Combine lentils, chopped hard-boiled egg, ham, and other ingredients for filling. Set aside. On lightly floured surface roll dough into a large rectangle, about 12 × 16"; and cut into 8 smaller rectangles. Place mound of filling (about ½ cup or more) in center of each rectangle. Gather corners together and pinch to seal. Place sealed-side down in a lightly greased baking pan. Cover and let rise again, until about double in volume (30+ minutes). Bake at 400°F for about 25 minutes, or until golden brown. Can be served cold or hot, and can be frozen if desired.

% RDAs (per serving)

Tryptophan	100	Leucine	108
Isoleucine	98	Phenylalanine, tyrosine	125
Lysine	106	Vitamin A	4
Valine	90	Vitamin D	5
Methionine, cysteine	80		
Threonine	108		

Vitamin K	36	Calcium	8
Vitamin C	30	Magnesium	26
Vitamin E	14	Copper	12
Riboflavin	15	Zinc	16
Vitamin B_6	20	Chromium	32
Vitamin B_{12}	12	Phosphorus	30
Thiamine	43	Potassium	28
Niacin	21	Iron	19
Folacin	28	Manganese	34
Pantothenic acid	33	Selenium	60
Biotin	13		

BAKED SOYBEANS WITH KOMBU
(3 Servings)

1 cup soybeans (mature)	200 gm.
1 cube vegetable bouillon	
4 fronds kombu	20 gm.
¼ cup millet	25 gm.
¼ cup wild rice	25 gm.
2 cloves garlic	6 gm.
¼ cup chopped celery	30 gm.
¼ cup chopped parsley	15 gm.
1½ tbsp. yeast	15 gm.
1 tbsp. dry ground sage	
1 tsp. freshly ground allspice	
2 tsp. dry ground oregano	
1 cup nonfat yogurt	240 gm.

NUTRITIONAL INFORMATION (per serving)

Total calories	434
% calories from fat	30
Total protein	31 gm.
Total carbohydrates	46 gm.
Total fat	14 gm.

Soak soybeans overnight and discard the soak water. Cook for 1 hour in double boiler with 3 cups water to which is added the vegetable bouillon cube. Cut or break kombu into ½-inch lengths, soak 10–15 minutes in water, drain, and add to beans. Add millet and wild rice, and cook an additional 30–45 minutes. Drain off most of any remaining water. Add remaining ingredients, mix, and place all in an oiled casserole. Cover and bake at 350° for about 1½ hours, adding more water if necessary to keep from becoming too dry.

% RDAs (per serving)

Tryptophan	257	Vitamin B_{12}	116
Isoleucine	253	Thiamine	120
Lysine	311	Niacin	25
Valine	235	Folacin	81
Methionine, cysteine	163	Pantothenic acid	60
Threonine	290	Biotin	46
Leucine	286	Calcium	32
Phenylalanine, tyrosine	321	Magnesium	85
		Copper	23
Vitamin A	10	Zinc	28
Vitamin D	90	Chromium	30
Vitamin K	181	Phosphorus	54
Vitamin C	18	Potassium	120
Vitamin E	104	Iron	46
Riboflavin	39	Manganese	85
Vitamin B_6	72	Selenium	89

BAKED STUFFED EGGPLANT
(2 Servings)

1 medium eggplant	500 gm.
1 tsp. olive oil	
1 medium onion, diced	110 gm.

1 bunch scallions, including the white part and half of the green, diced	**110 gm.**
4 cloves garlic, diced	**12 gm.**
½ cup mushrooms, chopped	**35 gm.**
1 medium green bell pepper	**40 gm.**
2 medium tomatoes, diced	**220 gm.**
4 tbsp. tomato paste	
¾ cup chopped parsley	**45 gm.**
2 tbsp. vermouth	
1 tsp. freshly grated ginger	
3 tbsp. finely chopped fresh basil	
½-inch cube cheddar cheese, grated	**15 gm.**

NUTRITIONAL INFORMATION (per serving)

Total calories	212
% calories from fat	17
Total protein	10 gm.
Total carbohydrates	34 gm.
Total fat	4 gm.

Wash and dry eggplant. Cut it in half lengthwise and scoop out the interior, taking care not to break the shell. Cut pulp into small cubes. Add oil to nonstick frying pan and sauté eggplant, onion, scallions, garlic, mushrooms, and bell pepper over medium-high heat until lightly browned. Add tomatoes, tomato paste, parsley, and vermouth; stir to blend and bring to simmering point. Stir in the ginger and basil. Fill the eggplant shells with the mixture and sprinkle cheese on top. Place shells in baking dish or dishes filled with ½ in. of hot water. Baked in preheated oven at 375°F for 20–25 minutes.

% RDAs (per serving)

Tryptophan	58	Valine	50
Isoleucine	55	Methionine, cysteine	32
Lysine	65	Threonine	56

Leucine	51	Folacin	45
Phenylalanine, tyrosine	61	Pantothenic acid	39
		Biotin	11
Vitamin A	62	Calcium	15
Vitamin D	4	Magnesium	22
Vitamin K	998	Copper	26
Vitamin C	190	Zinc	10
Vitamin E	12	Chromium	69
Riboflavin	24	Phosphorus	19
Vitamin B_6	28	Potassium	66
Vitamin B_{12}	2	Iron	26
Thiamine	20	Manganese	33
Niacin	20	Selenium	9

BEAN/MILLET-STUFFED PEPPER
(2 Servings)

½ cup soybeans (mature)	**100 gm.**
¼ cup garbanzo beans	**50 gm.**
½ cup millet	**50 gm.**
2 large green bell peppers	**600 gm.**
½ cup low-fat yogurt	**122 gm.**
1 small onion, chopped	**60 gm.**
½ cup chopped mushrooms	**35 gm.**
2 tbsp. yeast	**14 gm.**
2 tbsp. wheat germ	**12 gm.**
1 tbsp. fresh oregano	
1 tbsp. fresh basil	
1 tbsp. ketchup	
1 tsp. soy sauce	
1 whole nutmeg, grated	

NUTRITIONAL INFORMATION (per serving)

Total calories	557
% calories from fat	21
Total protein	34 gm.
Total carbohydrates	76 gm.
Total fat	13 gm.

Soak beans overnight. Discard soak water. Cook beans in 1½ cup water in double boiler for 2 hours. Cook millet in 1 cup boiling water in double boiler or covered saucepan for 45 minutes. Cut tops from peppers, remove seeds and stems, and steam for 10 minutes. Mix beans, millet, and yogurt in a bowl. Stir in remaining ingredients. Place peppers in oiled saucepan of size and shape to support them standing up. Spoon filling into them. Replace tops on peppers. Bake at 350° for 20 minutes.

% RDAs (per serving)

Tryptophan	262	Vitamin B_{12}	12
Isoleucine	294	Thiamine	167
Lysine	333	Niacin	42
Valine	251	Folacin	125
Methionine, cysteine	195	Pantothenic acid	89
Threonine	327	Biotin	47
Leucine	317	Calcium	26
Phenylalanine, tyrosine	366	Magnesium	79
		Copper	59
Vitamin A	27	Zinc	38
Vitamin D	3	Chromium	111
Vitamin K	169	Phosphorus	67
Vitamin C	647	Potassium	118
Vitamin E	134	Iron	64
Riboflavin	62	Manganese	129
Vitamin B_6	92	Selenium	92

BEER SLAW
(2 Servings)

4 cups sliced cabbage	**360 gm.**
1 large red bell pepper, diced	**100 gm.**
½ cup diced onion	**80 gm.**
1 cup low-fat yogurt	**244 gm.**
2 tbsp. chopped dill or chives	
½ tsp. pepper	
¼ cup beer	

NUTRITIONAL INFORMATION (per serving)

Total calories	167
% calories rom fat	16
Total protein	10 gm.
Total carbohydrates	25 gm.
Total fat	3 gm.

Combine cabbage, red pepper, onion, yogurt, dill (or chives), and pepper in a bowl. Add beer and mix well.

% RDAs (per serving)

Tryptophan	37	Vitamin C	328
Isoleucine	68	Vitamin E	31
Lysine	103	Riboflavin	23
Valine	70	Vitamin B_6	20
Methionine, cysteine	46	Vitamin B_{12}	24
Threonine	74	Thiamine	13
Leucine	77	Niacin	6
Phenylalanine,		Folacin	36
tyrosine	94	Pantothenic acid	32
		Biotin	10
Vitamin A	51		
Vitamin D	0	Calcium	27
Vitamin K	321	Magnesium	13

Copper	9	Potassium	46
Zinc	10	Iron	9
Chromium	47	Manganese	9
Phosphorus	21	Selenium	9

BORSCHT WITH GREENS
(2 Servings)

3 medium beets, grated	**200 gm.**
1 vegetable bouillon cube	
2 tbsp. tamari	
1 cup chopped beet greens	**150 gm.**
2 tbsp. chopped fresh dill	
1 scallion, chopped	**30 gm.**
1½ cups nonfat yogurt	**366 gm.**

NUTRITIONAL INFORMATION (per serving)

Total calories	184
% calories from fat	16
Total protein	13 gm.
Total carbohydrates	28 gm.
Total fat	3 gm.

Combine grated beets, vegetable bouillon cube, and tamari in 3 cups of water in a soup pot. Bring to a boil, cover, and simmer for 10 minutes. Add beet greens, dill, and scallion, and simmer another 5 minutes. Remove from heat and let cool to room temperature. Chill in refrigerator. Stir in yogurt just before serving.

% RDAs (per serving)

Tryptophan	52	Methionine, cysteine	63
Isoleucine	93	Threonine	100
Lysine	146	Phenylalanine, tyrosine	133
Valine	103		

Vitamin A	95	Calcium	37
Vitamin D	0	Magnesium	35
Vitamin K	0	Copper	11
Vitamin C	59	Zinc	19
Vitamin E	12	Chromium	19
Riboflavin	35	Phosphorus	27
Vitamin B_6	12	Potassium	64
Vitamin B_{12}	37	Iron	19
Thiamine	13	Manganese	78
Niacin	5	Selenium	0
Folacin	49		
Pantothenic acid	36		
Biotin	11		

BREAKFAST DRINK
(2 Servings)

1 cup blueberries	**150 gm.**
1½ cups strawberries	**200 gm.**
1 cup buttermilk	**244 gm.**
1 cup skim milk	**244 gm.**
1 medium banana	**150 gm.**

NUTRITIONAL INFORMATION (per serving)

Total calories	250
% calories from fat	7
Total protein	10 gm.
Total carbohydrates	47 gm.
Total fat	2 gm.

Blend all ingredients.

% RDAs (per serving)

Tryptophan	68	Vitamin B_{12}	24
Isoleucine	75	Thiamine	13
Lysine	102	Niacin	6
Valine	79	Folacin	12
Methionine, cysteine	54	Pantothenic acid	33
Threonine	90	Biotin	11
Leucine	95	Calcium	26
Phenylalanine, tyrosine	93	Magnesium	16
		Copper	13
Vitamin A	9	Zinc	9
Vitamin D	14	Chromium	31
Vitamin K	21	Phosphorus	23
Vitamin C	126	Potassium	49
Vitamin E	4	Iron	5
Riboflavin	31	Manganese	26
Vitamin B_6	30	Selenium	13

BROCCOLI/PASTA CASSEROLE
(2 Servings)

1½ cup pasta (whole-wheat elbow macaroni or noodles)	**150 gm.**
½ lb. broccoli	**225 gm.**
1 8-oz. can peeled tomatoes	**200 gm.**
1 medium-sized onion, chopped	**160 gm.**
2 cloves garlic, pressed	
2 tsp. oregano	
¼ cup chopped cilantro	
2 tbsp. wheat bran	**12 gm.**
¼ cup part-skim ricotta cheese	**62 gm.**
1 cup nonfat yogurt	**224 gm.**

NUTRITIONAL INFORMATION (per serving)

Total calories	470
% calories from fat	13
Total protein	27 gm.
Total carbohydrates	86 gm.
Total fat	7 gm.

Boil pasta about 12 minutes; drain and set aside. Steam broccoli until tender (not too long) and set aside. Simmer tomatoes (including the juice in the can), onion, garlic, and oregano for 20 minutes. Add cilantro and bran to sauce, and mix. In a small casserole layer the sauce, pasta, and broccoli, then repeat. Finely slice or chop the cheese into the yogurt, and spread on top. Bake in 400-degree oven for 25–30 minutes.

% RDAs (per serving)

Tryptophan	161	Vitamin B_{12}	27
Isoleucine	166	Thiamine	50
Lysine	217	Niacin	34
Valine	173	Folacin	51
Methionine, cysteine	133	Pantothenic acid	87
Threonine	190	Biotin	18
Leucine	204	Calcium	40
Phenylalanine, tyrosine	237	Magnesium	46
		Copper	9
Vitamin A	79	Zinc	28
Vitamin D	1	Chromium	80
Vitamin K	1,246	Phosphorus	59
Vitamin C	259	Potassium	77
Vitamin E	15	Iron	30
Riboflavin	44	Manganese	24
Vitamin B_6	40	Selenium	98

CALIFORNIA CORN SALAD
(2 Servings)

2 medium red bell peppers	**100 gm.**
2 medium green bell peppers	**100 gm.**
2 small yellow squash, sliced	**130 gm.**
2 small zucchini, sliced	**130 gm.**
2 small Japanese eggplants, diced	**200 gm.**
8 leaves romaine lettuce	**180 gm.**
1 cup cottage cheese dressing	
4 chopped basil leaves	
1 cup corn	**200 gm.**

NUTRITIONAL INFORMATION (per serving)

Total calories	299
% calories from fat	9
Total protein	18 gm.
Total carbohydrates	50 gm.
Total fat	3 gm.

Remove seeds and cut peppers into strips; drop into boiling water for 1 minute, then remove. Chill with cold water, and set aside. Drop squash, zucchini, and eggplant into boiling water for 2 minutes; remove and set aside. Tear lettuce leaves into pieces and mix these plus the cottage cheese dressing with all the above ingredients by hand. When serving, add a few chopped walnuts.

% RDAs (per serving)

Tryptophan	97	Phenylalanine, tyrosine	180
Isoleucine	121	Vitamin A	101
Lysine	156	Vitamin D	1
Valine	125	Vitamin K	164
Methionine, cysteine	98	Vitamin C	392
Threonine	162		
Leucine	172		

Vitamin E	17	Calcium	20
Riboflavin	38	Magnesium	31
Vitamin B_6	31	Copper	21
Vitamin B_{12}	16	Zinc	13
Thiamine	30	Chromium	64
Niacin	24	Phosphorus	30
Folacin	68	Potassium	76
Pantothenic acid	50	Iron	21
Biotin	7	Manganese	31
		Selenium	10

CAPE COD CHOWDER
(6 Servings)

3 potatoes	**750 gm.**
½ cup millet	**50 gm.**
1 tsp. butter	**4 gm.**
1 large leek, sliced	**160 gm.**
1 stalk celery, sliced	**60 gm.**
1 green bell pepper, diced	**50 gm.**
wakami, cut into small pieces	**15 gm.**
2 carrots, sliced	**160 gm.**
1 bay leaf	
small handful fresh basil (or 1 tsp. dried basil)	
½ tsp. paprika	
pinch of freshly ground nutmeg	
3 tbsp wheat germ	**15 gm.**
1½ lb. cod, cut into bite-sized pieces	**600 gm.**
2 cups skim milk	**500 gm**

NUTRITIONAL INFORMATION (per serving)

Total calories	260
% calories from fat	5
Total protein	23 gm.
Total carbohydrates	37 gm.
Total fat	1 gm.

Add the potatoes and millet to 3 cups of boiling water and boil 15 minutes. In the meantime, melt butter in nonstick skillet and sauté leek, celery, and green pepper for 2 to 3 minutes. Add contents of skillet to water containing the potatoes and millet. Soak wakami in water, drain, and add. Add carrots, bay leaf, basil, paprika, and nutmeg. Simmer for 10 minutes. Add wheat germ and fish and simmer another 20 minutes. Remove bay leaf and gradually stir in the milk.

% RDAs (per serving)

Tryptophan	159	Vitamin B_{12}	66
Isoleucine	155	Thiamine	22
Lysine	293	Niacin	26
Valine	150	Folacin	16
Methionine, cysteine	164	Pantothenic acid	26
Threonine	246	Biotin	5
Leucine	211	Calcium	13
Phenylalanine, tyrosine	210	Magnesium	27
		Copper	20
Vitamin A	64	Zinc	102
Vitamin D	55	Chromium	79
Vitamin K	36	Phosphorus	33
Vitamin C	74	Potassium	67
Vitamin E	25	Iron	13
Riboflavin	16	Manganese	10
Vitamin B_6	37	Selenium	97

CAULIFLOWER SOUP
(6 Servings)

1 cube vegetable bouillon	
2 small to medium cauliflowers cut in pieces	500 gm.
2 medium onions, chopped	200 gm.
2 cloves garlic, chopped	10 gm.

wakami, cut into small pieces	**15 gm.**
3 tbsp. whole-wheat flour	**26 gm.**
2 tbsp. yeast	**12 gm.**
2 cups skim milk	**488 gm.**
chives, chopped, as optional garnish	

NUTRITIONAL INFORMATION (per serving)

Total calories	80
% calories from fat	0
Total protein	6
Total carbohydrates	14
Total fat	0.5

Dissolve bouillon cube in 2 cups hot water in a large pan; add the cauliflower, onions and garlic, and simmer until cauliflower is soft. Soak wakami in water and drain. Stir in the flour and yeast, add wakami and milk, heat, and simmer for 25 minutes. Blend, reheat, and serve. May add chopped chives to the serving.

% RDAs (per serving)

Tryptophan	48	Vitamin B_{12}	30
Isoleucine	42	Thiamine	14
Lysine	54	Niacin	5
Valine	41	Folacin	15
Methionine, cysteine	30	Pantothenic acid	29
Threonine	50	Biotin	17
Leucine	49	Calcium	12
Phenylalanine, tyrosine	46	Magnesium	9
		Copper	8
Vitamin A	5	Zinc	7
Vitamin D	41	Chromium	14
Vitamin K	357	Phosphorus	13
Vitamin C	118	Potassium	24
Vitamin E	12	Iron	10
Riboflavin	13	Manganese	7
Vitamin B_6	13	Selenium	14

CHICKEN WITH ARTICHOKES
(4 Servings)

8 baby artichokes	**400 gm.**
½ cup whole-wheat flour	**200 gm.**
¼ cup freshly squeezed lemon juice	
3 cloves garlic, chopped	**15 gm.**
¼ cup chopped onions or shallots	**100 gm.**
1 tsp. olive oil	
3 chicken breasts	**600 gm.**
pepper, to taste	
1 cube vegetable bouillon	
1 cup vermouth	
⅛ cup chopped fresh marjoram	
½ lb. mushrooms	

NUTRITIONAL INFORMATION (per serving)

Total calories	412
% calories from fat	9
Total protein	45 gm.
Total carbohydrates	49 gm.
Total fat	4 gm.

Break off outer leaves from artichokes and cut off the lower ¼ to ½ of each artichoke. In large saucepan make paste with most of the flour and some cold water. Add about 1 quart of water plus lemon juice and bring to boil. Add artichokes and simmer for 25 minutes. Remove and set aside, leaving about ½ cup of sauce in the pan and discarding the rest. In nonstick frying pan sauté garlic and onions or shallots briefly in 1 tsp. olive oil. Add artichokes, sauté an additional 4–5 minutes, remove, and set aside. Sprinkle chicken with pepper; add to same frying pan and cook, with frequent turning, for about 5 minutes. Dissolve vegetable bouillon in 1 cup hot water. Now add all ingredients to the original saucepan containing the ½ cup original sauce. Add the vermouth, marjoram, and mushrooms. Simmer for about 15 minutes.

% RDAs (per serving)

Tryptophan	284	Vitamin B_{12}	22
Isoleucine	298	Thiamine	20
Lysine	455	Niacin	111
Valine	243	Folacin	9
Methionine, cysteine	274	Pantothenic acid	52
Threonine	350	Biotin	20
Leucine	319	Calcium	7
Phenylalanine, tyrosine	328	Magnesium	29
		Copper	20
Vitamin A	4	Zinc	20
Vitamin D	0	Chromium	49
Vitamin K	2	Phosphorus	43
Vitamin C	35	Potassium	48
Vitamin E	8	Iron	23
Riboflavin	26	Manganese	17
Vitamin B_6	56	Selenium	100

COLD GREEN SOUP
(2 Servings)

½ lb. spinach	**200 gm.**
2 cups chopped summer squash	**200 gm.**
1 medium cucumber, chopped	**180 gm.**
2 cups romaine lettuce	**150 gm.**
2 cups buttermilk	**488 gm.**
⅜ cup chopped parsley	**30 gm.**
½ small onion, chopped	**40 gm.**

NUTRITIONAL INFORMATION (per serving)

Total calories	299
% calories from fat	9
Total protein	15 gm.
Total carbohydrates	28 gm.
Total fat	3 gm.

Place spinach in 1 cup boiling water for 5 minutes, and squash in 1 cup boiling water for 10 minutes. Combine spinach, squash, plus cooking water, and cucumber, and puree in blender. Puree lettuce in 1 cup buttermilk. Combine all ingredients; add 1 cup buttermilk plus chopped parsley and onion. Chill.

% RDAs (per serving)

Tryptophan	98	Vitamin B_{12}	18
Isoleucine	102	Thiamine	22
Lysine	153	Niacin	14
Valine	109	Folacin	102
Methionine, cysteine	75	Pantothenic acid	45
Threonine	131	Biotin	12
Leucine	125	Calcium	24
Phenylalanine, tyrosine	120	Magnesium	40
		Copper	18
Vitamin A	230	Zinc	15
Vitamin D	0	Chromium	44
Vitamin K	243	Phosphorus	30
Vitamin C	211	Potassium	81
Vitamin E	23	Iron	35
Riboflavin	47	Manganese	47
Vitamin B_6	24	Selenium	37

COUNTRY COLE SLAW
(Yield: 4 Cups: 2 Servings)

3 cups finely sliced cabbage	**270 gm.**
½ cup finely sliced carrots	**80 gm.**
¼ cup finely sliced scallions	**40 gm.**
1 tbsp. pumpkin seeds (pepitas)	**10 gm.**
½ cup tofu	**100 gm.**
¼ cup yogurt	**60 gm.**
1 tbsp. sugar	
2 tbsp. lemon juice	
2 tbsp. Dijon mustard	

NUTRITIONAL INFORMATION (per serving)

Total calories	149
% calories from fat	30
Total protein	10 gm.
Total carbohydrates	16 gm.
Total fat	5 gm.

Mix cabbage, carrots, scallions, and pumpkin seeds in a large bowl. In a separate bowl, briefly blend tofu, yogurt, sugar, lemon juice, and mustard. Combine all ingredients and mix thoroughly.

% RDAs (per serving)

Tryptophan	67	Vitamin A	92
Isoleucine	60	Vitamin D	0
Lysine	76	Vitamin K	286
Valine	54	Vitamin C	121
Methionine, cysteine	43	Vitamin E	24
Threonine	60	Riboflavin	9
Leucine	69	Vitamin B_6	18
Phenylalanine,		Vitamin B_{12}	6
tyrosine	78	Thiamine	10

Niacin	5	Zinc	3
Folacin	25	Chromium	30
Pantothenic acid	14	Phosphorus	18
Biotin	5	Potassium	30
Calcium	17	Iron	14
Magnesium	21	Manganese	4
Copper	4	Selenium	8

CUCUMBER/FRUIT SALAD

(4 Servings)

¾ cup yogurt	183 gm.
¼ cup finely chopped fresh mint	
1 finely chopped jalapeño pepper	
½ tsp. cumin	
2 cups diced pineapple	280 gm.
2 cups sliced papaya	300 gm.
2 cups seedless grapes	300 gm.
1 medium cucumber, sliced	360 gm.
1 leaf seaweed (nori), cut into small (less than ½-inch) squares	10 gm.
¼ cup finely diced onion or scallion	40 gm.
romaine lettuce leaves	100 gm.

NUTRITIONAL INFORMATION (per serving)

Total calories	182
% calories from fat	8
Total protein	5 gm.
Total carbohydrates	37 gm.
Total fat	1.5 gm.

Mix yogurt, mint, jalapeño pepper, and cumin in a large bowl. Fold the pineapple, papaya, grapes, cucumber, nori, and onion (or scallion) into this. Serve on lettuce leaves.

% RDAs (per serving)

Tryptophan	23	Vitamin B_{12}	75
Isoleucine	29	Thiamine	15
Lysine	47	Niacin	6
Valine	36	Folacin	19
Methionine, cysteine	20	Pantothenic acid	21
Threonine	38	Biotin	4
Leucine	37	Calcium	13
Phenylalanine, tyrosine	38	Magnesium	23
		Copper	8
Vitamin A	50	Zinc	5
Vitamin D	33	Chromium	12
Vitamin K	43	Phosphorus	10
Vitamin C	126	Potassium	44
Vitamin E	3	Iron	21
Riboflavin	17	Manganese	79
Vitamin B_6	99	Selenium	1

DR. WALFORD'S ETERNAL YOUTH CHILI

(10 Servings)

6 large red chilis	**400 gm.**
1 cup pinto beans	**200 gm.**
1 tbsp. dry or ¼ cup fresh chopped oregano	
5 cups chicken broth	
5 cups beer	
8 medium tomatoes	**800 gm.**
1 cup sliced celery	**120 gm.**
6 large green bell peppers, coarsely chopped	**400 gm.**
3 medium onions	**600 gm.**
10 cloves garlic	**30 gm.**
½ cup chopped parsley	**30 gm.**
½ lb. hamburger	**200 gm.**

1 lb. beef, round	**400 gm.**
1 lb. pork, lean	**400 gm.**
⅓ cup chili powder	
¼ cup ground cumin	
1 tbsp. mole powder	
2 tbsp. coriander seeds	
one 8-oz. can tomato sauce	
one 6-oz. can tomato paste	
one 6- to 8-oz. portion prepared chili salsa	
1 tbsp. masa harina flour	
1 square unsweetened chocolate	

NUTRITIONAL INFORMATION (per serving)

Total calories	304
% calories from fat	24
Total protein	29 gm.
Total carbohydrates	29 gm.
Total fat	8 gm.

Prepare in five steps:

1) Remove stems and seeds from red chilis. Boil chilis for 30 minutes. Remove and discard skins. Blend pulp in blender.

2) Soak pinto beans overnight and discard water. Place oregano in boiling chicken broth plus beer for 5 minutes. Drain off oregano, saving the liquid. Simmer for 1 hour. Blend tomatoes and add to the pot. Add the cut celery.

3) Sauté the chopped green peppers in minimal amount of olive oil in nonstick pan until tender. Add onions and continue sautéing, with frequent stirring. Add garlic and parsley. Mix and remove from fire.

4) Brown all meat in a nonstick pan with minimal amount of olive oil.

5) Combine 1 + 2 + 3 + 4 in a large pot. Dissolve chili powder, ground cumin, mole powder, and coriander seeds in small quantity of beer to get lumps out; add to pot. Add and stir in tomato sauce, tomato paste, and chili salsa.

Dissolve masa harina flour in enough warm water to form a paste and add to pot. Add unsweetened chocolate (the chocolate is the "secret ingredient" of the chili). Simmer for 45 minutes and serve.

On the side, for garnishes, prepare: 1) chili salsa with cold chopped onions, 2) a plate of chopped cilantro, 3) a plate of finely chopped jalapeño peppers, 4) wedges of lime.

% RDAs (per serving)

Tryptophan	180	Vitamin B_{12}	46
Isoleucine	197	Thiamine	52
Lysine	312	Niacin	37
Valine	176	Folacin	27
Methionine, cysteine	152	Pantothenic acid	33
Threonine	254	Biotin	9
Leucine	222	Calcium	7
Phenylalanine, tyrosine	223	Magnesium	15
		Copper	9
Vitamin A	59	Zinc	24
Vitamin D	0	Chromium	98
Vitamin K	728	Phosphorus	30
Vitamin C	279	Potassium	56
Vitamin E	10	Iron	33
Riboflavin	24	Manganese	10
Vitamin B_6	40	Selenium	95

GREEN GRAIN SALAD WITH MUSTARD DRESSING
(2 Servings)

¼ cup brown rice	50 gm.
¼ cup bulgur wheat	50 gm.
½ cup brown lentils	50 gm.
2 tbsp. wheat or oat bran	12 gm.

½ cup sliced mushrooms	35 gm.
½ cup cubed green bell peppers	50 gm.
¼ cup chopped parsley	16 gm.
¼ cup chopped onion or scallions	40 gm.
¾ cup sliced celery	95 gm.
8 water chestnuts, sliced	50 gm.
1 tbsp. sunflower seeds	10 gm.

NUTRITIONAL INFORMATION (per serving, including dressing)

Total calories	380
% calories from fat	9
Total protein	16 gm.
Total carbohydrates	70 gm.
Total fat	4 gm.

Cook brown rice in ½ cup water. Let it cool. Soak the bulgur until soft, then drain. Wash the lentils. Cook them in 1½ cups water until done; drain and cool. Mix the grains, chopped vegetables, and lentils. Reserve some of the water chestnuts and mushrooms for garnish, if desired. Mix in the mustard dressing. Makes 2 portions.

Mustard Dressing:

1 egg white 15 gm.
1½ tbsp. Dijon mustard
½ cup wine or balsamic vinegar
¼ tsp. dried oregano
¼ tsp. cumin
dash of cayenne pepper

Blend the ingredients either by hand or in a blender.

% RDAs (per serving)

Tryptophan	94	Valine	98
Isoleucine	109	Methionine, cysteine	73
Lysine	101	Threonine	112

Leucine	114	Folacin	20
Phenylalanine, tyrosine	114	Pantothenic acid	43
		Biotin	8
Vitamin A	18	Calcium	7
Vitamin D	3	Magnesium	24
Vitamin K	11	Copper	33
Vitamin C	87	Zinc	17
Vitamin E	33	Chromium	43
Riboflavin	30	Phosphorus	34
Vitamin B_6	29	Potassium	49
Vitamin B_{12}	0	Iron	28
Thiamine	39	Manganese	45
Niacin	30	Selenium	37

HUMMUS

1 cup dry garbanzo beans
1 carrot
3 scallions
2 tbsp. parsley
⅓ cup (or more) of water
¼ cup lemon juice
2 tbsp. tamari
1 tbsp. Vegit seasoning
½ clove garlic, mashed (optional)
dash of cayenne pepper (optional)

NUTRITIONAL INFORMATION ***(per ¼ cup serving)***

Total calories	855
% calories from fat	12
Total protein	45 gm.
Total carbohydrates	144 gm.
Total fat	11 gm.
Total fiber	12 gm.

Soak the garbanzo beans overnight. Discard soak water. Put the beans in 2½ cups of fresh water in a saucepan. Bring to a boil. Reduce heat and simmer, partially covered, for 1 hour or until the beans are tender.

Shred the carrot and put it aside. (It is a good idea to use a food processor, if you have one, from here on.) Finely chop the scallions and parsley. Add the cooked and cooled garbanzos and grind them, with some water to help mash the beans. Also add the lemon juice, tamari, and Vegit, and mix. (Add more water if necessary to achieve the texture you desire.) By hand, mix in the shredded carrot. For added flavor, add garlic and cayenne.

Use this as a spread for sandwiches or as a dip for steamed vegetables.

% RDAs (per serving)

Tryptophan	194	Vitamin B_{12}	0
Isoleucine	338	Thiamine	52
Lysine	405	Niacin	26
Valine	244	Folacin	113
Methionine, cysteine	193	Pantothenic acid	77
Threonine	274	Biotin	23
Leucine	318	Calcium	31
Phenylalanine, tyrosine	363	Magnesium	85
		Copper	79
Vitamin A	184	Zinc	37
Vitamin D	0	Chromium	59
Vitamin K	91	Phosphorus	60
Vitamin C	117	Potassium	113
Vitamin E	12	Iron	86
Riboflavin	22	Manganese	101
Vitamin B_6	63	Selenium	29

INDIAN BROWN RICE
(1 Serving)

½ cup brown rice (brown basmati rice, if available) 100 gm.
1¼ cup warm water
2 tsp. unsalted butter
1 stick cinnamon
1 heaping tsp. cumin
1 heaping tsp. coriander
4 green cardamom, seeds only, or ½ tsp. ground cardamom

NUTRITIONAL INFORMATION (per serving)

Total calories	199
% calories from fat	14
Total protein	4 gm.
Total carbohydrates	39 gm.
Total fat	3 gm.

Rinse the rice and drain. If basmati rice is used, soak it for 30 minutes and then rinse and drain.

Melt the butter in a saucepan large enough for the rice and the water. Add the spices and the drained rice and mix thoroughly. Add the warm water, bring to a boil, lower the heat, cover, and simmer for 30 minutes or until done.

% RDAs (per serving)

Tryptophan	23	Phenylalanine, tyrosine	35
Isoleucine	21	Vitamin A	1
Lysine	21	Vitamin D	0
Valine	24	Vitamin K	0
Methionine, cysteine	20	Vitamin C	0
Threonine	31		
Leucine	34		

Vitamin E	8	Calcium	1
Riboflavin	1	Magnesium	11
Vitamin B_6	13	Copper	9
Vitamin B_{12}	0	Zinc	6
Thiamine	12	Chromium	8
Niacin	13	Phosphorus	9
Folacin	2	Iron	5
Pantothenic acid	13	Manganese	34
Biotin	6	Selenium	45

LIMA BEAN/CHESTNUT SALAD
(2 Servings)

½ cup dried lima beans	**100 gm.**
1 medium apple, diced	**150 gm.**
¼ lb. fresh chestnuts	**112 gm.**
1 tbsp. sunflower seeds	**20 gm.**
salad dressing (your choice)	
nori	**10 gm.**

NUTRITIONAL INFORMATION (per serving)

Total calories	411
% calories from fat	15
Total protein	16 gm.
Total carbohydrates	71 gm.
Total fat	7 gm.

Soak lima beans 2–4 hours. Drain. Add fresh water and bring to boil. Simmer for 1 hour, drain, and cool. Cut an X in the round side of each chestnut, add to boiling water, and simmer for 10 minutes. Cool and remove shells and outer skins from chestnuts. Cut into smaller pieces. Cut up nori. Mix all ingredients and chill.

% RDAs (per serving)

Tryptophan	92	Vitamin B_{12}	0
Isoleucine	115	Thiamine	41
Lysine	128	Niacin	10
Valine	115	Folacin	20
Methionine, cysteine	71	Pantothenic acid	24
Threonine	143	Biotin	6
Leucine	126	Calcium	6
Phenylalanine, tyrosine	115	Magnesium	54
		Copper	33
Vitamin A	7	Zinc	17
Vitamin D	67	Chromium	14
Vitamin K	0	Phosphorus	27
Vitamin C	33	Potassium	72
Vitamin E	58	Iron	50
Riboflavin	17	Manganese	103
Vitamin B_6	33	Selenium	15

MUSHROOM-AND-SPINACH VEAL ROLLS

(4 Servings)

½ lb. spinach, leaves only	**200 gm.**
½ cup chopped onion	**100 gm.**
½ pound mushrooms, chopped	**200 gm.**
1 tsp. olive oil	
3 cloves garlic, chopped	**15 gm.**
1 tsp. chopped fresh oregano	
pepper	
1 lb. thin veal strips	**400 gm.**
3 tbsp. white wine	

NUTRITIONAL INFORMATION (per serving)

Total calories	192
% calories from fat	38
Total protein	23 gm.
Total carbohydrates	7 gm.
Total fat	8 gm.

Steam spinach until just tender; pat dry on paper towel, chop, and set aside. Heat onions and mushrooms with 1 tsp. olive oil in nonstick frying pan about 5 minutes. Add garlic, oregano, and the chopped spinach, plus a small amount of pepper. Cook while stirring for 1–2 minutes. Flatten the already thin veal strips with thumbs until quite thin and spoon mushroom/spinach mixture into center. Roll and secure with toothpicks. Place in a small baking pan or aluminum foil with raised edges. Pour wine onto each roll. Bake uncovered at 350°F, with occasional basting, about 30 minutes.

% RDAs (per serving)

Tryptophan	153	Vitamin B_{12}	54
Isoleucine	192	Thiamine	18
Lysine	235	Niacin	47
Valine	153	Folacin	29
Methionine, cysteine	141	Pantothenic acid	54
Threonine	203	Biotin	14
Leucine	174	Calcium	6
Phenylalanine, tyrosine	171	Magnesium	18
		Copper	12
Vitamin A	81	Zinc	25
Vitamin D	48	Chromium	43
Vitamin K	75	Phosphorus	25
Vitamin C	49	Potassium	43
Vitamin E	10	Iron	31
Riboflavin	35	Manganese	14
Vitamin B_6	29	Selenium	33

175-DEGREE STEAK
(2 Servings)

1 pound beef loin/sirloin steak, ¾ to 1 inch thick, all fat trimmed off

NUTRITIONAL INFORMATION (per serving)

Total calories	334
% calories from fat	38
Total protein	52 gm.
Total carbohydrates	0
Total fat	14 gm.

Put water in both the top and bottom pots of a double boiler. Using a thermometer, bring water in the upper part of the double boiler to the 160°-to-180°F range. Wrap steak tightly in an oven cooking bag (Reynolds or other brand), expressing as much as possible all air bubbles so that the bag fits tightly around the steak. If you like, you may apply thin slices of onion or garlic to the surface of the steak before wrapping, but for best results they must be thin slices, not chunks, to ensure as tight and air-free a wrapping as possible. Close the bag securely with a tie to keep out the water. Place the steak in the water of the top pot and maintain the water at the above temperature. Ten to 12 minutes' cooking will yield a medium-rare steak, but you should experiment a little with the timing. As any residual air bubbles will rise to the top side of the cooking meat, turn the steak over midway through to ensure even cooking.

The above cooking procedure will not only give you the best-tasting steak you have ever eaten (Try it!), retaining *all* the flavor, but also the most healthful. The high temperatures of frying and broiling destroy some nutrients and, by searing the surfaces of the meat, cause the formation of carcinogens.

% RDAs (per serving)

Tryptophan	312	Vitamin B_{12}	77
Isoleucine	367	Thiamine	15
Lysine	613	Niacin	66
Valine	334	Folacin	4
Methionine, cysteine	307	Pantothenic acid	28
Threonine	398	Biotin	0
Leucine	431	Calcium	2
Phenylalanine, tyrosine	310	Magnesium	13
		Copper	5
Vitamin A	0	Zinc	64
Vitamin D	0	Chromium	31
Vitamin K	0	Phosphorus	38
Vitamin C	0	Potassium	44
Vitamin E	3	Iron	41
Riboflavin	26	Manganese	2
Vitamin B_6	26	Selenium	0

OYSTERS WITH MILLET
(2 Servings)

½ cup millet	**50 gm.**
½ lb. oysters	**200 gm.**
1 small onion	**40 gm.**
1 tbsp. ground sage	
½ tsp. cumin	
2 tbsp. Worcestershire sauce	
1 tbsp. chutney	

NUTRITIONAL INFORMATION (per serving)

Total calories	163
% calories from fat	14
Total protein	11 gm.

Total carbohydrates	23 gm.
Total fat	3 gm.

Place millet in 1 cup water in a covered double boiler and heat for 25 minutes. Add oysters, onion, sage, cumin, and Worcestershire sauce and cook another 5–10 minutes (5 if canned oysters, 10 if fresh), stirring several times. Garnish with chutney.

% RDAs (per serving)

Tryptophan	93	Vitamin B_{12}	600
Isoleucine	75	Thiamine	23
Lysine	106	Niacin	17
Valine	81	Folacin	4
Methionine, cysteine	81	Pantothenic acid	7
Threonine	102	Biotin	10
Leucine	108	Calcium	8
Phenylalanine, tyrosine	109	Magnesium	19
		Copper	165
Vitamin A	6	Zinc	270
Vitamin D	80	Chromium	34
Vitamin K	0	Phosphorus	19
Vitamin C	53	Potassium	14
Vitamin E	9	Iron	41
Riboflavin	17	Manganese	28
Vitamin B_6	13	Selenium	130

PASTA PRIMAVERA
(2 Servings)

¼ lb. whole-wheat noodles (fettuccine)	**130 gm.**
½ onion, chopped	**90 gm.**
1 clove elephant garlic, or 4–6 cloves regular garlic, finely chopped	**25 gm.**
1 tsp. olive oil	

4 to 5 French morel mushrooms, fresh, or 20 gm. dried (if dried, rehydrated for ½ to 1 hour), chopped	
½ medium red bell pepper	**50 gm.**
1 medium tomato	**120 gm.**
½ cup chopped parsley	**80 gm.**
4 tbsp. finely chopped fresh dill	**20 gm.**
⅓ to ½ cup Enrico's spaghetti sauce	
3 tbsp. Salsa*	
½-inch cube parmesan cheese, grated	**25 gm.**

NUTRITIONAL INFORMATION (per serving)

Total calories	358
% calories from fat	15
Total protein	16 gm.
Total carbohydrates	60 gm.
Total fat	6 gm.

Place noodles in briskly boiling water for 10 minutes. While they are cooking, fry onion and garlic in oil in nonstick skillet until onion is translucent. Add fresh or rehydrated mushrooms and cook for 1 minute; then add chopped pepper, tomato, parsley, and dill. Stir completely. Add spaghetti sauce and Salsa and simmer 3–5 minutes until parsley is thoroughly cooked. Place noodles on plate, cover with sauce, and sprinkle with Parmesan cheese.

% RDAs (per serving)

Tryptophan	117	Vitamin A	104
Isoleucine	103	Vitamin D	2
Lysine	126	Vitamin K	550
Valine	99	Vitamin C	234
Methionine, cysteine	87	Vitamin E	13
Threonine	95	Riboflavin	22
Leucine	118	Vitamin B_6	21
Phenylalanine,		Vitamin B_{12}	8
tyrosine	141	Thiamine	35

Niacin	25	Zinc	18
Folacin	30	Chromium	58
Pantothenic acid	40	Phosphorus	34
Biotin	12	Potassium	46
Calcium	22	Iron	31
Magnesium	28	Manganese	18
Copper	16	Selenium	91

PEANUT SAUCE

½ cup chopped red bell pepper	**50 gm.**
⅓ cup chopped onion	**40 gm.**
2 tbsp. olive oil	**28 gm.**
2 cloves crushed garlic	**6 gm.**
1 tbsp. chili powder	
⅓ tsp. turmeric	
½ cup finely ground roasted peanuts (grind in coffee grinder or food processor)	**72 gm.**
1 tbsp. lime juice	
⅓ cup dry white wine	
1 tbsp. tomato puree	
2 cups consommé	
1 tbsp. peanut butter	
½ tsp. cornstarch, blended with 1 tsp. cold water	

NUTRITIONAL INFORMATION (⅓ cup)

Total calories	188
% calories from fat	77
Total protein	5 gm.
Total carbohydrates	6 gm.
Total fat	16 gm.

Sauté the bell pepper and onion in olive oil until golden. Add garlic, chili powder, turmeric, and ground peanuts, and sauté an additional 2 minutes. Add lime juice and wine, and boil until mixture is almost dry. Add tomato puree and consommé, and simmer 15 minutes. Stir in peanut butter. Add cornstarch mixture; cook and stir until sauce is lightly thickened. Makes about 1⅓ cups of sauce. Serve hot, over vegetables.

% RDAs (per ⅓ cup)

Tryptophan	35	Vitamin B_{12}	0
Isoleucine	33	Thiamine	5
Lysine	29	Niacin	17
Valine	33	Folacin	5
Methionine, cysteine	20	Pantothenic acid	10
Threonine	31	Biotin	6
Leucine	36	Calcium	1
Phenylalanine, tyrosine	53	Magnesium	8
		Copper	4
Vitamin A	11	Zinc	3
Vitamin D	0	Chromium	4
Vitamin K	0	Phosphorus	6
Vitamin C	44	Potassium	8
Vitamin E	20	Iron	3
Riboflavin	2	Manganese	11
Vitamin B_6	3	Selenium	0

RUTH'S ITALIAN ZUCCHINI
(1 Serving)

1⅓ cups chopped onion	**120 gm.**
1 large clove garlic, chopped	
2 medium tomatoes, cubed	**130 gm.**
2 tbsp. chopped Italian parsley	
1½ tsp. dried oregano leaves	
Dash of pepper	
2 cups ¼-inch slices of zucchini	**130 gm.**

NUTRITIONAL INFORMATION (per serving)

Total calories	117
% calories from fat	4
Total protein	5 gm.
Total carbohydrates	23
Total fat	.5 gm.

Sauté the onion and garlic in a little water (enough to cover the bottom of the pan) in a nonstick pan until the onion is translucent. Add the tomatoes and herbs, mix, and cover for 2 minutes. (Add more water, if necessary.) Add the zucchini slices, mix, cover, and cook for 1 minute more. This is also good served as a cold salad.

% RDAs (per serving)

Tryptophan	26	Vitamin B_{12}	0
Isoleucine	15	Thiamine	12
Lysine	25	Niacin	13
Valine	15	Folacin	30
Methionine, cysteine	11	Pantothenic acid	26
Threonine	24	Biotin	9
Leucine	17	Calcium	7
Phenylalanine, tyrosine	20	Magnesium	13
		Copper	17
Vitamin A	48	Zinc	3
Vitamin D	0	Chromium	53
Vitamin K	1,170	Phosphorus	9
Vitamin C	140	Potassium	40
Vitamin E	7	Iron	12
Riboflavin	12	Manganese	13
Vitamin B_6	19	Selenium	4

SAFFRON SLS SOUP
(4 Servings)

2 large leeks (thoroughly rinsed to remove grit), sliced thin, including white and some green	**200 gm.**
1 medium onion, sliced thin	**160 gm.**
2 cloves garlic, minced	
1 tsp. grated fresh ginger	
4 cups broth (your choice)	
1 medium sweet potato, peeled and sliced	**180 gm.**
1 Hubbard or butternut squash, peeled and cut into 1-inch chunks	**300 gm.**
pepper (pinch)	
cinnamon (pinch)	
1 tsp. saffron threads (Get top-quality saffron in a gourmet store; expensive but worth it.)	
wakami, cut into small pieces	**20 gm.**
1 cup nonfat yogurt	

NUTRITIONAL INFORMATION (per serving)

Total calories	173
% calories from fat	8
Total protein	6 gm.
Total carbohydrates	34 gm.
Total fat	1.5 gm.

In a large nonstick pot stir-fry leeks, onion, garlic, and fresh ginger in a little broth until leeks are soft and onion is translucent. Add rest of broth plus sweet potato, squash, and a little pepper and cinnamon to taste (pinch of each). Heat saffron in a 400° oven for 2 minutes, powder it in a bowl, and dissolve it in a little broth. Add to pot. Soak wakami in water, drain, and add to pot. Cook 20 to 25 minutes until all is tender. Transfer to a blender (or food processor) and blend. Add yogurt and blend again. Return all ingredients to pot and reheat, if desired.

% RDAs (per serving)

Tryptophan	22	Vitamin B_{12}	46
Isoleucine	31	Thiamine	12
Lysine	49	Niacin	6
Valine	37	Folacin	20
Methionine, cysteine	21	Pantothenic acid	28
Threonine	35	Biotin	6
Leucine	38	Calcium	15
Phenylalanine, tyrosine	46	Magnesium	23
		Copper	10
Vitamin A	136	Zinc	6
Vitamin D	17	Chromium	39
Vitamin K	0	Phosphorus	14
Vitamin C	53	Potassium	40
Vitamin E	26	Iron	11
Riboflavin	15	Manganese	19
Vitamin B_6	19	Selenium	1

SCRAMBLED TOFU
(1 Serving)

3½ oz. tofu	100 gm.
3 medium mushrooms, chopped	25 gm.
½ small onion, chopped	80 gm.
½ medium red bell pepper, seeded and chopped	50 gm.
½ tsp. minced fresh thyme	
½ tsp. turmeric	
2 tbsp. Worcestershire sauce	

NUTRITIONAL INFORMATION

Total calories	145
% calories from fat	31
Total protein	11 gm.
Total carbohydates	14 gm.
Total fat	5 gm.

Drain and wash tofu. Poach mushrooms, onion, and pepper in small amount of water in nonstick frying pan until onions are translucent. Drain water from contents of pan and add tofu, along with remainder of ingredients. Cook while stirring until desired firmness is obtained (about 5 to 10 minutes). Garnish with small amount of salsa, and serve.

% RDAs

Tryptophan	86	Vitamin B_{12}	0
Isoleucine	76	Thiamine	10
Lysine	74	Niacin	8
Valine	60	Folacin	6
Methionine, cysteine	50	Pantothenic acid	19
Threonine	63	Biotin	6
Leucine	78	Calcium	13
Phenylalanine, tyrosine	94	Magnesium	30
		Copper	8
Vitamin A	46	Zinc	3
Vitamin D	4	Chromium	34
Vitamin K	6	Phosphorus	16
Vitamin C	184	Potassium	19
Vitamin E	1	Iron	17
Riboflavin	12	Manganese	5
Vitamin B_6	6	Selenium	8

SOY PASTE

(Yield: approx. 2 cups)

1 cup dry mature soybeans	**200 gm.**
Yogurt	**122 gm.**
Tomato	**25 gm.**
Lemon (peeled)	**25 gm.**

NUTRITIONAL INFORMATION (2 cups)

Total calories	962
% calories from fat	36
Total protein	75 gm.
Total carbohydrates	80 gm.
Total fat	38 gm.

Soak beans at least 2 hours in enough room-temperature water to keep them covered. Discard soak water. Add 4 cups fresh water, bring to a boil, cover, and simmer for 1½ to 2 hours. Drain. Make beans into a paste by using a food processor (the easiest) or a blender, or mash by hand with a fork. Add other ingredients and mix thoroughly. Store in a covered container in the refrigerator. Will keep for almost a week.

% RDAs (2 cups)

Tryptophan	604	Vitamin A	9
Isoleucine	609	Vitamin D	0
Lysine	734	Vitamin K	767
Valine	535	Vitamin C	33
Methionine, cysteine	386	Vitamin E	310
Threonine	671	Riboflavin	50
Leucine	668	Vitamin B_6	85
Phenylalanine,		Vitamin B_{12}	24
tyrosine	771	Thiamine	162

Niacin	26	Zinc	55
Folacin	91	Chromium	45
Pantothenic acid	106	Phosphorus	106
Biotin	125	Potassium	201
		Iron	90
Calcium	57	Manganese	224
Magnesium	140	Selenium	246
Copper	12		

SPLIT-PEA SOUP
(2 Servings)

1 cup split peas	**200 gm.**
1 tsp. thyme	
1 clove garlic	
2 cups vegetable or chicken bouillon	
2 medium carrots, sliced thin	**160 gm.**
½ cup chopped celery	**60 gm.**
¼ cup chopped onion	**40 gm.**
1 leek, chopped	**25 gm.**
½ tsp. freshly grated allspice	

NUTRITIONAL INFORMATION (per serving)

Total calories	409
% calories from fat	2
Total protein	26 gm.
Total carbohydrates	74 gm.
Total fat	1 gm.

Cook peas, thyme, garlic, and bouillon in double boiler for 30 minutes. Add remaining ingredients and cook an additional hour. Puree in blender.

% RDAs (per serving)

Tryptophan	130	Vitamin B_{12}	0
Isoleucine	188	Thiamine	32
Lysine	218	Niacin	15
Valine	165	Folacin	10
Methionine, cysteine	107	Pantothenic acid	10
Threonine	188	Biotin	3
Leucine	189	Calcium	4
Phenylalanine, tyrosine	195	Magnesium	28
Vitamin A	179	Copper	31
Vitamin D	0	Zinc	22
Vitamin K	91	Chromium	55
Vitamin C	22	Phosphorus	26
Vitamin E	6	Potassium	59
Riboflavin	17	Iron	47
Vitamin B_6	9	Manganese	2
		Selenium	4

STUFFED BELL PEPPERS IN BEER SAUCE
(2 Servings)

4 large green bell peppers	**240 gm.**
wakami, cut into small pieces	**10 gm.**
½ cup millet	**50 gm.**
1 cup Soy Paste*	**200 gm.**
½ cup finely chopped onions	**80 gm.**
1 medium carrot, grated	**50 gm.**
¼ cup chopped parsley	**20 gm.**
¼ cup chopped chives	**20 gm.**
⅓ cup natural ketchup	
½ tsp. freshly ground allspice	

Sauce:
½ cup finely chopped onion
⅔ cup natural ketchup
⅓ cup beer
2 tsp. Worcestershire sauce
Black pepper (to taste)

NUTRITIONAL INFORMATION (per serving)

Total calories	370
% calories from fat	26
Total protein	24 gm.
Total carbohydrates	106 gm.
Total fat	21 gm.
Total fiber	16 gm.

Cut tops off the bell peppers and reserve the tops. Clean out the inside seeds and membranes. Soak wakami in water and drain. Cook millet in 1½ cups of water for 45 minutes until all water is absorbed, adding wakami the last 15 minutes. In a large bowl combine Soy Paste, millet, chopped onion, carrot, parsley, chives, ketchup, and allspice. Stuff into the hollowed peppers until they bulge. Top with the reserved pepper caps. Steam in a steamer for 30 minutes and set aside while sauce is prepared.

Sauce:
Stir-fry onion in a nonstick frying pan until translucent (1–3 minutes). Add ketchup, beer, Worcestershire sauce, and pepper; simmer for about 3 minutes. Pour over the stuffed peppers and serve.

% RDAs (per serving)

Tryptophan	196	Threonine	203
Isoleucine	182	Leucine	215
Lysine	215	Phenylalanine, tyrosine	247
Valine	160		
Methionine, cysteine	127		

Vitamin A	84	Calcium	19
Vitamin D	34	Magnesium	75
Vitamin K	218	Copper	24
Vitamin C	305	Zinc	19
Vitamin E	89	Chromium	55
Riboflavin	27	Phosphorus	38
Vitamin B_6	53	Potassium	84
Vitamin B_{12}	66	Iron	48
Thiamine	64	Manganese	87
Niacin	16	Selenium	67
Folacin	37		
Pantothenic acid	39		
Biotin	39		

SUCCOTASH/BARLEY CHOWDER
(4 Servings)

⅔ cup dry lima beans	**140 gm.**
½ cup barley	**100 gm.**
5 cloves garlic	**18 gm.**
1 cup chopped onion	**140 gm.**
1 tsp. olive or corn oil	**9 gm.**
1 cup chopped celery	**40 gm.**
4 morel mushrooms	**20 gm.**
1½ cups raw corn	**220 gm.**
1 cup chopped Chinese cabbage	**150 gm.**
2 cups low-fat milk, warmed	**488 gm.**
¼ cup chopped parsley	**40 gm.**
kombu, cut into small pieces	**10 gm.**
⅓ cup yogurt	**100 gm.**
1 tsp. chopped fresh basil	
1 tsp. thyme	
½ to 1 tsp. black pepper	
2 cups buttermilk	**244 gm.**
2 tsp. tamari or 1 tbsp. miso	

NUTRITIONAL INFORMATION (per serving)

Total calories	442
% calories from fat	16
Total protein	22 gm.
Total carbohydrates	73 gm.
Total fat	8 gm.

Soak the beans for at least 2 hours in enough room-temperature water to keep them covered. Discard the water. Add the same amount of fresh water to the beans, bring to a boil, and reduce heat. Soak kombu in water, drain, and add. Cover the pan and simmer for 1 hour. Add the barley to the beans and continue cooking for 1 hour, being sure that the water doesn't boil away. Discard water. Meantime, in a large pot sauté the garlic and onion in the oil, stirring constantly with a rubber spatula until the onion is translucent. Add celery and mushrooms and continue stirring until they are cooked but still crisp. Add corn and Chinese cabbage, and cook 5 minutes. Add 2 cups of pre-warmed low-fat milk, then the parsley, yogurt, basil, thyme, black pepper, beans, and barley. Reheat but do not boil. Add buttermilk and tamari or miso, and continue to heat while stirring. Serve. Freeze what is not used.

% RDAs (per serving)

Tryptophan	128	Vitamin K	6
Isoleucine	165	Vitamin C	67
Lysine	207	Vitamin E	11
Valine	166	Riboflavin	39
Methionine, cysteine	119	Vitamin B_6	42
Threonine	196	Vitamin B_{12}	98
Leucine	200	Thiamine	31
Phenylalanine, tyrosine	203	Niacin	18
		Folacin	33
Vitamin A	30	Pantothenic acid	47
Vitamin D	73	Biotin	19

Calcium	35	Phosphorus	47
Magnesium	57	Potassium	76
Copper	13	Iron	28
Zinc	22	Manganese	30
Chromium	38	Selenium	35

SUSAN'S VEGGIE SAN
(1 Sandwich)

1 small bunch broccoli (¼ lb.)	**112 gm.**
¼ head cauliflower	**50 gm.**
2 brussels sprouts	**45 gm.**
1 tsp. Dijon mustard	
2 tbsp. balsamic vinegar (or use your favorite vinegar)	
1 whole-wheat pocket pita bread	**50 gm.**
1 portion of Hummus*	**¼ cup**
alfalfa sprouts	

NUTRITIONAL INFORMATION (per serving)

Total calories	429
% calories from fat	10
Total protein	23 gm.
Total carbohydrates	73 gm.
Total fat	5 gm.

Steam the vegetables for 10 minutes. Process the vegetables, mustard, and vinegar in a food processor, using the metal blade, until thoroughly ground up, or grind together by hand.

Open the pita bread and spread on a thin layer of Hummus. Put on a generous layer of the vegetable mixture (the amount of vegetables given here is for 1 sandwich). Put on a layer of alfalfa sprouts, and serve.

% RDAs (per serving)

Tryptophan	136
Isoleucine	161
Lysine	173
Valine	136
Methionine, cysteine	113
Threonine	172
Leucine	158
Phenylalanine, tyrosine	179
Vitamin A	106
Vitamin D	0
Vitamin K	927
Vitamin C	367
Vitamin E	11
Riboflavin	30
Vitamin B_6	42
Vitamin B_{12}	0
Thiamine	38
Niacin	24
Folacin	70
Pantothenic acid	83
Biotin	16
Calcium	22
Magnesium	43
Copper	25
Zinc	20
Chromium	61
Phosphorus	38
Potassium	74
Iron	42
Manganese	56
Selenium	91

TUNA CHUTNEY SPREAD
(3 Sandwiches)

One 7-oz. can tuna, packed in water	**200 gm.**
4 tbsp. chopped chutney	
3 tbsp. chopped green bell pepper	**15 gm.**
3 tbsp. minced scallions	**15 gm.**
½ cup tofu mayonnaise (page 237)	

NUTRITIONAL INFORMATION (per serving)

Total calories	112
% calories from fat	13
Total protein	22 gm.
Total carbohydrates	2 gm.
Total fat	1 gm.

Drain the tuna well and break it up into a bowl. Mix in remaining ingredients thoroughly.

% RDAs (per serving)

Tryptophan	135	Vitamin B_{12}	52
Isoleucine	128	Thiamine	3
Lysine	237	Niacin	48
Valine	159	Folacin	3
Methionine, cysteine	120	Pantothenic acid	8
Threonine	170	Biotin	2
Leucine	149	Calcium	5
Phenylalanine, tyrosine	158	Magnesium	9
		Copper	0
Vitamin A	1	Zinc	3
Vitamin D	41	Chromium	8
Vitamin K	0	Phosphorus	15
Vitamin C	11	Potassium	13
Vitamin E	0	Iron	8
Riboflavin	6	Manganese	1
Vitamin B_6	15	Selenium	173

VEGETABLE CURRY
(1 Serving)

¼ lb. kale, leaves and stems	**100 gm.**
¼ head of cauliflower, flowerettes separated	**100 gm.**
¼ lb. broccoli, flowers separated and stem diced	**100 gm.**
1 medium red potato	**200 gm.**
1 carrot, sliced	**80 gm.**
1 leaf of nori, finely cut	**5 gm.**
¾ cup yogurt	**180 gm.**
1 tsp. corn oil	**5 gm.**
3 tsp. cumin	
3 tsp. mustard seed	

3 tsp. turmeric
2 tsp. coriander
1½ tsp. cayenne

NUTRITIONAL INFORMATION (per serving)

Total calories	224
% calories from fat	16
Total protein	12 gm.
Total carbohydrates	35 gm.
Total fat	4 gm.

Boil or steam the vegetables and reserve the liquid. Dice the potato. In a pot large enough to hold the vegetables, heat the oil. Add the spices and mix well. Add the vegetables, nori, and about ¾ cup of the liquid. Mix well. Add the yogurt and mix well. Simmer over low heat for 20 minutes. If the curry gets too thick, add some more of the cooking water.

% RDAs (per serving)

Tryptophan	65	Vitamin B_{12}	18
Isoleucine	78	Thiamine	18
Lysine	107	Niacin	20
Valine	89	Folacin	33
Methionine, cysteine	48	Pantothenic acid	65
Threonine	102	Biotin	13
Leucine	93	Calcium	27
Phenylalanine, tyrosine	94	Magnesium	25
		Copper	5
Vitamin A	203	Zinc	9
Vitamin D	0	Chromium	66
Vitamin K	406	Phosphorus	24
Vitamin C	300	Potassium	66
Vitamin E	35	Iron	16
Riboflavin	31	Manganese	17
Vitamin B_6	34	Selenium	5

VEGETABLE SALAD #1
(4 Servings)

⅓ cup garbanzo beans	**70 gm.**
⅓ cup cowpeas	**60 gm.**
⅓ cup brown rice	**75 gm.**
4 tbsp. wild rice	**25 gm.**
⅓ cup bran	**20 gm.**
1 small sweet potato	**90 gm.**
1 spear broccoli	**85 gm.**
1 medium carrot	**85 gm.**
6 medium mushrooms, chopped	**60 gm.**
1 medium tomato	**85 gm.**
6 full leaves romaine lettuce	**125 gm.**
½ cup chopped parsley	**50 gm.**
1 medium green or red bell pepper	**75 gm.**
1 small squash (summer)	**65 gm.**
½ cup red cabbage	**45 gm.**
1 small onion, chopped	**55 gm.**
¾ cup nonfat yogurt	**183 gm.**
½ cup buttermilk	**122 gm.**
⅓ cup balsamic vinegar	

NUTRITIONAL INFORMATION (per serving)

Total calories	364
% calories from fat	10
Total protein	18 gm.
Total carbohydrates	64 gm.
Total fat	4 gm.

Soak garbanzos and cowpeas for several hours or overnight. Discard soak water. Add excess water, bring to a boil, reduce heat, cover, and simmer for ½ to 1 hour in a pot. Combine brown and wild rice, wash, and add to the beans. Cook for an additional hour, adding bran during last 10 minutes. Meantime, steam the sweet potato until soft (about 15 minutes) and steam the broccoli and carrot about 10 minutes. Cool and peel the sweet potato. Cut the potato, broccoli, and carrot into pieces and place them in a large bowl. Cut up mushrooms, tomato, lettuce, parsley, bell pepper, squash, cabbage, and onion and add to bowl. Drain beans and rice from the pan in a sieve, cool with water, and add to the bowl. Blend yogurt, buttermilk, and vinegar and add to the bowl. Mix thoroughly by hand.

% RDAs *(per serving)*

Tryptophan	98	Vitamin B_{12}	12
Isoleucine	123	Thiamine	37
Lysine	152	Niacin	27
Valine	122	Folacin	50
Methionine, cysteine	83	Pantothenic acid	57
Threonine	132	Biotin	15
Leucine	133	Calcium	23
Phenylalanine, tyrosine	137	Magnesium	40
		Copper	21
Vitamin A	139	Zinc	21
Vitamin D	3	Chromium	50
Vitamin K	332	Phosphorus	36
Vitamin C	165	Potassium	62
Vitamin E	22	Iron	32
Riboflavin	30	Manganese	56
Vitamin B_6	33	Selenium	21

VEGETABLE STIR-FRY WITH ALMONDS AND OYSTERS

(1 Serving)

¼ cup millet	**25 gm.**
2–4 raw oysters	**100 gm.**
½ cup diced summer squash	**65 gm.**

1 medium stalk broccoli	**180 gm.**
½ cup diced green bell pepper	**50 gm.**
½ cup chopped onions	**80 gm.**
½ cup chopped mushrooms	**35 gm.**
½ cup peas	**70 gm.**
2 tsp. almonds	**16 gm.**
Worcestershire sauce, to taste	
½ cup vegetable bouillon	

NUTRITIONAL INFORMATION (per serving)

Total calories	327
% calories from fat	30
Total protein	24 gm.
Total carbohydrates	58 gm.
Total fat	11 gm.

Roast the millet in a nonstick skillet. Let brown, stirring occasionally, until a nutty fragrance can be detected. Add remaining ingredients and stir-fry in bouillon with constant tossing for 5 to 10 minutes.

% RDAs (per serving)

Tryptophan	162	Vitamin C	532
Isoleucine	161	Vitamin E	57
Lysine	168	Riboflavin	66
Valine	160	Vitamin B_6	51
Methionine, cysteine	131	Vitamin B_{12}	300
Threonine	185	Thiamine	60
Leucine	182	Niacin	47
Phenylalanine,		Folacin	59
tyrosine	181	Pantothenic acid	102
Vitamin A	112	Biotin	22
Vitamin D	46	Calcium	27
Vitamin K	522	Magnesium	50

Copper	117	Potassium	90
Zinc	154	Iron	56
Chromium	101	Manganese	51
Phosphorus	46	Selenium	78

WHOLE-WHEAT SPAGHETTI WITH CLAM SAUCE
(1 Serving)

Whole-grain spaghetti	**65 gm.**
2 cloves garlic, minced	
2 tbsp. olive oil	**14 gm.**
2 tbsp. chopped parsley	**7 gm.**
8 clams	**140 gm.**
⅓ cup clam juice	
½ tbsp. sherry	
⅛ tsp. (more or less, depending on your taste) Italian hot red pepper flakes	

NUTRITIONAL INFORMATION (per serving)

Total calories	470
% calories from fat	34
Total protein	27 gm.
Total carbohydrates	50 gm.
Total fat	18 gm.

Bring 3 quarts of water to a boil. Put the pasta in for about 8 minutes or until desired doneness. While the pasta is cooking, sauté the minced garlic in the olive oil until very lightly browned. Add the parsley, clams, clam juice, sherry, and hot pepper, and bring to a simmer. Simmer for 3 minutes. Drain the pasta, top with the clam sauce, and serve.

% RDAs (per serving)

Tryptophan	192	Vitamin B_{12}	891
Isoleucine	170	Thiamine	36
Lysine	240	Niacin	26
Valine	182	Folacin	10
Methionine, cysteine	177	Pantothenic acid	28
Threonine	229	Biotin	5
Leucine	206	Calcium	11
Phenylalanine, tyrosine	236	Magnesium	19
Vitamin A	14	Copper	2
Vitamin D	0	Zinc	24
Vitamin K	3	Chromium	126
Vitamin C	43	Phosphorus	39
Vitamin E	19	Potassium	28
Riboflavin	20	Iron	61
Vitamin B_6	17	Manganese	2
		Selenium	81

WILD RICE/SCALLOP CASSEROLE
(2 Servings)

½ cup wild rice	80 gm.
¼ cup brown rice	50 gm.
Dried morel mushrooms	20 gm.
½ lb. scallops	200 gm.
1 medium red onion, chopped	80 gm.
3 cloves garlic, finely chopped	18 gm.
1 8-oz. can tomato sauce	
1 medium tomato, diced	100 gm.
6 oz. nonfat yogurt	168 gm.
1 small jar pimentos	
¼ cup chopped fresh basil	
⅛ cup chopped fresh chives	

NUTRITIONAL INFORMATION (per serving)

Total calories	393
% calories from fat	5
Total protein	28 gm.
Total carbohydrates	66 gm.
Total fat	2 gm.

Wash and combine rice; simmer in 2 cups water for 45 minutes. Soak mushrooms in cold water for ½ hour. Discard water. Chop the mushrooms. Mix all ingredients except chives and bake in casserole in 350° preheated oven for 30 minutes. Mix in chives, and serve.

% RDAs (per serving)

Tryptophan	190	Vitamin B_{12}	55
Isoleucine	186	Thiamine	33
Lysine	270	Niacin	33
Valine	212	Folacin	15
Methionine, cysteine	115	Pantothenic acid	42
Threonine	247	Biotin	10
Leucine	231	Calcium	16
Phenylalanine, tyrosine	231	Magnesium	35
		Copper	9
Vitamin A	12	Zinc	27
Vitamin D	2	Chromium	46
Vitamin K	452	Phosphorus	46
Vitamin C	28	Potassium	51
Vitamin E	6	Iron	26
Riboflavin	33	Manganese	19
Vitamin B_6	14	Selenium	26

Appendix B

NUTRITIVE VALUES OF THE BEST FOODS

	WEIGHT OF NORMAL PORTION		NUTRITIVE VALUES OF FOODS (VALUES PER 100 GM)						
FOOD Category and Substance	Normal Portion	Amt. Grams	Calories	Protein (GM)	Fat	Carbohydrate	Fiber	% Satd. Fat	Cholesterol (MG)
VEGETABLES									
Artichoke—Boiled	base & ends—leaves	100	26	3	0.2	10	2.5	0	0
Asparagus	4 large spears	100	26	2.5	0.2	5	0.7	0	0
Beets (greens)	cooked 1 cup	150	24	2.2	0.3	5	1.3	0	0
Beets—Red Raw	1 cup diced	140	43	1.6	0.1	10	0.8	0	0
Broccoli	1 med. stalk	180	32	3.6	0.3	6	1.5	0	0
Brussels Sprouts	2 large	140	45	5	0.4	8	1.6	0	0
Cabbage	1 cup finely shredded	90	24	1.3	0.2	5	0.1	0	0
Cabbage—Chinese	cup 1 inch pcs.	75	14	1.2	0.1	3	0.6	0	0
Cabbage—Red	1 cup shredded	100	31	2	0.2	7	1	0	0
Carrots	1 carrot 7.5 x 1.125	80	42	1.1	0.2	10	1	0	0
Cauliflower	1 cup whole flowerettes	100	27	2.7	0.2	5	1	0	0
Celeriac	1/4 of 1 large	100	40	2	0.3	8.5	1.3	0	0
Celery	1 cup chopped	120	17	.9	0.1	4	0.6	0	0
Chard	1/4 lb.	115	25	2.4	0.3	4.5	0.8	0	0
Corn	1 cob 5 x 1.75 (kernels)	140	96	3.5	1	22	0.7	0	0
Cucumber	1 small 6.5 x 1.5	180	15	.9	0.1	3.4	0.6	0	0
Eggplant	1 cup diced	200	25	1.2	0.2	6	0.9	0	0
Garlic	1 clove (1.3 x .5 x .3)	3	137	6.2	0.2	31	1.5	0	0
Kale	1/4 lb.	115	38	4.2	0.8	6	1.3	0	0
Leeks	3–4 (5 inches)	100	52	2.2	0.3	11.2	1.3	0	0
Lettuce—Iceberg	wedge .125 of head	90	13	9	0.1	3	0.5	0	0
Lettuce—Romaine	1 cup chopped	55	18	1.3	0.3	3.5	0.7	0	0
Mushrooms	1 cup sliced or diced	70	28	2.7	0.3	4.4	0.8	0	0
Mushrooms—Shiitake	2 oz.	55	275	12.5	1.6	65	5.5	0	0
Onions	1 cup chopped	160	38	1.5	0.1	9	0.6	0	0
Parsley	1 T chopped	4	44	3.6	0.6	9	1.5	0	0

Peppers—Green	1 cup strips	100	22	1.2	0.2	5	1.4	0	0
Pepper (red—sweet)	1 large or 1 cup strips	100	31	1.4	0.3	7.1	1.7	0	0
Potato—White	2.75 x 4.25	250	77	2	0.1	17	0.5	0	0
Potato—Sweet	5 x 2	180	114	1.7	0.4	27	0.7	0	0
Radishes (red)	10 small (1 in. diam.)	100	17	1	0.1	3.6	0.7	0	0
Spinach	1 cup chopped	55	26	3.2	0.3	4	0.6	0	0
Squash (summer)	1 cup—cubed	130	19	1.1	0.1	4.2	0.6	0	0
Squash (winter)	1 cup baked	205	50	1.4	0.3	12.4	1.4	0	0
Tomato	2.5 inch diam.	100	22	1.1	0.2	5	0.5	0	0
Turnip Greens	¼ lb.	115	28	3	0.3	5	0.8	0	0
Waterchestnut	4 chstnts	25	80	1.4	0.2	19	0.8	0	0
Yams	¼ lb.	115	100	2.1	0.2	23.2	0.9	0	0
LEGUMES									
Beans—Garbanzos	¼ cup	50	360	21	5	61	5	9	0
Beans—Green	1 cup	100	32	1.9	0.2	7	1	0	0
Beans—Lima	½ cup	100	345	20.4	1.6	64	4.3	0	0
Beans—Pinto	½ cup	100	349	23	1.2	63.7	4.3	0	0
Cowpeas	½ cup	70	343	23	1.5	62	4.4	0	0
Lentils—Brown	½ cup	100	340	25	1.1	60	4	0	0
Peas	1 cup	140	84	6	0.4	14	2	0	0
Soybeans (mature)	¼ cup	50	403	34	18	34	5	15	0
Soybean Curd (tofu)	1 piece 2.5 x 1 x 2.75	120	72	8	4.2	2.4	0.1	0	0
Split Peas	½ cup	100	345	24.7	0.9	61.8	1.7	0	0
SEAWEED									
Hijiki	¼ cup	8	256	7.5	0.5	46	0	0	0
Kombu	¼ cup	8	219	6	1.2	42	6.7	0	0
Nori	¼ cup	8	235	27	0.8	40	4.7	0	0
Wakami	¼ cup	8	227	12.4	0.3	47.4	3.6	0	0
FISH AND SHELLFISH									
Bass—Black Sea	3.5 oz.	100	93	19	1	0	0	0	55
Bass—White Sea	3.5 oz.	100	98	18	2	0	0	50	55
Catfish	3.5 oz.	100	103	18	3	0	0	33	55

FOOD Category and Substance	WEIGHT OF NORMAL PORTION: Normal Portion	Amt. Grams	NUTRITIVE VALUES OF FOODS (VALUES PER 100 GM): Calories	Protein (GM)	Fat	Carbohydrate	Fiber	% Satd. Fat	Cholesterol (MG)
Clams	4 cherrystone	70	76	13	1.6	2	0	0	50
Cod	3.5 oz.	100	78	18	0.3	0	0	0	50
Crab (steamed)	3.5 oz.	100	93	17	2	0.5	0	0	100
Haddock	3.5 oz.	100	79	18	0.1	0	0	0	60
Halibut	3.5 oz.	100	100	21	1.2	0	0	0	50
Herring (Pacific)	1 herring	50	98	17.5	2.6	0	0	0	85
Lobster	1 cup cubed	145	91	19	1.5	0.5	0	0	77
Mackerel (Atlantic)	3.5 oz.	100	191	19	12	0	0	33	95
Ocean Perch	3.5 oz.	100	88	18	1.2	0	0	0	55
Oysters	med.—2 selects	25	66	8.4	1.8	3.4	0.1	0	50
Perch—White	3.5 oz.	100	118	19	4	0	0	25	55
Red Snapper	3.5 oz.	100	93	20	1	0	0	0	55
Salmon (Atlantic)	3.5 oz.	100	217	23	13	0	0	31	39
Salmon (Atlantic can)	1 can 6.5 oz	185	203	22	12	0	0	25	37
Sardines (Pacific)	3.5 oz	100	157	19	9	0	0	22	112
Sardines (Atlantic can)	3.5 oz.	100	203	24	11	0	0	0	130
Scallops—Raw	1 large	25	80	15	0.2	3	0	0	35
Shark	3.5 oz	100	103	24	0.1	0	0	0	33
Shrimp—Raw	3.5 oz	100	91	18	0.8	1.5	0	0	150
Sole	3.5 oz.	100	79	17	0.8	0	0	0	50
Squid	3.5 oz	100	84	16.5	1	0	0	0	56
Swordfish	3.5 oz	100	118	19	4	0	0	25	55
Tuna (canned)	0.5 cup	115	127	28	0.8	0	0	0	63
MEAT AND POULTRY									
Beef—Loin/Sirloin	3.5 oz.	100	143	22	6	0	0	46	65
Beef—Round	3.5 oz	100	135	22	5	0	0	45	65
Calves Liver	3.5 oz	100	140	19	5	4	0	20	300

Chicken (dark meat)	3.5 oz	100	130	20	4.3	0	0	25	80
Chicken (light meat)	3.5 oz	100	117	23	2	0	0	25	58
Ham (canned)	3.5 oz.	100	193	18	12	0.9	0	37	89
Hamburger	3.5 oz.	100	179	21	10	0	0	50	68
Lamb (choice)	3.5 oz.	100	263	17	21	0	0	57	71
Lamb—Loin	3.5 oz	100	138	20	6	0	0	55	70
Pork (thin)	3.5 oz.	100	165	20	9.1	0	0	36	60
Rabbit (domestic)	3.5 oz.	100	162	21	8	0	0	38	0
Turkey (light meat)	3.5 oz.	100	114	23.4	2	0	0	32	60
Turkey (dark meat)	3.5 oz.	100	123	20	4	0	0	33	75
Veal	3.5 oz	100	156	20	8	0	0	48	71
Veal—Loin	3.5 oz.	100	156	19.7	8	0	0	48	71
FRUIT									
Apples	1 med. 2.75 in. diam.	150	59	.2	0.4	15	0.8	0	0
Applesauce—Unsweetened	½ cup	100	40	.2	5	11	0.5	0	0
Apricots	1 med.	40	51	1.4	0.4	11	0.6	0	0
Avocado	1 cup	150	167	2	17	7	2.1	0	0
Banana	1 med.	150	85	1	0.5	23	0.5	0	0
Blueberries	1 cup	140	56	7	0.5	15	1.5	0	0
Cantaloupe	0.5 med.	400	30	.9	0.3	8	0.4	0	0
Cranberries	1 cup	100	49	.4	0.2	13	1.2	0	0
Dates—Nat'l & Dried	5 w/o pits	40	274	2.2	0.5	73	2.3	0	0
Figs—Raw	2 large/3 small	100	74	.8	0.3	19	1.2	20	0
Grapefruit	sections 1 cup	190	41	.7	0.1	8.4	0.2	0	0
Grapes	1 cup	150	67	.6	0.4	17	0.8	0	0
Lemon (peeled)	1 med.	100	29	1.1	0.3	9.3	0.4	0	0
Lime	1 med.	100	30	.7	0.2	10.5	0.5	0	0
Nectarine	2 med.	100	49	.9	0.5	12	0.4	0	0
Orange	1 med.	180	47	.9	0.1	12	0.4	0	0
Papaya	⅓ med.	100	39	.6	0.1	10	0.8	0	0
Peaches	1 med.	100	38	.7	0.1	11	0.6	0	0
Pears	1 small	75	61	.4	0.4	15	1.4	0	0

FOOD Category and Substance	WEIGHT OF NORMAL PORTION Normal Portion	Amt. Grams	NUTRITIVE VALUES OF FOODS (VALUES PER 100 GM) Calories	Protein (GM)	Fat	Carbohydrate	Fiber	% Satd. Fat	Cholesterol (MG)
Persimmon—Native	1 med.	100	127	.8	0.4	33.5	1.5	0	0
Pineapple	1 cup diced	140	52	.4	0.4	12	0.5	0	0
Plums	2 med.	100	55	.79	0.6	13	0.6	0	0
Raisins	2 T	18	289	3.2	0.5	79	1.3	0	0
Raspberries—Red	3/4 cup	100	50	.9	0.6	12	3	0	0
Strawberries	1 cup whole	150	37	.6	0.4	7	0.5	0	0
Watermelon	1 cup diced	160	26	.6	0.4	7	0.3	0	0
Orange Juice	1 cup	248	45	7	0.2	10.4	0.1	0	0
CEREAL									
Buckwheat	1 cup	100	335	11.7	2.4	73	10	0	0
Grape Nuts	1 cup	224	357	11.7	0.4	82	4.8	0	0
Cereals—Rolled Oats	1 cup	80	391	14	7	68	1.2	29	0
Cereals—Rye	1 cup	80	355	12	1.7	73	2	0	0
Shredded Wheat	1 biscuit	25	360	11	2.2	80	9.3	0	0
Wheat Flakes	1 cup	30	355	10	1.6	81	1.6	0	0
Whole Wheat Hot	1 cup	125	342	11.2	2	75	2	0	0
GRAIN									
Grains—Barley	1/4 cup	50	349	8	1	79	0.5	0	0
Bulgar Wheat	1/2 cup	100	361	11	1.5	76	1.7	0	0
Cornmeal	1/4 cup	30	355	9.2	3.9	74	1.6	11	0
Gluten Flour	1 cup	140	378	41.4	1.9	47	0 4	0	0
Millet	1/4 cup	25	327	10	2.9	73	3.2	34	0
Popcorn (plain—popd)	3 cups	42	386	12.7	5	77	2.2	20	0
Rice (brown—raw)	short grain—1/4 cup	50	356	7.5	2	77	0.9	0	0
Rye Flour	1 cup—sifted	88	357	9.4	1	78	0.4	0	0
Wheat Bran	1 T	6	213	16	4.6	62	9	21	0
Wheat Flour (enr)	1/2 cup sifted	55	364	10.5	1	76.1	0.3	0	0

Wheat Flour (wh)	½ cup sifted	55	333	13.3	2	71	2.3	0	0
Wheat Germ	1 T	6	395	27	11	47	2.5	18	0
Wild Rice	¼ cup	40	353	14.1	0.7	75.3	1	0	0
DAIRY									
Butter Milk	1 cup	244	41	3.3	0.9	4.8	0	67	4
Lowfat Milk (2%)	1 cup	244	50	3.3	1.9	4.8	0	63	8
Skim Milk	1 cup	244	35	.84	0.2	4.9	0	55	2
Whole Milk	1 cup	244	62	3.3	3.3	4.7	0	61	14
Yogurt (lowfat)	1 cup	244	64	5.3	1.6	7	0	63	6
CHEESE									
Cheese—American	1 slice 2.25 x 2.25 x .25	25	375	22	31	1.6	0	64	94
Cheese—Cheddar	1 inch cubed	30	402	25	33	1.3	0	64	105
Cheese (cottage)—Dry Curd	1 cup	200	85	17	0.4	1.9	0	64	7
Cheese—Cottage (1% fat)	¼ cup	60	72	12	1	2.7	0	64	4
Cheese (feta)	1 inch cube	17	264	14	21	4	0	71	89
Cheese—Monterey Jack	1 inch cube	30	373	24	30	0.7	0	62	112
Mozzarella (part skim)	1 inch cube	30	252	24	16	3	0	63	58
Ricotta (part skim)	½ cup	124	140	11	8	5	0	62	31
Cheese—Swiss	1 inch cube	30	369	28	27	3.4	0	66	92
BREAD									
Pumpernickel	1 slice	32	247	9.1	1.3	53	1.3	0	0
Bread—Rye—Amer	1 slice	25	243	9	1.1	52	0.4	0	1
Bread—Wheat	1 slice	25	241	9	2.6	49	1.5	20	3
EGGS									
Eggs—White	1 med.	15	49	10	0	1.2	0	0	0
Eggs—Whole	1 whole med. refuse 12%	50	158	13	12	1.2	0	28	548
Eggs—Yolk	1 med.	29	369	16	33	0.2	0	30	1602
NUTS & SEEDS									
Almonds	1 T.	8	598	19	54	20	2.6	8	0
Cashew	14 large	28	561	17	46	29	1.4	17	0
Chestnuts (fresh)	2 lrge or 3 smll	15	194	3	1.5	42	1	0	0
Peanuts (roasted)	1 T. chpd or 15 whl	9	582	26	49	21	2.7	22	0

FOOD Category and Substance	WEIGHT OF NORMAL PORTION: Normal Portion	Amt. Grams	NUTRITIVE VALUES OF FOODS (VALUES PER 100 GM): Calories	Protein (GM)	Fat	Carbohydrate	Fiber	% Satd. Fat	Cholesterol (MG)
Pecans	10 large	9	687	9.2	71	14.6	2.3	7	0
Pumpkin Seeds	1/8 cup	17	553	29	47	15	1.9	18	0
Sunflower Seeds	1/8 cup	18	560	24	47	20	4	12	0
OILS									
Butter—Salted	1 T	14	717	.9	81	0.1	0-	62	219
Corn Oil	1 T	14	900	0	100	0	0	12.7	0
Olive Oil	1 T	14	900	0	100	0	0	13.5	0
Safflower Oil	1 T	14	900	0	100	0	0	9.1	0
Sesame Oil	1 T	14	884	.8	100	0	0	14.2	0
Soy Oil	1 T	14	900	0	100	0	0	14.4	0
MISCELLANEOUS									
Melba Toast	1 slice	4	475	16.7	15	67.5	0	0	0
Yeast	1 oz	28	283	39	1	38	1.7	0	0

FOOD Category and Substance	WEIGHT OF NORMAL PORTION Normal Portion	Amt Grams	NUTRITIVE VALUES OF FOODS (VALUES PER 100 GM) ESSENTIAL AMINO ACIDS (MG) Tryptophan	Threonine	Isoleucine	Leucine	Lysine	Phenylalan	Tyrosine	Valine	Methionine/ Cysteine
VEGETABLES											
Artichoke—Boiled	base & ends—leaves	100	0	0	0	0	0	0	0	0	0
Asparagus	4 large spears	100	30	75	90	110	120	78	45	120	55
Beets (greens)	cooked 1 cup	150	26	84	90	140	120	128	0	110	70
Beets—Red Raw	1 cup diced	140	14	34	52	55	86	27	86	49	48
Broccoli	1 med. stalk	180	45	133	137	177	160	175	0	185	90
Brussels Sprouts	2 large	140	50	170	206	216	219	162	100	215	137
Cabbage	1 cup finely shredded	90	10	36	50	53	61	27	30	40	38
Cabbage—Chinese	cup 1 inch pcs	75	10	34	35	49	57	25	25	37	35
Cabbage—Red	1 cup shredded	100	16	56	78	80	94	42	0	60	59
Carrots	1 carrot 7.5 x 1 125	80	8	33	33	50	45	30	25	50	36
Cauliflower	1 cup whole flowerettes	100	40	120	135	200	160	100	34	155	68
Celeriac	1/4 of 1 lrge	100	0	0	0	0	0	0	0	0	0
Celery	1 cup chopped	120	14	40	45	75	27	50	16	55	25
Chard	1/4 lb.	115	25	100	100	130	95	80	0	95	7
Corn	1 cob 5 x 1.75 (kernels)	140	21	144	130	390	130	200	170	220	110
Cucumber	1 small 6.5 x 1.5	180	6	21	25	35	35	20	0	28	8
Eggplant	1 cup diced	200	12	45	50	70	32	50	45	60	20
Garlic	1 clove (1.3 x .5 x .3)	3	0	0	0	0	0	0	0	0	0
Kale	1/4 lb.	115	50	150	150	280	130	170	0	200	70
Leeks	3–4 (5 inches)	100	0	0	0	0	0	0	0	0	0
Lettuce—Iceberg	wedge .125 of head	90	10	54	50	83	50	67	102	71	29
Lettuce—Romaine	1 cup chpd	55	13	54	50	83	75	67	35	71	42
Mushrooms	1 cup sliced or diced	70	8	100	600	320	0	0	0	425	190
Mushrooms—Shiitake	2 oz.	55	0	0	0	0	0	0	0	0	0
Onions	1 cup chopped	160	20	20	20	35	60	40	46	30	26

FOOD Category and Substance	WEIGHT OF NORMAL PORTION		NUTRITIVE VALUES OF FOODS (VALUES PER 100 GM) ESSENTIAL AMINO ACIDS (MG)								
	Normal Portion	Amt. Grams	Tryptophan	Threonine	Isoleucine	Leucine	Lysine	Phenylalan	Tyrosine	Valine	Methionine/ Cysteine
Parsley	1 T chpd	4	75	0	0	0	530	0	0	0	18
Peppers—Green	1 cup strips	100	8	50	46	46	50	55	55	32	35
Pepper (red—sweet)	1 large or 1 cup strips	100	10	58	53	53	60	70	60	38	40
Potato—White	2.75 x 4.25	250	21	86	72	105	111	92	43	111	25
Potato—Sweet	5 x 2	180	30	80	82	97	80	90	80	127	58
Radishes (red)	10 small (1 in. diam)	100	4	49	54	75	28	48	0	25	2
Spinach	1 cup chopped	55	51	141	150	245	200	130	110	176	120
Squash (summer)	1 cup—cubed	130	9	35	35	50	42	30	0	41	14
Squash (winter)	1 cup baked	205	0	0	0	0	0	0	0	0	0
Tomato	2.5 inch diam.	100	9	36	32	45	46	28	14	31	13
Turnip Greens	1/4 lb	115	47	127	106	210	133	142	86	154	54
Waterchestnut	4 chstnts	25	0	0	0	0	0	0	0	0	0
Yams	1/4 lb	115	27	76	79	136	86	84	84	98	58
LEGUMES											
Beans—Garbanzos	1/4 cup	50	165	750	1200	1500	1415	1000	700	1000	560
Beans—Green	1 cup	100	26	70	90	110	100	100	80	91	47
Beans—Lima	1/2 cup	100	184	960	1180	1700	1370	1200	535	1290	630
Beans—Pinto	1/2 cup	100	210	1000	1310	1980	1710	1270	890	1400	460
Cowpeas	1/2 cup	70	250	850	1094	1710	1480	1200	600	1530	645
Lentils—Brown	1/2 cup	100	220	900	1320	1760	1530	1100	670	1360	384
Peas	1 cup	140	65	250	275	455	480	290	200	300	157
Soybeans (mature)	1/4 cup	50	525	1470	2010	2900	2350	2050	1300	2000	1065
Soybean Curd (tofu)	1 piece 2.5 x 1 x 2 75	120	132	233	359	616	458	440	330	363	215
Split Peas	1/2 cup	100	220	860	1310	1750	1510	1140	660	1330	604
SEAWEED											
Hijiki	1/4 cup	8	40	180	350	405	160	320	170	570	180
Kombu	1/4 cup	8	130	615	205	230	160	0	0	780	0

Nori	1/4 cup	8	280	1030	870	1510	800	0	0	1950	0
Wakami	1/4 cup	8	120	550	290	860	375	0	0	700	0
FISH AND SHELLFISH											
Bass—Black Sea	3.5 oz	100	190	830	980	1460	1690	710	620	1020	712
Bass—White Sea	3.5 oz	100	180	770	920	1370	1580	670	574	950	668
Catfish	3.5 oz	100	180	790	830	1440	1600	650	600	1160	670
Clams	4 cherrystone	70	170	610	610	1000	1040	540	540	810	545
Cod	3.5 oz	100	197	900	800	1450	1700	850	650	900	800
Crab (steamed)	3.5 oz	100	200	730	745	1400	1250	650	600	750	720
Haddock	3.5 oz	100	180	790	920	1370	1600	680	490	970	775
Halibut	3.5 oz	100	200	890	1078	1500	1760	750	540	1070	860
Herring (Pacific)	1 herring	50	180	870	1000	1500	1530	740	190	1040	760
Lobster	1 cup cubed	145	220	870	890	1650	1500	770	700	910	780
Mackerel (Atlantic)	3.5 oz.	100	186	810	950	1410	1640	690	500	1000	670
Ocean Perch	3.5 oz	100	200	700	800	1200	1600	650	625	1100	740
Oysters	med—2 selects	25	110	390	400	650	670	350	350	530	360
Perch—White	3.5 oz	100	225	750	840	1290	1630	640	680	1250	780
Red Snapper	3.5 oz	100	200	850	1010	1490	1740	730	0	1050	570
Salmon (Atlantic)	3.5 oz	100	225	970	1125	1690	1960	832	700	1200	815
Salmon (Atlantic can)	1 can 6.5 oz.	185	200	875	1025	1500	1800	750	550	1100	785
Sardines (Pacific)	3.5 oz.	100	190	820	960	1430	1660	700	510	1010	750
Sardines (Atlantic can)	3.5 oz.	100	240	1040	1220	1820	2110	890	650	1280	898
Scallops—Raw	1 large	25	190	680	680	1120	1160	600	600	910	673
Shark	3.5 oz.	100	220	820	1390	1710	1930	830	740	1100	570
Shrimp—Raw	3.5 oz.	100	200	800	820	1530	1390	740	840	840	920
Sole	3.5 oz.	100	220	800	800	1350	1650	650	625	900	550
Squid	3.5 oz.	100	347	1368	2096	2900	3280	1500	1500	2665	4293
Swordfish	3.5 oz.	100	220	770	840	1300	1610	630	700	1260	676
Tuna (canned)	0.5 cup	115	320	1100	1200	1850	2300	900	1000	1800	985
MEAT & POULTRY											
Beef—Loin/Sirloin	3.5 oz.	100	260	970	1150	1800	1920	900	750	1220	800
Beef—Round	3.5 oz.	100	260	970	1150	1800	1930	910	750	1220	810
Calves Liver	3.5 oz.	100	300	900	1000	1750	1450	950	700	1200	700

	WEIGHT OF NORMAL PORTION		NUTRITIVE VALUES OF FOODS (VALUES PER 100 GM) ESSENTIAL AMINO ACIDS (MG)								
FOOD Category and Substance	Normal Portion	Amt. Grams	Tryptophan	Threonine	Isoleucine	Leucine	Lysine	Phenylalan	Tyrosine	Valine	Methionine/ Cysteine
Chicken (dark meat)	3.5 oz.	100	235	850	1060	1500	1700	800	680	1000	815
Chicken (light meat)	3.5 oz.	100	285	992	1235	1740	2055	920	780	1150	940
Ham (canned)	3.5 oz.	100	200	700	910	1325	1477	710	640	930	740
Hamburger	3.5 oz.	100	242	914	1083	1700	1810	860	710	1150	775
Lamb (choice)	3.5 oz.	100	200	750	800	1200	1275	625	500	800	610
Lamb—Loin	3.5 oz.	100	220	780	890	1320	1380	700	600	840	740
Pork (thin)	3.5 oz.	100	250	900	1000	1435	1600	790	700	1014	710
Rabbit (domestic)	3.5 oz.	100	0	1020	1080	1640	1820	790	0	1020	540
Turkey (light meat)	3.5 oz.	100	270	1040	1220	1870	2210	930	930	1240	1020
Turkey (dark meat)	3.5 oz.	100	230	890	1040	1600	1890	800	790	1070	866
Veal	3.5 oz.	100	250	850	1030	1400	1600	800	700	1000	685
Veal—Loin	3.5 oz.	100	260	850	1040	1440	1645	790	720	1020	685
FRUIT											
Apples	1 med 2.75 in. diam.	150	2	7	8	12	12	5	4	9	5
Applesauce—Unsweetened	½ cup	100	2	6	6	10	10	5	3	8	4
Apricots	1 med.	40	15	47	44	77	97	52	29	47	9
Avocado	1 cup	150	22	70	75	131	100	72	52	103	61
Banana	1 med	150	12	34	33	71	48	38	24	47	28
Blueberries	1 cup	140	3	18	21	40	12	24	8	28	18
Cantaloupe	0.5 med	400	6	1	25	34	20	30	20	28	12
Cranberries	1 cup	100	0	0	0	0	0	0	0	0	0
Dates—Nat'l & Dried	5 w/o pits	40	50	52	47	88	60	56	30	66	67
Figs—Raw	2 large/3 small	100	6	25	23	33	30	18	32	28	18
Grapefruit	sections 1 cup	190	2	0	0	0	18	0	0	0	2
Grapes	1 cup	150	3	17	5	13	14	13	11	17	31
Lemon (peeled)	1 med	100	0	0	0	0	0	0	0	0	0
Lime	1 med	100	3	0	0	0	14	0	0	0	2

Nectarine	2 med.	100	0	0	0	0	0	0	0	0	0
Orange	1 med.	180	9	15	25	23	47	31	16	40	30
Papaya	⅓ med.	100	8	11	8	16	25	9	5	10	2
Peaches	1 med.	100	2	27	20	40	23	22	18	38	23
Pears	1 small	75	6	10	11	20	14	10	3	14	9
Persimmon—Native	1 med.	100	14	41	35	58	45	36	23	42	25
Pineapple	1 cup diced	140	5	12	13	19	25	12	12	16	13
Plums	2 med.	100	0	16	16	21	17	17	6	19	10
Raisins	2 T	18	0	0	0	0	0	0	0	0	0
Raspberries—Red	¾ cup	100	0	0	0	0	0	0	0	0	0
Strawberries	1 cup whole	150	7	19	14	31	25	18	21	18	6
Watermelon	1 cup diced	160	7	27	19	18	62	15	12	16	8
Orange Juice	1 cup	248	2	8	8	13	9	9	4	11	8
CEREAL											
Buckwheat	1 cup	100	146	420	400	690	450	450	280	780	430
Grape Nuts	1 cup	224	210	370	480	830	860	590	360	590	306
Cereals—Rolled Oats	1 cup	80	175	460	500	1000	500	700	450	700	520
Cereals—Rye	1 cup	80	137	400	400	700	400	500	225	560	400
Shredded Wheat	1 biscuit	25	210	370	430	760	340	530	320	540	284
Wheat Flakes	1 cup	30	115	330	470	840	340	450	290	540	318
Whole Wheat Hot	1 cup	125	130	303	457	706	289	457	457	488	392
GRAIN											
Grains—Barley	¼ cup	50	100	279	343	570	280	429	247	411	323
Bulgur Wheat	½ cup	100	127	340	390	750	300	480	350	450	392
Cornmeal	¼ cup	30	60	370	430	1190	270	420	560	470	170
Gluten Flour	1 cup	140	440	1100	1900	3100	790	2250	1340	1980	1612
Millet	¼ cup	25	220	400	560	1540	340	450	900	600	480
Popcorn (plain—popd)	3 cups	42	80	510	590	1670	370	580	0	660	400
Rice (brown—raw)	short grain—¼ cup	50	84	300	300	650	300	400	275	400	250
Rye Flour	1 cup—sifted	88	110	350	400	630	380	440	300	490	310
Wheat Bran	1 T.	6	256	500	650	900	600	550	425	680	560
Wheat Flour (enr)	½ cup sifted	55	130	305	485	810	240	580	360	450	320

FOOD Category and Substance	WEIGHT OF NORMAL PORTION Normal Portion	Amt. Grams	NUTRITIVE VALUES OF FOODS (VALUES PER 100 GM) ESSENTIAL AMINO ACIDS (MG) Tryptophan	Threonine	Isoleucine	Leucine	Lysine	Phenylalan	Tyrosine	Valine	Methionine/ Cysteine
Wheat Flour (wh)	½ cup sifted	55	160	380	580	890	370	660	500	620	460
Wheat Germ	1 T.	6	260	1430	1270	1700	1600	1000	800	1460	740
Wild Rice	¼ cup	40	240	550	633	1140	660	400	400	930	390
DAIRY											
Butter Milk	1 cup	244	35	160	200	330	280	175	140	250	110
Lowfat Milk (2%)	1 cup	244	47	150	200	320	260	160	160	220	120
Skim Milk	1 cup	244	50	150	200	330	270	165	165	230	120
Whole Milk	1 cup	244	45	150	200	300	250	160	160	220	115
Yogurt (lowfat)	1 cup	244	30	210	300	500	475	300	275	400	150
CHEESE											
Cheese—American	1 slice 2.25 x 2.25 x .25	25	325	700	1025	2000	2100	1100	1200	1300	715
Cheese—Cheddar	1 inch cubed	30	320	900	1550	2400	2100	1300	1200	1700	780
Cheese (cottage)—Dry Curd	1 cup	200	190	770	1015	1770	1400	930	920	1070	680
Cheese—Cottage (1% fat)	.25 cup	60	140	550	700	1300	1000	670	660	770	490
Cheese (feta)	1 inch cube	17	0	0	0	0	0	0	0	0	0
Cheese—Monterey Jack	1 inch cube	30	300	875	1500	2350	2036	1300	1200	1600	765
Mozzarella (part skim)	1 inch cube	30	310	900	1200	2400	2500	1300	1400	1500	820
Ricotta (part skim)	½ cup	124	145	520	600	1240	1350	560	600	700	385
Cheese—Swiss	1 inch cube	30	400	1000	1500	3000	2600	1700	1700	2100	1025
BREAD											
Pumpernickel	1 slice	32	100	330	390	610	370	425	350	470	390
Bread—Rye—Amer	1 slice	25	100	400	400	600	290	500	225	475	360
Bread—Wheat	1 slice	25	130	310	475	720	325	550	380	490	385
EGGS											
Eggs—White	1 med	15	155	450	620	880	625	650	400	760	650
Eggs—Whole	1 whole med refuse 12%	50	195	600	760	1070	820	700	500	875	680
Eggs—Yolk	1 med	29	240	890	940	1400	1110	700	700	1000	600

NUTS & SEEDS											
Almonds	1 T	8	175	500	700	1300	450	1000	600	1100	635
Cashew	14 large	28	375	650	1100	1400	730	870	650	1460	690
Chestnuts (fresh)	2 lrge 3 smll	15	40	100	110	170	180	60.	60	150	30
Peanuts (roasted)	1 T chpd or 15 whl	9	340	800	1300	1900	1100	1600	1100	1500	825
Pecans	10 large	9	140	390	550	770	440	560	320	530	300
Pumpkin Seeds	1/8 cup	17	530	880	1630	2290	1330	1640	0	1580	780
Sunflower Seeds	1/8 cup	18	360	940	1320	1820	910	1270	380	1410	950
OILS											
Butter—Salted	1 T.	14	12	40	50	80	70	40	40	60	30
Corn Oil	1 T.	14	0	0	0	0	0	0	0	0	0
Olive Oil	1 T.	14	0	0	0	0	0	0	0	0	0
Safflower Oil	1 T	14	0	0	0	0	0	0	0	0	0
Sesame Oil	1 T	14	0	0	0	0	0	0	0	0	0
Soy Oil	1 T	14	0	0	0	0	0	0	0	0	0
MISCELLANEOUS											
Melba Toast	1 slice	4	190	440	700	1170	350	700	650	660	505
Yeast	1 oz.	28	700	2300	2400	3200	3300	1900	1900	2700	1380

NUTRITIVE VALUES OF FOODS (VALUES PER 100 GM)

VITAMINS

FOOD Category and Substance	Normal Portion	Amt. Grams	(I.U.) A	(MG) C	(I.U.) D	(I.U.) E	(Mcg) K	(MG) Thiamine	(MG) Riboflavin	(MG) Niacin	(Mcg) B-6	(Mcg) Folacin	(Mcg) B-12	(MG) Pantothenic	(Mcg) Biotin
VEGETABLES															
Artichoke—Boiled	base & ends—leaves	100	150	8	0	0.28	0	0.07	0.04	0.700	0.100	0	0	0.300	4.100
Asparagus	4 large spears	100	900	33	0	3	60	0.18	0.20	1.500	0.150	64	0	0.600	1.700
Beets (greens)	cooked 1 cup	150	6100	30	0	2.20	0	0.10	0.22	0.400	0.100	110	0	0.250	2.700
Beets—Red Raw	1 cup diced	140	20	10	0	0.04	0	0.03	0.05	0.400	0.055	90	0	0.150	2
Broccoli	1 med. stalk	180	2500	110	0	0.69	200	0.10	0.23	0.900	0.200	70	0	1.200	0.500
Brussels Sprouts	2 large	140	550	100	0	1.30	570	0.10	0.16	0.900	0.230	78	0	0.700	0.400
Cabbage	1 cup finely shredded	90	130	50	0	2.50	125	0.05	0.05	0.300	0.160	66	0	0.200	2.400
Cabbage—Chinese	cup 1 inch pcs	75	150	25	0	0	0	0.05	0.04	0.600	0.780	83	0	0	0
Cabbage—Red	1 cup shredded	100	40	60	0	0.20	0	0.09	0.06	0.400	0.200	34	0	0.320	0.100
Carrots	1 carrot 7.5 x 1.125	80	11000	8	0	0.70	80	0.06	0.05	0.600	0.150	32	0	0.280	2.500
Cauliflower	1 cup whole flowerettes	100	60	80	0	0.04	300	0.11	0.10	0.700	0.210	55	0	1	17
Celeriac	¼ of 1 lrge	100	0	8	0	4	100	0.05	0.06	0.700	0.170	7	0	0	0
Celery	1 cup chopped	120	240	9	0	0.54	0	0.03	0.03	0.300	0.060	12	0	0.430	0.100
Chard	¼ lb.	115	6500	32	0	0	0	0.06	0.17	0.500	0	0.700	0	0.170	0
Corn	1 cob 5 x 1 75 (kernels)	140	400	12	0	0.73	2	0.15	0.12	1.700	0.160	33	0	0.540	6
Cucumber	1 small 6.5 x 1.5	180	250	11	0	0.22	5	0.03	0.04	0.200	0.040	15	0	0.250	0.400
Eggplant	1 cup diced	200	10	5	0	0.04	0	0.05	0.05	0.600	0.080	30	0	0.220	0
Garlic	1 clove (1.3 x .5 x .3)	3	0	15	0	0.02	0	0.25	0.08	0.500	0	0	0	0	0
Kale	¼ lb	115	8900	125	0	8	0	0	0.26	2.100	0.300	60	0	1	0.500
Leeks	3–4 (5 inches)	100	40	17	0	1.40	0	0.11	0.06	0.500	0.200	36	0	0.120	1.400
Lettuce—Iceberg	wedge 125 of head	90	330	6	0	0.80	129	0.06	0.06	0.300	0.055	37	0	0.200	3

Lettuce—Romaine	1 cup chpd	55	1900	18	0	0.50	103	0.05	0.08	0.400	0.055	179	0	0.200	0.700
Mushrooms	1 cup sliced or diced	70	0	3	78	0.10	17	0.10	0.46	4.200	0.130	23	0	2.200	16
Mushrooms—Shiitake	2 oz	55	0	0	0	0	0	0.32	0.74	10	0	0	0	0	0
Onions	1 cup chopped	160	40	10	0	0.18	0	0.03	0.04	0.200	0.130	25	0	0.130	3.500
Parsley	1 T chpd	4	8500	172	0	2.60	0	0.12	0.26	1.200	0.160	120	0	0.300	0.400
Peppers—Green	1 cup strips	100	420	128	0	1	0	0.08	0.08	0.500	0.260	19	0	0.230	0
Pepper (red—sweet)	1 large or 1 cup strips	100	4450	204	0	0	0	0.08	0.08	0.500	0	0	0	0.270	0
Potato—White	2.75 x 4.25	250	0	20	0	0.09	3	0.10	0.04	1.500	0.250	19	0	0.380	0.400
Potato—Sweet	5 x 2	180	8800	21	0	6.80	0	0.10	0.06	0.600	0.220	50	0	0.820	4.300
Radishes (red)	10 small (1 in. diam)	100	10	26	0	0	0	0.03	0.03	0.300	0.075	24	0	0.180	0
Spinach	1 cup chopped	55	8100	51	0	2.80	89	0.10	0.20	0.600	0.280	193	0	0.300	7
Squash (summer)	1 cup—cubed	130	410	22	0	0.18	0	0.05	0.09	1	0.080	31	0	0.360	0
Squash (winter)	1 cup baked	205	3700	13	0	0	0	0.05	0.11	0.600	0.150	34	0	0.400	0
Tomato	2.5 inch diam.	100	900	23	0	0.51	630	0.06	0.04	0.700	0.100	39	0	0.330	4
Turnip Greens	¼ lb.	115	7600	139	0	3.30	650	0.20	0.40	0.800	0.260	95	0	0.380	0.400
Waterchestnut	4 chstnts	25	0	4	0	0	0	0.14	0.20	1	0	0	0	0	0
Yams	¼ lb.	115	0	9	0	0	0	0.10	0.04	0.500	0	50	0	0.390	0
LEGUMES															
Beans—Garbanzos	¼ cup	50	50	0	0	0	0	0.31	0.15	2	0.500	200	0	1.300	10
Beans—Green	1 cup	100	600	20	0	0.03	14	0.08	0.11	0.500	0.080	44	0	0.200	0.400
Beans—Lima	½ cup	100	0	0	0	0.66	0	0.48	0.17	1.900	0.600	110	0	1	9.800
Beans—Pinto	½ cup	100	0	0	0	0	0	0.84	0.21	2.200	0.531	216	0	0	0
Cowpeas	½ cup	70	30	6	0	0	0	1	0.20	2.200	0.560	70	0	1	21
Lentils—Brown	½ cup	100	60	0	0	1.90	0	0.37	0.22	2	0.600	36	0	1.400	0
Peas	1 cup	140	640	27	0	0.22	0	0.35	0.14	3	0.160	50	0	0.750	9
Soybeans (mature)	¼ cup	50	80	0	0	23	190	1.10	0.30	2.200	0.800	170	0	1.700	80
Soybean Curd (tofu)	1 piece 2.5 x 1 x 2.75	120	0	0	0	0	0	0.06	0.03	0.100	0	0	0	0	0
Split Peas	½ cup	100	60	0	0	0	0	0.37	0.22	2	0	0	0	0	0

NUTRITIVE VALUES OF FOODS (VALUES PER 100 GM)
VITAMINS

FOOD Category and Substance	Normal Portion	Amt. Grams	(I.U.) A	(MG) C	(I.U.) D	(I.U.) E	(Mcg) K	(MG) Thia-mine	(MG) Ribo-flavin	(MG) Niacin	(Mcg) B-6	(Mcg) Folacin	(Mcg) B-12	(MG) Panto-thenic	(Mcg) Biotin
SEAWEED															
Hijiki	¼ cup	8	0	0	0	0	0	0	0	0	0	45	80	0.630	0
Kombu	¼ cup	8	190	13	5400	0	0	0.07	0.26	2.100	10	45	45	0.630	0
Nori	¼ cup	8	6474	14	5400	0	0	0.28	1.20	5.500	70	45	80	0.630	0
Wakami	¼ cup	8	255	15	5400	0	0	0.11	0.14	10	0	45	80	0.630	0
FISH AND SHELLFISH															
Bass—Black Sea	3.5 oz.	100	0	0	0	0	0	0.10	0.08	1.900	0	9	0	0	0
Bass—White Sea	3.5 oz.	100	0	0	0	0	0	0.10	0.03	2.100	0	9	0	0	0
Catfish	3.5 oz.	100	217	0	0	0	0	0.04	0.03	1.500	0.290	20	2.200	0.470	0
Clams	4 cherrystone	70	100	10	0	0	0	0.10	0.18	1.300	0.080	0	19.100	0.300	0
Cod	3.5 oz	100	33	2	52	0.33	0	0.06	0.07	2.200	0.230	18	0.800	0.140	3
Crab (steamed)	3.5 oz.	100	2200	2	0	0	0	0.16	0.08	2.800	0.300	15	10	0.600	0
Haddock	3.5 oz	100	0	0	0	0.58	0	0.04	0.07	3	0.180	10	1.300	0.130	5
Halibut	3.5 oz.	100	440	0	44	1.27	0	0.07	0.07	8.300	0.430	15	1	0.280	8
Herring (Pacific)	1 herring	50	100	3	315	1.60	0	0.02	0.16	3.500	0.370	11	2	1	4.500
Lobster	1 cup cubed	145	0	0	0	2.20	0	0.10	0.05	1.500	0	17	0.500	1.500	5
Mackerel (Atlantic)	3.5 oz.	100	450	3	1100	2.26	0	0.15	0.33	8.200	0.500	9	9	0.240	18
Ocean Perch	3.5 oz	100	40	0.80	3	1.86	0	0.10	0.08	1.900	0.230	9	1	0.360	0
Oysters	med—2 selects	25	300	30	320	1 30	0	0.14	0 18	2.500	0.050	10	18	0.250	9
Perch—White	3.5 oz	100	170	1	0	0	0	0.01	0.04	1.500	0	0	0	0	0
Red Snapper	3 5 oz	100	0	0	0	0	0	0.17	0.02	3.500	0	0	0	0	0
Salmon (Atlantic)	3.5 oz	100	310	9	154	2	0	0.18	0.08	7	0.700	26	4	1.300	0.900
Salmon (Atlantic can)	1 can 6.5 oz	185	230	0	220	1.50	0	0.03	0.16	7.400	0.300	20	7	0.550	15
Sardines (Pacific)	3 5 oz	100	110	3	1150	0	0	0.02	0.15	3.600	0.240	16	17	1	24
Sardines—(Atlantic can)	3.5 oz	100	220	0	0	2 50	0	0.03	0.20	5.400	0.180	16	10	0.850	5
Scallops—Raw	1 large	25	100	0	0	0	0	0.10	0.06	1.300	0	16	1.200	0.130	0

Shark	3 5 oz	100	2417	0	0	0	0	0.02	0.03	6.600	0.250	0	0	0	0
Shrimp—Raw	3 5 oz	100	0	1 90	150	6	0	0.02	0.03	3.200	0.100	11	0.900	0.280	1
Sole	3 5 oz	100	0	0	0	0	0	0.05	0.05	1 700	0	11	0.800	0.300	0
Squid	3 5 oz	100	616	0	0	1.80	0	0.02	0.12	3.200	0.060	10	0	0	0
Swordfish	3 5 oz	100	1600	0	0	0	0	0.05	0.05	8	0	8	1	0.190	0
Tuna (canned)	½ cup	115	90	0	250	0	0	0.04	0.10	13	0.430	15	2.200	0.300	3
MEAT & POULTRY															
Beef—Loin/Sirloin	3 5 oz	100	10	0	0	0.20	0	0.09	0.19	5.200	0.230	7	1	0.500	0
Beef—Round	3.5 oz	100	10	0	0	0	0	0.09	0.19	5.200	0.400	6	1.850	0.660	5
Calves Liver	3.5 oz	100	22500	36	15	2	90	0.20	2 70	11	0.700	220	60	8	100
Chicken (dark meat)	3.5 oz.	100	70	3	0	0.40	0	0.08	0.20	6.200	0.330	10	0.360	1.200	10
Chicken (light meat)	3.5 oz	100	28	1.20	0	0.43	0	0.07	0.09	11	0.540	4	0.380	0.800	11
Ham (canned)	3.5 oz	100	0	0	0	1	15	0.50	0.20	4	0.400	8	0.600	0.680	5
Hamburger	3.5 oz	100	20	0	0	0.90	7	0.09	0.18	5	0.400	7	1.800	0.600	0
Lamb (choice)	3.5 oz.	100	0	0	0	0.90	0	0.15	0.20	5	0.280	4	2	0.550	6
Lamb—Loin	3.5 oz	100	0	0	0	0	0	0.18	0.25	5.800	0 280	4	2.200	0.280	0
Pork (thin)	3.5 oz.	100	0	0	0	0.90	11	0.95	0.20	5.100	0.450	8	0.700	0.800	5
Rabbit (domestic)	3.5 oz.	100	0	0	0	0.60	0	0.08	0.06	12.800	0.440	0	0	0.780	0
Turkey (light meat)	3.5 oz.	100	40	0	0	0.13	0	0.07	0.11	6	0.550	8	0.450	0.680	0
Turkey (dark meat)	3.5 oz.	100	140	0	0	0.95	0	0.09	0.22	3.300	0.360	11	0.400	1.200	0
Veal	3.5 oz	100	0	0	152	0	0	0.14	0.25	6	0.340	5	1.600	0.900	2
Veal—Loin	3.5 oz.	100	0	0	0	0	0	0.14	0.26	6.600	0.340	5	1.750	0.900	0
FRUIT															
Apples	1 med 2 75 in. diam.	150	52	6	0	0.90	0	0.02	0.01	0.077	0.048	2.800	0	0.061	0.900
Applesauce—Unsweetened	½ cup	100	30	1	0	0.20	2	0.01	0.03	0.200	0.026	0.600	0	0.100	0.300
Apricots	1 med.	40	2612	10	0	0.75	0	0.03	0.04	0.600	0.054	8.600	0	0.240	0
Avocado	1 cup	150	612	8	0	2	8	0.11	0.12	1.900	0.280	62	0	1	5.500
Banana	1 med	150	81	9	0	0.40	2	0.05	0.10	0.500	0.580	19	0	0.260	4.400
Blueberries	1 cup	140	100	13	6.40	0	0	0.05	0.05	0.400	0.036	6.400	0	0.090	0
Cantaloupe	0.5 med	400	3220	42	0	0.20	0	0.04	0.02	0.600	0.120	17	0	0.130	3
Cranberries	1 cup	100	46	14	0	0	0	0.03	0.02	0.100	0.065	1.700	0	0.220	0

NUTRITIVE VALUES OF FOODS (VALUES PER 100 GM)

VITAMINS

FOOD Category and Substance	Normal Portion	Amt. Grams	(I.U.) A	(MG) C	(I.U.) D	(I.U.) E	(Mcg) K	(MG) Thiamine	(MG) Riboflavin	(MG) Niacin	(Mcg) B-6	(Mcg) Folacin	(Mcg) B-12	(MG) Pantothenic	(Mcg) Biotin
Dates—Nat'l & Dried	5 w/o pits	40	50	3	0	0	0	0.09	0.10	2.200	0.190	12.600	0	0.780	0
Figs—Raw	2 large/3 small	100	142	2	0	0	0	0.06	0.05	0.400	0.110	6.700	0	0.390	0.300
Grapefruit	sections 1 cup	190	10	33	0	0.37	0	0.04	0.02	0.200	0.043	10	0	0.280	3
Grapes	1 cup	150	100	4	0	0	0	0.09	0.06	0.300	0.110	4	0	0.024	1.600
Lemon (peeled)	1 med.	100	30	53	0	1.20	0	0.04	0.02	0.100	0.080	10.600	0	0.190	0
Lime	1 med.	100	10	29	0	0	0	0.03	0.02	0.200	0	8.200	0	0.220	0
Nectarine	2 med.	100	736	5.40	0	0	0	0.02	0.04	1	0.025	3.700	0	0.160	0
Orange	1 med.	180	200	53	0	0.36	1	0.09	0.04	0.300	0.060	30	0	0.250	1.900
Papaya	1/3 med.	100	2010	62	0	0	0	0.03	0.03	0.400	0.019	0	0	0.220	0
Peaches	1 med.	100	535	7	0	0.90	8	0.02	0.04	1	0.018	3.400	0	0.170	1.700
Pears	1 small	75	20	4	0	0.80	0	0.02	0.04	0.100	0.018	7.300	0	0.070	0.100
Persimmon—Native	1 med.	100	0	66	0	0	0	0.02	0.03	0.200	0	0	0	0	0
Pineapple	1 cup diced	140	25	15	0	0.15	0	0.09	0.04	0.400	0.080	11	0	0.160	0
Plums	2 med.	100	320	9.50	0	0.70	0	0.04	0.10	0.500	0.080	2.200	0	0.180	0.100
Raisins	2 T	18	8	3	0	1	6	0.16	0.09	0.800	0.250	3.300	0	0.045	4.500
Raspberries—Red	3/4 cup	100	130	25	0	0.45	0	0.03	0.09	0.900	0.057	0	0	0.240	1.900
Strawberries	1 cup whole	150	27	57	0	0.18	13	0.02	0.07	0.200	0.054	17.700	0	0.340	4
Watermelon	1 cup diced	160	370	9.60	0	0	0	0.08	0.02	0.200	0.140	2.200	0	0.200	3.600
Orange Juice	1 cup	248	200	50	0	0.06	0	0.09	0.03	0.400	0.040	55	0	0.190	0.800
CEREAL															
Buckwheat	1 cup	100	0	0	0	5.50	0	0.60	0.15	4.400	0.300	0	0	1.500	0
Grape Nuts	1 cup	224	4409	0	143	1.60	0	1.30	1.50	17.600	1.800	353	5.300	0.950	0
Cereals—Rolled Oats	1 cup	80	0	0	0	1.60	20	0.60	0.14	1	0.140	52	0	1.090	24
Cereals—Rye	1 cup	80	0	0	0	1.80	0	0.40	0.22	1.600	0.350	78	0	1	6
Shredded Wheat	1 biscuit	25	0	0	0	0.54	0	0.26	0.28	5.300	0.250	50	0	0.830	0
Wheat Flakes	1 cup	30	0	0	0	0.63	0	0.64	0.14	4.900	0.300	0	0	0.470	0
Whole Wheat Hot	1 cup	125	0	0	0	1.60	17	0.40	0.30	4.900	0.019	78	0	0.920	0

GRAIN															
Grains—Barley	1/4 cup	50	0	0	0	0.85	0	0.12	0.05	3	0.220	20	0	0.500	31
Bulgur Wheat	1/2 cup	100	0	0	0	0.09	0	0.30	0.15	4	0.200	46	0	0.700	0
Cornmeal	1/4 cup	30	510	0	0	0.22	0	0.38	0.11	2	0.250	24	0	0.580	6.600
Gluten Flour	1 cup	140	0	0	0	0	0	0.03	0.03	0.500	0	25	0	0	0
Millet	1/4 cup	25	0	0	0	0.07	0	0.73	0.38	2 300	0.750	0	0	0	0
Popcorn (plain—popd)	3 cups	42	0	0	0	0	0	0.37	0.12	2.200	0.200	0	0	0	0
Rice (brown—raw)	short grain—1/4 cup	50	0	0	0	2	0	0.34	0.05	5	0.550	16	0	1.100	12
Rye Flour	1 cup—sifted	88	0	0	0	0.64	0	0.15	0.07	0.600	0.090	12	0	0.720	6
Wheat Bran	1 T	6	0	0	0	2.20	80	0.70	0.35	20	0.800	260	0	3	14
Wheat Flour (enr)	1/2 cup sifted	55	0	0	0	0.04	0	0.44	0.26	3.500	0.060	21	0	0.470	1
Wheat Flour (wh)	1/2 cup sifted	55	0	0	0	0.37	4	0.55	0.12	4.300	0.340	54	0	1.100	9
Wheat Germ	1 T	6	0	0	0	90	350	2	0.70	4	1.200	330	0	1.200	17
Wild Rice	1/4 cup	40	0	0	0	0	0	0.45	0.63	6.200	0	0	0	1.020	0
DAIRY															
Butter Milk	1 cup	244	33	1	0	0.07	0	0.03	0.15	0.100	0.034	5	0.220	0.280	1.500
Lowfat Milk (2%)	1 cup	244	210	1	42	0	2	0.04	0.17	0.100	0.040	5	0.360	0.320	0
Skim Milk	1 cup	244	210	1	42	0.01	0	0.04	0.14	0.100	0.040	5	0.380	0.330	1.500
Whole Milk	1 cup	244	210	0.90	42	0.09	3	0.04	0.16	0.100	0.040	5	0.360	0.310	5
Yogurt (lowfat)	1 cup	244	70	0.80	1 12	0.06	0	0.04	0.20	0.200	0.050	11	0.600	0.600	3.300
CHEESE															
Cheese—American	1 slice 2.25 x 2.25 x .25	25	1200	0	12	1	35	0.03	0.35	0.100	0.070	8	0.700	0.500	0
Cheese—Cheddar	1 inch cubed	30	1100	0	12	1	35	0.03	0.38	0.100	0.070	18	0.800	0.400	3.600
Cheese (cottage)—Dry Curd	1 cup	200	30	0	12	1	35	0.03	0.14	0.200	0.080	15	0.830	0.160	0
Cheese—Cottage (1% fat)	1/4 cup	60	37	0	12	1	35	0.02	0.17	0.130	0.070	12	0.600	0.200	0
Cheese (feta)	1 inch cube	17	0	0	12	1	35	0	0	0	0	0	0	0	0
Cheese—Monterey Jack	1 inch cube	30	950	0	12	1	35	0	0.40	0	0	0	0	0	0
Mozzarella (part skim)	1 inch cube	30	600	0	12	1	35	0.02	0.30	0.100	0.070	9	0.800	0.080	0

NUTRITIVE VALUES OF FOODS (VALUES PER 100 GM)

VITAMINS

FOOD Category and Substance	Normal Portion	Amt. Grams	(I.U.) A	(MG) C	(I.U.) D	(I.U.) E	(Mcg) K	(MG) Thia-mine	(MG) Ribo-flavin	(MG) Niacin	(Mcg) B-6	(Mcg) Folacin	(Mcg) B-12	(MG) Panto-thenic	(Mcg) Biotin
Ricotta (part skim)	½ cup	124	430	0	12	1	35	0.02	0.19	0.080	0.020	0	0.290	0	0
Cheese—Swiss	1 inch cube	30	800	0	12	1	35	0.02	0.37	0.090	0.080	6	1.700	0.400	0
BREAD															
Pumpernickel	1 slice	32	0	0	0	0	4	0.22	0.13	1.250	0.160	0	0	0.500	0
Bread—Rye—Amer	1 slice	25	0	0	0	0	4	0.18	0.07	1.400	0.100	23	0	0.450	0
Bread—Wheat	1 slice	25	0	0	0	0.15	4	0.30	0.10	2.800	0.180	58	0	0.800	2
EGGS															
Eggs—White	1 med	15	0	0.30	0	0	0	1	0.29	0.100	0.003	16	0.070	0.240	7
Eggs—Whole	1 whole med refuse 12%	50	520	0	56	1	11	0.09	0.30	0.062	0.120	65	1.500	1.700	23
Eggs—Yolk	1 med	29	1839	0	100	3 10	0	0.25	0.44	0.070	0.300	152	3.800	4.400	52
NUTS & SEEDS															
Almonds	1 T	8	0	0	0	36	0	0.24	0.90	3.500	0.100	100	0	0.500	18
Cashew	14 large	28	100	0	0	0.28	0	0.43	0.25	1.800	0	70	0	1.300	0
Chestnuts (fresh)	2 lrge 3 smll	15	0	27	0	0 70	0	0.22	0.22	0.600	0.330	0	0	0.470	1.500
Peanuts (roasted)	1 T chpd or 15 whl	9	0	0	0	10	0	0.32	0.13	17	0.300	100	0	2	35
Pecans	10 large	9	130	2	0	1.80	0	0.86	0.13	0 900	0.180	24	0	1.710	27
Pumpkin Seeds	⅛ cup	17	70	0	0	0	0	0.24	0.19	2.400	0.090	0	0	0	0
Sunflower Seeds	⅛ cup	18	50	0	0	74	0	2	0.23	5.400	1 300	234	0	1.400	0
OILS															
Butter—Salted	1 T	14	3000	0 20	35	2 40	30	0.01	0.03	0.042	0.003	3	0	0.050	0
Corn Oil	1 T	14	0	0	0	21	0	0	0	0	0	0	0	0	0
Olive Oil	1 T	14	0	0	0	17 80	0	0	0	0	0	0	0	0	0
Safflower Oil	1 T	14	0	0	0	50	0	0	0	0	0	0	0	0	0
Sesame Oil	1 T	14	0	0	0	1 40	0	0	0	0	0	0	0	0	0
Soy Oil	1 T	14	0	0	0	16	0	0	0	0	0	0	0	0	0
MISCELLANEOUS															
Melba Toast	1 slice	4	0	0	0	0	0	0 16	0 16	0	0	0	0	0	0

NUTRITIVE VALUES OF FOODS (VALUES PER 100 GM)
MINERALS

FOOD Category and Substance	Normal Portion	Amt Grams	(MG) Ca	(MG) P	(MG) Mg	(MG) K	(MG) Na	(MG) Fe	(MG) Cu	(MG) Mn	(MG) Zn	(Mcg) Se	(Mcg) Cr
VEGETABLES													
Artichoke—Boiled	base & ends—leaves	100	50	70	12	300	30	1 100	0.310	0.360	0.350	0	0
Asparagus	4 large spears	100	22	60	20	280	2	1	0.210	0.180	0.800	0	4
Beets (greens)	cooked 1 cup	150	120	40	106	570	130	3.300	0.090	0.900	0	0	4
Beets—Red Raw	1 cup diced	140	16	33	29 500	335	60	0 700	0 130	1.260	1.090	0	5
Broccoli	1 med stalk	180	100	80	24	380	15	1 100	0.011	0.056	0.270	0	11
Brussels Sprouts	2 large	140	36	80	30	390	14	1 500	0.011	0.110	0.370	18	10
Cabbage	1 cup finely shredded	90	50	30	13	230	20	0.560	0.060	0.060	0.140	2.300	8
Cabbage—Chinese	cup 1 inch pcs	75	43	40	14	253	23	0.600	0	0	0.270	0	5
Cabbage—Red	1 cup shredded	100	40	35	13	270	25	0.800	0.090	0	0.460	0	5
Carrots	1 carrot 7 5 x 1 125	80	37	36	23	340	47	0.510	0.011	0.020	0.120	2.200	5
Cauliflower	1 cup whole flowerettes	100	25	56	24	300	13	0 580	0.011	0.160	0.460	0.700	3
Celeriac	¼ of 1 lrge	100	43	115	0	300	100	0.600	0.020	0.150	0.310	10	4
Celery	1 cup chopped	120	40	28	22	340	130	0.480	0.010	0.020	0.070	0.600	8
Chard	¼ lb	115	90	40	65	550	145	3.200	0.110	0.800	0	0	6
Corn	1 cob 5 x 1 75 (kernels)	140	3	110	50	280	0.300	0.700	0.011	0.020	0.400	0.400	9
Cucumber	1 small 6.5 x 1.5	180	25	27	11	160	6	1 100	0.010	0.060	0.100	0	1
Eggplant	1 cup diced	200	12	26	16	200	2	0.700	0.090	0.190	0.280	0	2
Garlic	1 clove (1.3 x .5 x .3)	3	30	200	27	530	19	1.500	0.170	0.330	1.330	27.600	4
Kale	¼ lb	115	180	70	37	380	75	2.200	0.090	0.550	0	2.300	4
Leeks	3–4 (5 inches)	100	50	50	23	350	5	1 100	0.100	0	0.100	0	8
Lettuce—Iceberg	wedge 125 of head	90	20	22	11	175	9	0.500	0.037	0.070	0.250	0.800	4
Lettuce—Romaine	1 cup chpd	55	68	26	11	264	9	1.100	0.040	0.310	0.260	0	7
Mushrooms	1 cup sliced or diced	70	6	120	13	400	15	1.700	0.260	0.030	1.100	13	14
Mushrooms—Shiitake	2 oz.	55	16	240	0	2590	100	3.900	0	0	0	0	14
Onions	1 cup chopped	160	27	36	12	160	10	0.500	0.100	0.080	0.110	1.500	11
Parsley	1 T chpd	4	200	60	40	700	45	6.200	0.520	0.940	0.900	0	4

NUTRITIVE VALUES OF FOODS (VALUES PER 100 GM)
MINERALS

FOOD Category and Substance	Normal Portion	Amt. Grams	(MG) Ca	(MG) P	(MG) Mg	(MG) K	(MG) Na	(MG) Fe	(MG) Cu	(MG) Mn	(MG) Zn	(Mcg) Se	(Mcg) Cr
Peppers—Green	1 cup strips	100	9	22	18	210	13	0.700	0.070	0.150	0.100	0.600	10
Pepper (red—sweet)	1 large or 1 cup strips	100	13	30	9.460	213	0	0.600	0.040	0.150	0.210	0	10
Potato—White	2.75 x 4.25	250	7	50	35	400	3	0.760	0.050	0.040	0.200	0.500	21
Potato—Sweet	5 x 2	180	30	50	30	240	10	0.700	0.060	0.620	0.160	0.700	20
Radishes (red)	10 small (1 in. diam)	100	30	30	15	320	18	0	0.130	0.040	0.180	4	3
Spinach	1 cup chopped	55	90	50	90	470	70	3	0.080	0.600	0.400	18	10
Squash (summer)	1 cup—cubed	130	28	29	16	200	1	0.400	0.140	0.100	0.300	0	1
Squash (winter)	1 cup baked	205	22	38	17	370	1	0.600	0.100	0.220	0.440	0	3
Tomato	2 5 inch diam.	100	13	27	14	240	3	0.500	0.010	0.020	0.046	0.500	9
Turnip Greens	1/4 lb	115	250	60	60	470	71	1.800	0.090	1.420	0	0	5
Waterchestnut	4 chstnts	25	4	65	0	500	20	0.600	0	0	0	0	4
Yams	1/4 lb	115	20	70	40	600	10	0.600	0.160	0	0.400	0	20
LEGUMES													
Beans—Garbanzos	1/4 cup	50	150	330	144	800	26	7	0.740	1.220	2.700	0	10
Beans—Green	1 cup	100	56	44	30	240	7	0.800	0.040	0.270	0.300	0.600	4
Beans—Lima	1/2 cup	100	72	385	180	1530	4	7.800	0.180	0.540	2.800	0	10
Beans—Pinto	1/2 cup	100	135	457	0	984	10	6.400	0	0	4.400	0	17
Cowpeas	1/2 cup	70	75	430	230	1000	35	5.800	0	0	2.800	0	10
Lentils—Brown	1/2 cup	100	80	377	80	790	30	6.800	0.660	0	3.100	11	11
Peas	1 cup	140	26	120	35	300	2	2	0.130	0.110	1.300	0.300	4
Soybeans (mature)	1/4 cup	50	230	550	265	1700	5	8	0.110	2.800	3.600	60	10
Soybean Curd (tofu)	1 piece 2 5 x 1 x 2 75	120	130	130	110	40	7	2	0	0	0	0	0
Split Peas	1/2 cup	100	0	260	80	670	36	7.600	0.580	0	3.100	0	18
SEAWEED													
Hijiki	1/4 cup	8	0	0	0	0	0	60	0	0	0	0	0
Kombu	1/4 cup	8	950	360	1670	10600	2500	7	0	0	0	3.500	0
Nori	1/4 cup	8	350	510	2040	3300	1290	74	0	4	0	1.300	0
Wakami	1/4 cup	8	1162	195	3050	4200	2500	43	0	0	0	5.900	0

FISH AND SHELLFISH													
Bass—Black Sea	3 5 oz	100	20	207	0	255	70	1	0	0	0.700	0	0
Bass—White Sea	3 5 oz	100	20	212	0	256	68	1	0	0	0.700	0	0
Catfish	3 5 oz	100	37	187	19.060	330	60	0.400	0.100	0.060	0.700	0	0
Clams	4 cherrystone	70	70	160	0	180	120	6	0	0	1.500	0	40
Cod	3 5 oz	100	10	200	28	400	70	0.400	0.230	0.010	14.600	43	7
Crab (steamed)	3 5 oz	100	43	175	34	180	210	0.800	0.270	0.020	3.600	0	0
Haddock	3 5 oz	100	25	200	24	300	60	0.700	0.011	0.020	0.320	20	5
Halibut	3 5 oz	100	13	211	23	449	54	0.700	0.230	0.010	0.700	0	1
Herring (Pacific)	1 herring	50	45	225	0	420	74	1.300	0	0	0.700	143	0
Lobster	1 cup cubed	145	29	200	22	180	210	0.600	0.730	0.040	1.800	63	2
Mackerel (Atlantic)	3.5 oz	100	5	230	28	420	100	1	0.160	0.020	0.500	120	4
Ocean Perch	3.5 oz	100	20	200	32	270	80	1	0	0	0.700	196	0
Oysters	med—2 selects	25	90	140	32	120	70	5.500	3.070	0.210	40	65	13
Perch—White	3.5 oz	100	50	192	0	286	50	0.900	0	0	0.700	0	0
Red Snapper	3 5 oz	100	16	214	28	323	67	0.800	0	0	0.700	0	0
Salmon (Atlantic)	3 5 oz	100	80	190	29	420	74	0.900	0.200	0	0.930	0	1
Salmon (Atlantic can)	1 can 6 5 oz	185	154	300	30	400	74	0.900	0.080	0.020	1 100	0	0
Sardines (Pacific)	3.5 oz	100	33	215	24	420	74	1.800	0.170	0	2.300	85	20
Sardines (Atlantic can)	3.5 oz	100	437	500	52	590	823	2.900	0.040	0	3	0	20
Scallops—Raw	1 large	25	26	210	38	396	255	1.800	0	0	0.850	0	11
Shark	3.5 oz	100	14	204	27.300	549	79	1 100	0.030	0.020	0.310	0	0
Shrimp—Raw	3.5 oz	100	60	170	50	220	140	1.600	0.240	0.030	1.500	60	12
Sole	3.5 oz	100	12	200	73	340	80	0.800	0.010	0.020	0.300	0	16
Squid	3.5 oz	100	12	120	20.460	223	158	0.500	1.670	0.050	1.560	0	0
Swordfish	3 5 oz	100	19	200	0	449	54	0.900	0	0	0.700	0	0
Tuna (canned)	½ cup	115	16	200	23	280	40	1.600	0.010	0.020	0.400	130	5
MEAT AND POULTRY													
Beef—Loin/Sirloin	3 5 oz	100	12	200	22	355	65	3.200	0.040	0.020	4.200	0	7
Beef—Round	3.5 oz	100	13	220	16	355	65	3.200	0.050	0.020	3	36	44
Calves Liver	3.5 oz	100	8	330	16	280	70	9	5	0.170	4	43	40
Chicken (dark meat)	3.5 oz	100	12	160	23	220	85	1	0.063	0.021	2	12	13

NUTRITIVE VALUES OF FOODS (VALUES PER 100 GM)
MINERALS

FOOD Category and Substance	Normal Portion	Amt. Grams	(MG) Ca	(MG) P	(MG) Mg	(MG) K	(MG) Na	(MG) Fe	(MG) Cu	(MG) Mn	(MG) Zn	(Mcg) Se	(Mcg) Cr
Chicken (light meat)	3.5 oz	100	12	187	27	240	68	0.730	0.040	0.020	0.970	11	11
Ham (canned)	3.5 oz	100	11	160	19	340	1100	2.700	0.340	0.020	1 700	0	26
Hamburger	3.5 oz	100	12	200	21	350	65	3	0.060	0.020	3.400	20	6
Lamb (choice)	3 5 oz	100	10	150	15	295	75	1.200	0.060	0.020	3	18	8
Lamb—Loin	3.5 oz	100	6.800	185	16	300	75	1.300	0.045	0.020	2.400	0	9
Pork (thin)	3 5 oz	100	11	226	22	285	70	2.900	0.011	0.020	1.400	24 -	10
Rabbit (domestic)	3.5 oz	100	20	350	25	385	43	1.300	0.540	0	1.400	0	0
Turkey (light meat)	3 5 oz	100	12	210	27	314	67	1	0.060	0.020	1 700	0	11
Turkey (dark meat)	3 5 oz	100	17	185	21	290	80	1.600	0.140	0.020	3.400	0	11
Veal	3 5 oz	100	11	200	15	320	90	3	0.050	0.020	3	0	7
Veal—Loin	3 5 oz	100	11	200	16	320	90	0.670	0	0	2.160	0	7
FRUIT													
Apples	1 med 2 75 in diam	150	7	7	5	115	1	0.200	0.040	0.045	0.040	0.300	2
Applesauce—Unsweetened	½ cup	100	3	7	3	75	2	0 120	0.030	0.080	0.030	0.200	8
Apricots	1 med	40	14	19	12	296	1	0.500	0.040	0.080	0.260	0	0
Avocado	1 cup	150	11	42	39	634	10	1.020	0.270	0.230	0.420	0	0
Banana	1 med	150	6	20	29	400	1	0.300	0 100	0.150	0.160	1	9
Blueberries	1 cup	140	6	10	5	90	6	0.200	0.060	0.300	0.110	0	5
Cantaloupe	½ med	400	11	17	11	310	9	0.200	0.042	0.047	0.160	0	2
Cranberries	1 cup	100	7	10	5	70	1	0.200	0.060	0.160	0.130	0	0
Dates—Nat'l & Dried	5 w o pits	40	32	40	35	650	3	1 200	0.290	0.300	0.300	0	19
Figs—Raw	2 large 3 small	100	35	14	17	230	1	0.370	0.070	0.130	0.200	0	0
Grapefruit	sections 1 cup	190	12	8	9	148	1	0.060	0.050	0.010	0.070	0	0.500
Grapes	1 cup	150	14	10	5	190	2	0 300	0.040	0.718	0.040	0	3
Lemon (peeled)	1 med	100	26	16	28	140	2	0 600	0.040	0	0.060	12	1
Lime	1 med	100	33	18	0	100	2	0 600	0 070	0	0 110	0	1
Nectarine	2 med	100	4	16	8	212	0	0 150	C 070	0.044	0.090	0	0

Orange	1 med	180	40	14	10	180	1	0.100	0.045	0.025	0.070	1.300	3
Papaya	1/3 med	100	24	5	10	260	3	0.100	0.016	0.011	0.070	0	0
Peaches	1 med	100	5	12	7	200	1	0.110	0.070	0.050	0.140	0.400	2
Pears	1 small	75	11	11	6	130	2	0.300	0.110	0.080	0.120	0.600	2
Persimmon—Native	1 med	100	27	26	0.800	310	1	2.500	0	0	0	0	0
Pineapple	1 cup diced	140	7	7	14	110	1	0.400	0.110	1.700	0.080	0.600	0
Plums	2 med	100	4	10	7	172	2	0.100	0.043	0.049	0.100	0	2
Raisins	2 T	18	50	100	33	750	12	2.100	0.310	0.310	0.270	0	6
Raspberries—Red	3/4 cup	100	22	12	18	150	0	0.900	0.074	1.010	0.460	0	0
Strawberries	1 cup whole	150	14	19	10	170	1	0.400	0.120	0.290	0.130	0	3
Watermelon	1 cup diced	160	8	9	11	116	2	0.200	0.032	0.037	0.070	0	2
Orange Juice	1 cup	248	11	17	11	200	1	0.200	0.044	0.014	0.050	0	12
CEREAL													
Buckwheat	1 cup	100	114	280	253	450	0	3.100	0.430	2.090	0.870	18	38
Grape Nuts	1 cup	224	38	250	67	334	695	4.300	0.330	0	2.200	0	0
Cereals—Rolled Oats	1 cup	80	50	400	140	350	2	4.500	0.343	3.630	3.400	0	9
Cereals—Rye	1 cup	80	40	375	115	470	1	3.700	0.420	0	2.800	0	4
Shredded Wheat	1 biscuit	25	38	353	132	360	10	4.200	0.660	2.390	3.300	0	0
Wheat Flakes	1 cup	30	40	310	111	0	1032	4.400	0.450	1.500	2.300	0	0
Whole Wheat Hot	1 cup	125	40	380	122	390	2	3.400	0.460	3.200	2.700	0	0
GRAIN													
Grains—Barley	1/4 cup	50	16	200	37	160	3	2	0.370	1.600	2	66	8
Bulgur Wheat	1/2 cup	100	30	350	0	230	4	3	0	0	0	0	8
Cornmeal	1/4 cup	30	20	256	47	284	1	2.400	0.200	0.280	1.840	0	10
Gluten Flour	1 cup	140	40	140	0	60	2	0.400	0	0	1.650	0	8
Millet	1/4 cup	25	20	311	162	430	1	6.800	0.850	1.900	1.800	0	8
Popcorn (plain—popd)	3 cups	42	11	281	0	256	3	2.700	0	0	3.900	0	9
Rice (brown—raw)	short grain—1/4 cup	50	30	220	90	210	9	1.800	0.360	1.700	1.800	39	8
Rye Flour	1 cup--sifted	88	22	185	92	156	1	1.100	0.420	1.940	2.800	0	9
Wheat Bran	1 T	6	120	1300	490	1100	9	10.800	1.170	9.110	9.800	0	29
Wheat Flour (enr)	1/2 cup sifted	55	16	87	27	95	2	2.900	0.130	0.400	0.700	19.200	5
Wheat Flour (wh)	1/2 cup sifted	55	41	372	113	370	3	3.300	0	0	2.400	63	11

NUTRITIVE VALUES OF FOODS (VALUES PER 100 GM)
MINERALS

FOOD Category and Substance	Normal Portion	Amt. Grams	(MG) Ca	(MG) P	(MG) Mg	(MG) K	(MG) Na	(MG) Fe	(MG) Cu	(MG) Mn	(MG) Zn	(Mcg) Se	(Mcg) Cr
Wheat Germ	1 T	6	70	1100	340	800	3	5.600	0.950	9.300	14.300	111	14
Wild Rice	¼ cup	40	19	339	130	220	7	4.200	0	0	4.650	0	0
DAIRY													
Butter Milk	1 cup	244	116	89	11	150	50	0.050	0.005	0.010	0.400	0	1
Lowfat Milk (2%)	1 cup	244	120	95	14	150	50	0.050	0.010	0.003	0.400	9	0
Skim Milk	1 cup	244	120	100	11	166	52	0.040	0.005	0.010	0.400	4.800	1
Whole Milk	1 cup	244	120	90	13	150	50	0.050	0.005	0.010	0.400	1.200	1
Yogurt (lowfat)	1 cup	244	180	140	17	230	70	0.080	0.009	0.002	0.900	0	0
CHEESE													
Cheese—American	1 slice 2.25 x 2.25 x .25	25	600	750	22	160	1400	0.400	0.110	0.400	3	9	56
Cheese—Cheddar	1 inch cubed	30	720	500	28	100	620	0.700	0.050	0.110	3	0	29
Cheese (cottage)—Dry Curd	1 cup	200	32	100	4	32	13	0.230	0	0	0.470	0	3
Cheese—Cottage (1% fat)	¼ cup	60	60	130	5	90	400	0.140	0.020	0	0.400	5.400	0
Cheese (feta)	1 inch cube	17	490	340	19	60	1115	0.650	0	0	2.900	0	36
Cheese—Monterey Jack	1 inch cube	30	750	440	27	80	500	0.700	0	0	3	0	36
Mozzarella (part skim)	1 inch cube	30	650	460	23	84	470	0.200	0	0	3	0	36
Ricotta (part skim)	½ cup	124	270	180	15	125	125	0.440	0	0	1.300	0	0
Cheese—Swiss	1 inch cube	30	960	600	36	110	260	0.170	0.110	0.040	4	11	36
BREAD													
Pumpernickel	1 slice	32	84	230	72	450	570	2.500	0	0	1 100	0	7
Bread—Rye—Amer	1 slice	25	75	150	40	145	560	2.700	0.017	0.500	1.600	0	7
Bread—Wheat	1 slice	25	80	250	80	260	530	3.200	0.170	1.200	1.800	70	8
EGGS													
Eggs—White	1 med	15	11	11	9	140	150	0.030	0.005	0.010	0.020	5	8
Eggs—Whole	1 whole med refuse 12%	50	55	200	12	130	140	2.100	0.050	0.020	1.400	10.400	22
Eggs—Yolk	1 med	29	152	500	16	90	50	6	0.010	0.020	3.400	18	30

NUTS & SEEDS													
Almonds	1 T	8	230	500	270	775	4	5	1.240	1.900	3.570	2	0
Cashew	14 large	28	40	375	270	460	15	6.400	2 170	0.840	5.120	0	0
Chestnuts (fresh)	2 lrge 3 smll	15	30	90	33	454	6	1 700	0.060	3.670	0	0	0
Peanuts (roasted)	1 T chpd or 15 whl	9	70	400	175	700	5	2.200	0.400	1.500	3	0	0
Pecans	10 large	9	70	290	110	600	0	2.600	1 100	1.500	4.100	3	0
Pumpkin Seeds	⅛ cup	17	50	1140	0	0	0	10	0	0	0	0	7
Sunflower Seeds	⅛ cup	18	120	800	40	920	30	4.500	5	0.400	11	71	7
OILS													
Butter—Salted	1 T	14	24	23	2	26	800	0.160	0.030	0.040	0.050	146	17
Corn Oil	1 T	14	0	0	0	0	0	0	0	0	0.200	0	47
Olive Oil	1 T	14	0 180	1 200	0.010	0	0.040	0.400	0.070	0	0.060	0	0
Safflower Oil	1 T	14	0	0	0	0	0	0	0	0	0.200	0	7
Sesame Oil	1 T	14	0	0	0	0	0	0	0	0	0	0	0
Soy Oil	1 T	14	0.040	0 250	0.030	0.250	0	0.020	0	0	0.200	0	0
MISCELLANEOUS													
Melba Toast	1 slice	4	84	100	0	225	75	1.600	0	0	0	0	0
Yeast	1 oz	28	210	1750	230	1900	120	17	5.300	0.400	11	71	136

References and Notes

Chapter 1

1. P. Starr, *The Social Transformation of American Medicine.* New York: Basic Books, 1982.
2. *Ibid.*
3. T. S. Eliot, interview in *The New York Times*, September 21, 1958.
4. C. P. Snow, *The New Physicists.* Boston: Little, Brown, 1981.
5. R. L. Walford, in *Trends in U.S. Life Expectancy*, Hearing before Committee on Finance, U.S. Senate, 98th Congress, July 15, 1983. Washington, D.C.: Senate Hearing 98-359, 1983, pp. 116–31.
6. "Death and Taxes: The Public Policy of Living Longer." Washington, D.C.: Population Reference Bureau, Inc., September, 1984.
7. Cited by R. L. Walford, *Maximum Life Span.* New York: W. W. Norton, 1983, p. 99.
8. "Dr. Alexander Leaf's New Views on the Very Old," interview in *East West Journal*, September, 1984, p. 39.
9. R. A. Good, personal comunication. (Dr. Good is currently Chairman of Pediatrics at the University of South Florida College of Medicine.)
10. Quoted by Claudia Wallis, "Hold the Eggs and Butter," *Time*, March 26, 1984, p. 61.

11. Quoted by Joan Arehart-Treichel, "Eating Your Way Out of High Blood Pressure," *Science News*, 1983, p. 233.
12. S. B. Eaton and M. Konner, *New England Journal of Medicine* 312:283, 1985.
13. *Ibid.*

Chapter 2

1. S. Whittingham, J. Irwin, and I. MacKay, *Australian J. Medicine* 18:30, 1969.
2. R. Weindruch and R. L. Walford. *The Retardation of Aging by Dietary Restriction*. New York: Raven Press (scheduled for 1987).
3. The just-released *Normal Human Aging: The Baltimore Longitudinal Study of Aging* (ed. N. W. Shock *et al.*), NIH Publication No. 84-2450, November 1984, is of course a gold mine for the human biomarker area. Other useful books on human biomarkers are R. F. Morgan's *The Adult Growth Examination*. Fresno, Calif.: Internat. Assn. Applied Psychology, 1986; and particularly W. Dean's *Biological Aging Measurement*, El Toro, Calif.: The Aging Research Inst., 1986.
4. J. W. Hollingsworth *et al.*, *Yale J. Biol. Med* 38:11, 1965.
5. R. A. Defronzo, in *Biological Markers of Aging* (ed. M. E. Reff and E. L. Schneider), NIH Publication No. 82-2221, 1982, p. 98.
6. Whittingham *et al.*, *op. cit.*
7. R. Weindruch *et al.*, *Age* 5:111, 1982.

Chapter 3

1. C. M. McCay, in *Cowdry's Problems of Aging, Biological and Medical Aspects* (ed. A. I. Lansing). Baltimore: Williams and Wilkins, 1952, p. 130.
2. B. J. Merry and A. M. Holehan, 13th Internat. Congr. Gerontol., New York, July 12–17, 1985.

3. In the 1940s two University of Chicago professors (Carlson and Hoelzel, 1946) introduced the technique of intermittent fasting. Beginning at 42 days of age, and using a high-quality diet, rats were fasted 1 day in 4, 1 day in 3, and every other day. Maximum life span was increased by 20 to 30 percent in all instances, and *there was no stunting of growth on any of the regimens.*
A. H. Carlson and F. Hoelzel, *J. Nutrition* 31:363, 1946.
4. R. Weindruch and R. L. Walford, *The Retardation of Aging by Dietary Restriction.* New York: Raven Press (scheduled for 1987).
5. With caloric restriction beginning at time of weaning, scientists at the University of Texas (Yu *et al.*, 1982; Bertrand *et al.*, 1980) extended average life spans in rats from 32 months out to 47 months. In similar experiments scientists at the National Institute on Aging extended average life spans in rats by more than 83 percent (Goodrick *et al.*, 1982).
B. P. Yu *et al.*, *J. Gerontology* 37:130, 1982.
H. A. Bertrand, *J. Gerontology* 35:827, 1980.
C. L. Goodrick *et al.*, *Gerontology* 28:233, 1982.
6. G. Fernandes *et al.*, in *Immunology and Aging* (ed. T. Makinodan and E. J. Yunis). New York: Plenum Press, 1977, p. 111.
C. Kubo, B. C. Johnson, *et al.*, *J. Nutrition*, 114:1884, 1984.
R. A. Good, 13th Internat. Congress Gerontol., New York, July 12–17, 1985.
7. E. J. Masoro, *J. Nutrition* 115:842, 1985.
8. Goodrick *et al.*, *op. cit.*
9. C. Kubo, N. K. Day, *et al.*, *Proceedings Natl. Acad. Sci., USA*, 81:5831, 1984.
Kubo, Johnson, *et al.*, *op cit.* 1984.
10. R. Weindruch and R. L. Walford, *Science* 215:1415, 1982.
11. M. H. Ross, *Am. J. Clin. Nutr.* 25:834, 1972.

12. D. E. Harrison *et al.*, *Proceedings Natl. Acad. Sci., U.S.A.* 81:1835, 1984.
C. L. Goodrick *et al.*, AGE 6:145, 1983.
13. McCay, *op. cit.*
14. A. Tannenbaum, *Am J. Cancer* 38:335, 1940.
15. C. H. Barrows, Jr., and G. C. Kokkonen, in *Nutritional Approach to Aging Research* (ed. G. B. Moment). Boca Raton, Fla.: CRC Press, 1982, p. 219.
16. N. H. Sarkar *et al.*, *Proceedings Natl. Acad. Sci., U.S.A.* 79:7758, 1982.
17. Yu, *ibid.*
18. K. E. Cheney *et al.*, *J. Gerontology* 38:420, 1983.
M. H. Ross and G. J. Bras, *J. Nutrition* 103:944, 1973.
19. Weindruch and Walford, *op. cit.*
20. McCay, *op. cit.*
21. B. N. Berg and H. S. Simms in *Biological Aspects of Aging* (ed. N. Shock). New York: Columbia University Press, 1962, p. 35.
22. J. B. Young *et al.*, *Metabolism* 27:1711, 1978.
23. A. V. Everitt, *Mechanisms of Ageing and Development* 12:161, 1980.
24. M. T. R. Subbiah and R. G. Siekert, Jr., *J. Nutrition* 41:1, 1979.
25. J. E. Johnson, Jr., and C. H. Barrows, Jr., *Anatomical Record* 196:145, 1980.
A. V. Everitt, in *Nutritional Approach to Aging Research* (ed. G. B. Moment). Boca Raton, Fla: CRC Press, 1982, p. 245.
J. R. Wyndham *et al.*, *Archives of Gerontology and Geriatrics* 2:317, 1983.
26. R. L. Walford, *The Immunologic Theory of Aging*. Copenhagen: Munksgaard, 1969.
R. L. Walford, *Maximum Life Span*. New York: W. W. Norton, 1983.
S. R. S. Gottesman and R. L. Walford, in *Methods in Aging Research* (ed. R. C. Adelman and G. S. Roth). Boca Raton, Fla: CRC Press, 1982, p. 233.

27. Sufai-Kutti *et al.*, *Clinical Immunology and Immunopathology*, 15:293, 1980.
R. Weinruch *et al.*, AGE, 5:111, 1982.
G. Fernandes *et al.*, *Proceedings Natl. Acad. Sci. U.S.A.* 80:874, 1983.
J. A. Levy and W. J. W. Morrow,.*Immunology Today* 4:249, 1983.

28. K. Nandy, *Mechanisms of Ageing and Development* 18:97, 1982.

29. Caloric restriction not only will slow the rate of immune-system aging, but may even bring about some *rejuvenation*. One good test measures the response of white blood cells (lymphocytes) to certain plant extracts. At UCLA we have investigated the extracts known as PHA and Con-A. They stimulate lymphocytes to produce fresh DNA (the hereditary double-helix material in each cell) and then to divide into two new cells. We have found that the lymphocytes of 16-month-old mice that had been on the high/low diet since 12 months of age respond to PHA and Con-A *to the same degree as 6–8-month-old fully fed mice* (Weindruch *et al.*, 1979). Evidently this rejuvenation does not involve *all* bodily systems, since the maximum life span of this lot of mice was extended by only 20 percent. Nevertheless, the results—actual rejuvenation of at least one important age-deteriorating function—are highly encouraging. Rejuvenation is even better than retardation.
R. Weindruch and R. L. Walford, *Federation Proceedings* 38:2007, 1979.

30. D. N. Kalu *et al.*, *Mechanisms of Ageing and Development* 26:103, 1984.
D. N. Kalu *et al.*, *Endocrinology* 115:1239, 1984.

31. *Ibid.*

32. P. J. Leveille *et al.*, *Science* 224:1247, 1984.

33. S. Chipalkatti *et al.*, *J. Nutrition* 113:944, 1983.

34. D. E. Harrison and J. R. Archer, *Experimental Aging Research* 9:245, 1984.

35. G. M. Reavan and E. P. Reaven, *Metabolism* 30:982, 1981.
36. R. J. M. Carter *et al.*, *Am. J. Physiol.* 242: R89–93, 1982.
37. E. J. Masoro, "Food Restriction and the Aging 'Process." *J. Am. Geriatric Soc.* 32:296, 1984.
38. *Ibid.*

39. Two of these features deserve an illustration. We see in the left panel of the figure below that the cholesterol level of a 24-month-old rat on a high/low diet is the same as that of a fully fed rat merely 12 months old; and in the right panel, the response of fat cells to the hormone glucagon falls to zero by 6 months of age in fully fed rats, but on a high/low diet the response is held at a very youthful level until 12 months, and then declines slowly.

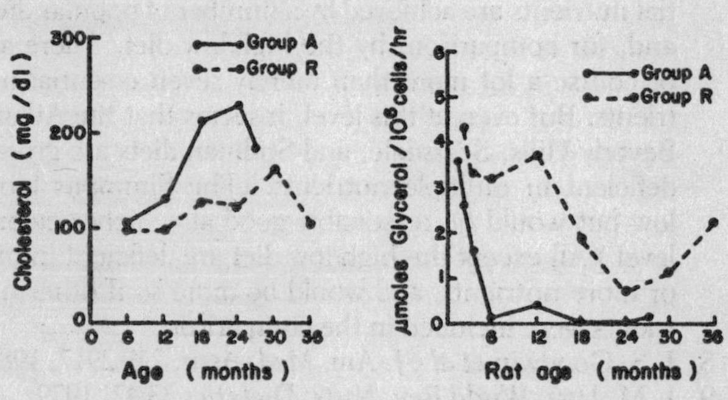

Effect of a high/low diet on blood cholesterol in rats, and on the response of fat cells to the hormone glucagon.
Left Panel, Cholesterol: The age-related rise which occurs in rats on a regular diet is much less in rats on the high/low diet.
Right Panel, Response to the hormone glucagon: In rats fed a regular diet the response falls rapidly after birth, and is negligible by 6 months; on the high/low diet even 12-month-old animals are responding like weanlings, and 18-month-old animals like 3-month-old animals (adapted from E. J. Masoro, *J. Am. Geriatrics Soc.* 32:296, 1984).

40. J. A. Joseph *et al. Neurobiology of Aging* 4:191, 1983.
41. R. F. Mervis *et al.*, AGE 7:144, 1984.
42. R. L. Walford, *Maximum Life Span*. New York: W. W. Norton, 1983.
43. C. L. Goodrick *et al.*, AGE 7:1, 1984.
44. D. K. Ingram *et al.*, *J. Gerontology* (in press).

Chapter 4

1. W. Edmundson, *Ecology Food Nutr.* 8:189, 1979.
2. R. R. Recker and R. P. Heanen, *Am. J. Clin. Nutr.* 41:254, 1985.
3. *Consumer Reports*, February, 1981, p. 68.
4. P. B. Swan, *Annual Review of Nutrition* 3:413, 1983.
5. W. Mertz, *Nutrition Today* 19:22, 1984.
6. M. A. Walker and L. Page, *Journal of the American Dietetic Association* 66:146, 1975.
7. The table given opposite shows what percentages of the Recommended Daily Allowances for seven essential nutrients are achieved by a number of popular diets and, for comparison, by the high/low diet. There are of course a lot more than merely seven essential nutrients. But even at this level, it seems that the Atkins, Beverly Hills, Scarsdale, and Stillman diets are grossly deficient in multiple nutrients. (The Simmons looks low but would be reasonably good at a higher caloric level.) All except the high/low diet are deficient in one or more nutrients, and would be more so if other nutrients were included in the comparison.
8. J. S. Goodwin *et al.*, *J. Am. Med. Assn.* 249:2917, 1983.
9. J. M. Hsu, *World Rev. Nutr. Dietetics* 33:42, 1979.
10. M. H. Ross and G. J. Bras, *Nature* 250:263, 1974.
11. M. H. Ross, in *Nutrition and Aging* (ed. M. Winick). New York: Wiley & Sons, 1976, p. 43.
12. R. Weindruch and R. L. Walford, *Science* 215:1415, 1982.
13. A. Keys *et al.*, *Biology of Human Starvation*. Minneapolis: Univ. of Minnesota Press, 1950.

Values in Percentage of Recommended Daily Allowances

Diet	Average Calories	Thiamine	Vit. B_6	Vit. B_{12}	Calcium	Magnesium	Iron	Zinc
Atkins	2,136	73	80	145	80	53	69	92
Beverly Hills	1,058	60	65	0	33	72	64	25
Carbohydrate Cravers	1,190	93	70	63	97	87	76	71
California	1,240	107	70	45	97	90	77	65
F-plan	1,256	153	145	58	85	160	146	138
I Love America	1,256	87	60	55	93	77	70	75
I Love New York	1,490	93	80	177	100	108	102	93
Pritikin	1,304	120	110	40	112	126	114	86
Simmons	888	60	55	108	67	56	57	53
Scarsdale	1,014	60	65	37	52	74	56	52
Stillman	1,304	60	65	753	45	55	84	117
High/Low	1,358	185	181	417	108	143	115	115

(Values for the first 11 diets adapted from M. C. Fisher and P. A. Lachance, *Journal of American Dietetic Association* 85:450, 1985. Values for high/low diet are averages from the 20 days of food combinations, Appendix A, this book.)

14. T. J. Thomson *et al*, *Lancet* 2:992, 1966.
15. But in some cases body-protein loss during prolonged dieting has resulted in cardiac-muscle loss and sudden death.
16. H. L. Taylor, *Am. J. Physiol.* 143:148, 1945.
17. A. J. Stunkard, *Nutrition, Longevity, and Aging* (ed. M. Rockstein and M. L. Sussman). New York: Academic Press, 1976, p. 253.
18. K. H. Duncan *et al.*, *Am. J. Clin. Nutr.* 37:763, 1983.
19. *Ibid.*
20. M. Krotkiewski, *Brit. J. Nutr.* 52:97, 1984.
21. A. S. Levine and J. E. Morley, *Nutrition Today*, January/February, 1983, p. 6.
22. S. D. Morrison, *Nutrition Reviews* 41:133, 1983.
23. R. Carmena *et al.*, *Internatl. J. Obesity* 8:135, 1984.
    T. A. Hughes *et al.*, *Am. J. Med.* 77:7, 1984.
    J. Zimmerman *et al.*, *Arteriosclerosis* 4:115, 1984.
24. M. J. Pertshuk *et al.*, *Am. J. Clin. Nutr.* 35:968, 1982.
25. N. A. Ricotti *et al.*, *New Eng. J. Med.* 34:1601, 1984.
26. J. A. Golla *et al.*, *Am. J. Clin. Nutr.* 34:2756, 1981.
27. R. Weindruch *et al.*, *Proceedings Natl. Acad. Sci., U.S.A.* 79:898, 1982.
28. Y. Kagawa, *Preventive Medicine* 7:205, 1978.
29. Y. Kagawa *et al.*, *J. Nutr. Sci. Vitaminol.* 28:441, 1982.
30. Y. Kagawa, *Preventive Medicine*, *op. cit.*
31. E. Schneider and J. A. Brody, *New Eng. J. Med.* 309:854, 1983.
32. L. A. Gavrilov *et al.*, *Gerontology* 29:176, 1983.
33. E. A. Vallejo, *Revista Clinica Española* 63:25, 1957.

Chapter 5

1. R. S. Goor *et al.*, *Am. J. Clin. Nutr.* 4:299,1985.
2. E. S. Horton, *Am. J. Med.* 30:32, 1983.
   D. Blair et al., *Amer. J. Epidemiology* 119:526, 1984.
3. R. Andres, in *Aging, Cancer and Cell Membranes*, Vol. 7 of *Adv. Pathobiology* (ed. C. Borek, C. M. Fenoglio,

and D. W. King). New York: Thieme-Stratton, 1980, p. 238.
4. A. J. Stunkard, *Internatl. J. Obesity* 7:201, 1983.
5. W. P. Catelli (Director of Framingham Heart Study), cited by *Wall Street Journal*, Dec. 1, 1982, p. 32.
6. G. G. Roads and A. Kagan, *Lancet* 1:492, 1983.
7. A. J. Stunkard, *J. Psychedelic Drugs* 10:331, 1978.
8. R. L. Leibel and J. Hirsch, *Metabolism* 33:164, 1984.
9. *Nutrition Reviews* 43:61, 1985.
10. A. P. Simopoulos, *Nutrition Reviews* 2:33, 1985.
G. Kolata, *Science* 227:1019, 1985.
11. D. P. Burkitt in *Nutrition and Killer Diseases* (ed. J. Rose), Park Ridge, N.J.: Noyes Pub., 1982, p. 1.
12. M. J. Gibney and P. G. Burstyn, *Atherosclerosis* 35:339, 1980.
13. W. Dock, *New Eng. J. Med.* 285:58, 1971.
14. *Nutrition Reviews* 9:317, 1984.
15. M. S. Brown and J. L. Goldstein, *Scientific American* November, 1984, p. 58.
16. A. Keys, *Am. J. of Epidemiology* 121:870, 1985.
17. The diet of Paleolithic man derived 20 percent of its calories from fat (See p. 31).
18. A. Keys, *Am. J. Clin. Nutr.* 40:351, 1984.
19. M. Liebman and T. L. Bazzarre, *Amer. J. Clin. Nutr.* 38:612, 1983.
20. R. S. Goor and B. M. Rifkind in *Nutrition and Killer Diseases* (ed. J. Rose), Park Ridge, N.J.: Noyes Pub., 1982, p. 84.
21. E. Hietanen (ed.), *Regulation of Serum Lipids by Physical Exercise*. Boca Raton, Fla.: CRC Press, 1982.
22. R. Saynor *et al.*, *Atherosclerosis* 50:3, 1984.
23. B. E. Phillipson *et al.*, *New Eng. J. Med.* 312:1210, 1985.
24. D. Kromhout *et al.*, *New Eng. J. Med.* 312:1205, 1985.
25. K. K. Carroll, *Federation Proceedings* 41:2792, 1982.
26. R. A. Anderson and A. S. Kozlovsky, *Am. J. Clin. Nutr.* 41:1177, 1985.

27. M. S. Seelig in *Intervention in the Aging Process.* Part A: *Quantitation, Epidemiology and Clinical Research* (ed. W. Regelson and F. M. Sinex). New York: Alan R. Liss, 1983, p. 279.
28. R. J. Morin, *Longevity Letter*, April, 1985, p. 2.
29. H. Trowell *et al.*, *Lancet* 1:967, 1976.
M. A. Eastwood and R. Passmore, *Nutrition Today* 19:6, 1984.
30. *Consumer Reports*, February, 1980, p. 68.
31. J. H. Zavoral *et al.*, *Am. J. Clin. Nutr.* 38:285, 1983.
R. Sarathy and G. Saraswathi, *Am. J. Clin. Nutr.* 38:295, 1983.
K. M. Behall *et al.*, *Am. J. Clin. Nutr.* 39:209, 1984.
A. Aro *et al.*, *Am. J. Clin. Nutr.* 39:911, 1984.
32. D. R. Swanson, *Longevity Letter*, April, 1985, p. 4.
33. H. B. Hubert, *Circulation* 67:968, 1983.
34. J. L. Marx, *Science* 219:158, 1983.
35. National Research Council, *Diet, Nutrition, and Cancer.* Washington, D.C.: National Academy Press, 1982.
36. *Ibid.*
37. *Nutr. Rev.* 43:170, 1985.
C. Garland *et al.*, *Lancet* 1:307, 1985.
38. On the other hand, certain *pro*carcinogens such as the chemicals benzo(a)pyrene, AAF, and DMBA are actually *activated* into carcinogens by the mixed-function oxidases. And the Brassicaceae family effect might equally be due to stimulation of the enzyme glutathione transferase. So the beneficial anticancer effect of these vegetables seems real, but the mechanism is not yet clear.
39. D. W. Winn *et al.*, *Cancer Research* 44:1216, 1984.
40. D. A. Denton, in *Mechanisms of Hypertension* (ed. M. P. Sambhi), *Excerpta Medica Amsterdam*, 1973, p. 46.
H. Blackburn and R. Prineas, *Karger Gazette* 44–45:1, 1983.
41. *Nutr. Action*, March, 1985.
42. J. Z. Miller *et. al.*, *Hypertension* 5:790, 1983.

43. G. Berglund, *Acta Medica Scandinavia* (Suppl.) 672: 117, 1983.
44. A. J. Stunkard, in *Nutrition, Longevity and Aging* (ed. M. Rockstein & M. L. Sussman). New York: Academic Press, 1976, p. 253.
45. J. M. Iacono *et al.*, *Am. J. Clin. Nutr.* 38:860, 1983.
46. P. Puska, *Lancet* 1:1, 1983.
47. K. T. Khaw *et al.*, *Lancet* 2:1127, 1982.
48. D. A. McCarron *et al*, *Science* 224:1392, 29 June, 1984.
49. Swanson, *op. cit.*
50. H. W. Gruchow *et al.*, *J. Am. Med. Assn.* 253:1567, 1985.
51. M. R. Sowers *et al.*, *Am. J. Clin. Nutr.* 42:135, 1985.
52. J. Villar *et al.*, *Internatl. J. Gynaecol. & Obstet.* 21:271, 1984.
53. J. M. Belizan *et al.*, *J. Am. Med. Assn.* 249:1161, 1983.
54. R. T. Jarrett, in *Nutrition and Killer Diseases* (ed. J. Rose). Park Ridge, N.J.: Noyes Pub., 1982, p. 107.
55. S. Goldstein, *Pathologie Biologie* (Paris), 32:99, 1984.
R. Vracko and E. P. Benditt, *Federation Proceedings* 34:68, 1975.
56. G. Kolata, *Science* 203:1098, 1979.
57. S. Pongor *et al.*, *Proceedings Natl. Acad. Sci. U.S.A.* 81:2684, 1984.
58. J. Olefsky, *J. Clinical Investigation* 53:64, 1974.
59. E. Reaven *et al.*, *Diabetes* 32:175, 1983.
60. J. W. Anderson in *Dietary Fiber in Health and Disease* (ed. G. V. Vahouny and D. Kritchevsky). New York: Plenum Press, 1982, p. 151.
G. Ricardi *et al.*, *Diabetologia* 26:116, 1984.
61. D. J. A. Jenkins, in *Nutritional Pharmacology* (ed. G. A. Spiller). New York: Alan R. Liss, 1982, pp. 117–145.
62. J. F. Halter and M. Chen, in *Nutritional Approaches to Aging Research* (ed. G. B. Moment). Boca Raton, Fla.: CRC Press, 1982, p. 14.
63. J. M. Hsu, *World Rev. Nutr. & Diet* 33:42, 1979.
64. J. F. Potter, *Metabolism* 34:199, 1985.

65. T. A. Hughes *et al.*, *Am. J. Med.* 77:7, 1984.
66. R. Marcus *et al.*, *J. Clinical Endocrinology and Metabolism* 58:223, 1984.
67. C. C. Johnson, Jr., and S. Epstein, *Orthopedic. Clinics of North America* 12:559, 1981.
68. H. Spencer, *Clinical Orthopaedics and Related Research* 184:270, 1984.
69. E. L. Radin and L. E. Lanyon, in *Lectures on Gerontology*, Vol. I, Part B (ed. A. Viidik). New York: Academic Press, 1982, p. 379.
70. *Nutrition Action*, December, 1984, p. 12.
71. R. R. Recker and R. P. Heaner, *Am. J. Clin. Nutr.* 41:254, 1985.
72. D. Kalu *et al.*, AGE 6:141, 1983.

Chapter 6

1. They need to be paired because in addition to swirling around the central nucleus, each electron spins on its own axis; and to maintain stability in the universe, for reasons known best to the high priests of physics, every electron spinning to the right must be balanced by one spinning to the left. Atmospheric oxygen is a rare exception to this rule, having two *un*paired electrons, a phenomenon exploited by all aerobic (oxygen-using) organisms.
2. W. A. Pryor, *Annals of N.Y. Acad. Sci.* 1:393, 1982; and Pryor in *Free Radicals in Molecular Biology, Aging, and Disease* (ed. D. Armstrong *et al.*). New York: Raven Press, 1984, pp. 13–41.
3. By John Crowe Ransom, "Captain Carpenter."
4. Many antioxidants, or "scavengers," are enzymes which change the free radicals into stable compounds. Superoxide dismutase, catalase, and glutathione peroxidase are examples of free-radical scavengers, and they guard against the superoxide anion radical, against hydrogen peroxide, and against the hydroxyl radical, respectively. Some vitamins (E and C) also have antioxidant properties.

5. J. Marx, *Science* 219:158, 1983.
B. N. Ames. *Science* 221:1256–64, 1983.

6. The relationship holds for superoxide dismutase, uric acid, the carotenes, and vitamin E (Cutler, 1983; Cutler, 1984). However, a number of other free-radical scavengers do *not* show such a relationship: vitamin C, glutathione, and glutathione peroxidase (the enzyme that requires selenium). And if some free-radical scavengers do and just as many do not correlate with maximum life span, one could interpret the data in either of two directions. Dr. Richard Cutler of the National Institute of Aging tends to dismiss the noncorrelating antioxidants as not being important in aging. Whether the cart is before the horse is difficult to say because they are going in a circle.
R. G. Cutler, in *Intervention in the Aging Process. Part B: Basic Research and Preclinical Screening* (ed. W. Regelson and F. M. Sinex). New York: Alan R. Liss, 1983, p. 69.
R. G. Cutler, *Proceedings Natl. Acad. Sci. U.S.A.* 81:7627, 1984.

7. More fully, the pigment is a degradation product resulting from the reactions of a cross-linking agent (malondialdehyde) with cell membranes. And malondialdehyde comes from free-radical processes involving lipid peroxidation. It has been shown that the peroxide levels in serum and brain bear a roughly inverse relation to maximum life span in mammals, right on up from mouse to monkey to man (Cutler, 1983). But again we have a paradox: certain drugs will greatly slow down or inhibit the development of the pigment in mammals, but exert little or no effect on maximum life span. So what is the real relevance of the pigment?
Cutler, in *Intervention in the Aging Process*, *op. cit.*

8. A. Tappel *et al.*, *J. Gerontology* 28:415, 1973.
D. G. Hafeman and W. G. Hoekstra, *J. Nutrition* 107:656, 1977.
R. D. Lippman, *Review of Biological Research in Aging*

(ed. M. Rothstein). New York: Alan R. Liss, 1982, 1:315.

9. Antioxidants such as vitamin E or the chemical agent Santoquin were reported to improve the immune response of mice (Harman *et al.*, 1977). The height of the response was greater in antioxidant-treated animals. That sounds like a favorable result. However, examination of the data reveals that the time at which the immune response peaked was *later* in the treated mice. If aging were really being retarded, the peak should come *sooner*, as that would represent reversal of what is seen in normal aging. When rich and not-so-rich antioxidant mixtures were fed to mice, the former but not the latter inhibited the buildup of age pigment; but only the latter improved the biomarkers represented by treadmill performance and kidney function, and neither antioxidant mixture improved survival (Tappel *et al.*, 1973). Thus a clear picture does not emerge.

   D. H. Harman *et al.*, *J. Am. Geriatrics Soc.* 25:400, 1977.

   A. Tappel *et al.*, *op. cit.*

10. Some extension of species maximum life span may have been achieved by antioxidant therapy in invertebrate species such as fruit flies.

11. E. L. Schneider and J. D. Reed, *New Eng. J. Med.* 312:1159, 1985.

12. Below are reproduced, adjusted to the same scale, the seven "best" survival-curve studies using antioxidants which I can find in the biological literature. Even where some differences were detected between antioxidant-fed and normally fed animals (chart F in the figure), neither population exceeded the maximal life spans for the species.

    Compare these curves with those of Figure 3.1 from high/low diet studies in naturally long-lived mouse strains (page 59). The difference is striking.

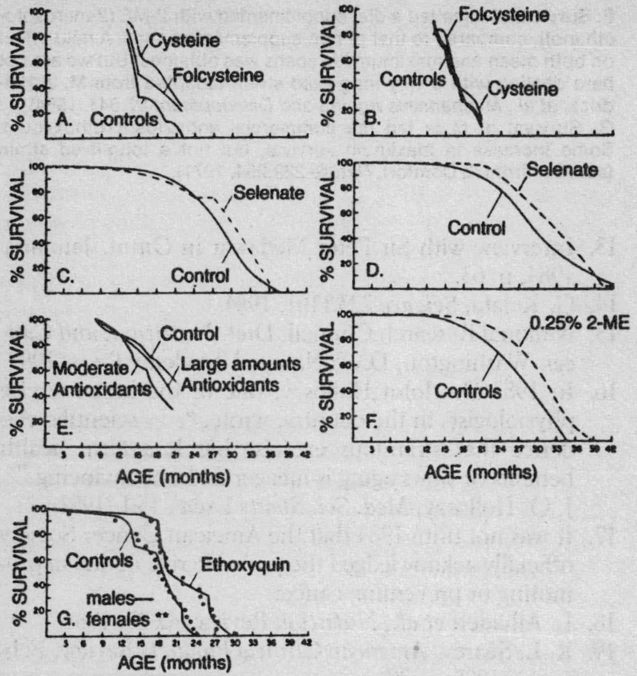

Survival curves of long-lived strains of mice and rats given various antioxidants throughout part or all of their lives.
A&B: In male mice (A), treatment by injection with large doses of cysteine or folcysteine (folic acid + thiazolidincarboxylic acid) on alternate days for 42 days led to increased survival; but (B) in female rats no effect at all was seen (adapted from S. Oeriu and E. Vochitsu, *J. Gerontology* 20:417, 1965).
C&D: Survival curves of male (C) and female (D) rats fed either a normal diet or a diet supplemented with selenium (as selenate). We see mild increases in mean life spans in the supplemented animals, but no significant differences in maximum life spans (adapted from N. A. Schroeder and M. Mitchner, *J. Nutrition* 101:1531, 1971).
E: Survival curves of mice fed normally or given a cocktail containing moderate amounts of vitamin E, BHT, vitamin C, methionine, and selenium, or large amounts of these same compounds. Either there was no effect, or the antioxidants slightly decreased survival (adapted from A. Tappel *et al.*, *J. Gerontology* 2:415, 1973).

F: Survival of mice fed a diet supplemented with 2-ME (2-mercaptoethanol), compared to that of non-supplemented mice. A mild effect on both mean and maximum life spans was obtained. But we are not here dealing with a very long-lived strain (adapted from M. J. Heidrick, *et al.*, *Mechanisms Ageing and Development* 27:341, 1984).

G: Survival of mice fed the commercial antioxidant Ethoxyquin. Some increase in maximum survival, but not a long-lived strain (adapted from A. Comfort, *Nature* 229:254, 1971).

13. Interview with Sir Peter Medawar in *Omni*, January, 1984, p. 63.
14. G. Kolata, *Science* 223:1161, 1984.
15. National Research Council, *Diet, Nutrition, and Cancer.* Washington, D.C.: National Academy Press, 1982.
16. In 1983 Dr. John Holloszy, one of the best exercise physiologists in the country, wrote, ". . . scientific evidence that strenuous exercise has long-term health benefits or slows aging is meager and unconvincing." J. O. Holloszy, *Med. Sci. Sports Exerc.* 15:1, 1983.
17. It was not until 1984 that the Ameican Cancer Society officially acknowledged the probable role of diet in promoting or preventing cancer.
18. L. Alhadeff *et al.*, *Nutrition Reviews* 42:33, 1984.
19. R. L. Searcy, *American Clinical Products Review*, February, 1985, p. 20.
20. H. F. Carroll and S. Emerson, *Nutrition Reviews* 42:265, 1984.
    D. B. Roll, *Nutrition Reviews* 42:265, 1984.
21. Both an increase and a decrease in cholesterol have been attributed to intake of vitamin C, but in none of the studies in humans was the effect statistically significant (Klevay, 1976). Very large doses of ascorbic acid given over a six-month period have not been toxic in experimental mice (Deschner *et al.*, 1983). One short article reports that vitamin C given to pregnant rats in dosages equivalent to 20 gm. per day in humans may cause kidney damage (Lavender, 1978). However, at least a few humans have taken doses of vitamin C up to 15 gm. per day without known ill effects (White,

1981). Convincing evidence of severe vitamin C toxicity has been found in guinea pigs. When kept on an unfortified wheat diet and given large doses of vitamin C, the guinea pigs experienced a high death rate within 25 days (Nandi *et al.*, 1973). But when milk casein was added to the wheat diet, thus supplying the essential amino acid lysine, no toxicity at all was seen. Thus, large doses of vitamin C might be harmful to a person on a meatless, amino acid–imbalanced diet. But this is *reductio ad absurdum.* There seems to be reasonable evidence that vitamin C may interfere with the absorption of copper, an essential trace element, from the gastrointestinal tract (Solomons *et al.*, 1979; Finley, 1983). This is the only untoward effect that rests on solid evidence.

L. Klevay, *Proceedings of the Society for Experimental Biology and Medicine* 151:579, 1976.
D. Deschner, *Nutrition and Cancer* 4:241, 1983.
L. M. Lavender, *Federation Proceedings* 37:321, 1978.
J. D. White, *New Eng. J. Med.* 304:1491, 1981.
B. K. Nandi *et al.*, *J. Nutr.* 103:1688, 1973.
N. W. Solomons, *Am. J. Clin. Nutr.* 32:856, 1979.
E. B. Finley, *Am. J. Clin. Nutr.* 37:553, 1983.

22. H. J. Roberts, *J. Am. Med. Assn.* 246:129, 1981.
23. H. J. Roberts, *Angiology* 30:169, 1979.
24. Bieri *et al.*, *New Eng. J. Med.* 308:1063, 1983.
25. The *Federal Register* of 1979, a publication of the Food and Drug Administration, states that the maximum safe dose of vitamin E is certainly greater than 400 International Units, and that doses up to 3,000 units for up to eleven years have had no detrimental effect.
26. W. M. Ringsdorf and E. Chereskin, *J. Holistic Medicine* 6:49, 1984.
27. Nutrient-balance studies have forced an increase in RDAs for calcium from the previous 800 mg./day up to 1,200 mg./day. At the lower figure, 30–40 percent of men were found to be in negative calcium balance.
28. H. Kamin, *Am. J. Clin. Nutr.* 41:165, 1985.

29. Only a single and limited study has addressed this problem. While mice fed ½ RDA levels of (all) vitamins lived 12 percent less long than controls, there was no difference in survival between mice fed regular RDA and those fed 4 times the RDA amounts of (all) vitamins (Kokkonen and Barrows, 1985). Of course 4-times-RDA amounts of vitamin E, for example, would still be quite small in terms of an antioxidant effect.

C. C. Kokkonen and C. H. Barrows, *AGE* 8:13, 1985.

30. R. Anderson *et al.*, *Am J. Clin. Nutr.* 33:71, 1980.

31. L. M. Corwin and R. K. Gordon, *Annals of N.Y. Acad. Sci.* 393:437, 1982.

32. Ames, *Ibid.*

Chapter 7

1. P. J. Hornsby and J. F. Crivello, *Molecular and Cellular Endocrinology* 30:1, 1983.

2. Vitamin E works mainly on the cell membranes, where it protects polyunsaturated fatty acids against free-radical attacks (Lippman, 1983). It may also to some degree protect the DNA of cells against radiation-induced damage, mutation, and chemically induced cancer (Beckman and Roy, 1982; Ames, 1983). And it has been reported to markedly increase the endurance of rats during exercise sufficiently strenuous to cause extensive free-radical damage to tissues (Davies *et al.*, 1982).

R. D. Lippman, in *Rev. Biol. Research in Aging* (ed. M. Rothstein). New York: Alan R. Liss, 1983, 1:315.

C. Beckman and R. M. Roy, *Mutation Research* 105:73, 1982.

B. N. Ames, *Science* 221:1256, 1983.

K. J. A. Davies *et al.*, *Biochemical Biophysical Research Communications* 107:1198, 1982.

3. J. Epstein and D. Gershon, *Mechanisms of Ageing and Development* 1:257, 1972.

H. E. Enesco and C. Verdon-Smith, *Experimental Gerontology* 15:335, 1980.
M. Kahn and H. E. Enesco, *AGE* 4:109, 1981.
J. E. Fleming and L. S. Yengoyan, *AGE* 4:132, 1981.
M. Sawada and H. E. Enesco, *Experimental Gerontology* 19:179, 1984.

4. In the worm C. *briggsae*, the maximum normal life span of 56 days was incrased to 69 days by vitamin E (Epstein and Gershon, 1972). However—and now we must look at the evidence critically—in this and a similar experiment with another worm, *Turbatrix aceti* (Kahn and Enesco, 1981), the effect was obtained only if vitamin E was present very early in life. If it was present for the first 6 days and then withdrawn, a big effect was obtained; but very little benefit accrued if the vitamin was added after 10 days and kept in the diet for the rest of the life of the worms. An effect limited to an early phase of development does not suggest simple protection against free radicals, which of course are generated *throughout* life.

Yet another interpretive problem can be illustrated by these invertebrate studies. It is possible that the effects of antioxidants which are so glibly attributed to free-radical "scavenging" are really due to straightforward repression of oxygen metabolism. In fruit flies, a significant inverse correlation exists between simple oxygen consumption and average life span; those flies on antioxidants, including vitamin E, consume much *less* oxygen than control flies (Fleming and Yengoyan, 1981; Miquel *et al.*, 1982). This decreased consumption might lead to an enhanced metabolic efficiency, so positive effects could be due to such an alteration, rather than an antioxidant effect (Weber *et al.*, 1982).

Finally, a number of the effects attributed to free-radical scavenging might be due to interaction in prostaglandin pathways (Ball *et al.*, 1986). Indeed, vitamin E may enhance the immune response by suppressing prostaglandin E_2 synthesis (Meydani *et al.*, 1986).

M. Kahn and H. E. Enesco, *AGE* 4:109, 1981.

J. E. Fleming and L. S. Yengoyan, *AGE* 4:132, 1981.

J. Miquel *et al.*, *Archives of Gerontology and Geriatrics* 1:159, 1982.

H. U. Weber *et al.*, *Archives of Gerontology and Geriatrics* 1:299, 1982.

S. Ball *et al.*, in *Free Radicals, Aging and Degenerative Disease* (ed. J. E. Johnson and R. L. Walford). New York: Plenum Press, 1986 (in press).

S. N. Meydani *et al.*, *Mechanisms of Ageing and Development*, 1986 (in press).

5. D. Harman, *The Gerontologist* 8:13, 1968.
A. Tappel *et al.*, *J. Gerontology* 28:415, 1973.
A. D. Blackett and D. A. Hall, *J. Gerontology* 36:529, 1981.

6. A. Tappel *et al*, *J. Gerontology* 28:415, 1973.
A. S. Csallany *et al.*, *J. Nutrition* 107:1792, 1977.
Blackett and Hall, *op. cit.*
B. M. Zuckerman and M. A. Geist in *Age Pigments* (ed. R. S. Sohal). North Holland: Elsevier, 1981, p. 283.

7. Age pigment is the insoluble end product of free-radical damage to certain components of the cell, which have been further digested, degraded, and stored in vacuoles within the cell. The rate of accumulation of pigment in dog hearts is 5.5 times as fast as in human hearts and humans live about 5.5 times as long as dogs. The same relationship holds, albeit less proportionately, with other animal species. (See note 6, Chapter 6.)

8. R. P. Tengerdy in *Vitamin E: A Comprehensive Treatise* (ed. L. J. Machlin). New York: Marcel Dekker, 1980, pp. 429–44.
L. M. Corwin and R. K. Gordon, *Annals of N.Y. Acad. Sci.* 393:437, 1982.

W. R. Beisel, *Am. J. Clin. Nutr.* 35:Suppl. #2, 417, 1982.

9. T. Yasanaga *et al.*, *J. Nutrition* 112:1075, 1982.
10. Almost every aspect of the immune system, including resistance to infection, specific antibody responses, responses to mitogens, and "clearance" of particles from the blood, has been shown to be enhanced by moderate increases in vitamin E intake (Stinnett, 1983).
    J. D. Stinnett (ed.), *Nutrition and the Immune Response.* Boca Raton, Fla: CRC Press, 1983.
11. J. J. Barboriak *et al.*, *Am. J. Clin. Path.* 77:371, 1982.
12. N. J. Serfontein *et al.*, *Am. J. Clin. Path.* 79:604, 1983.
13. J. G. Bieri *et al.*, *New Eng. J. Med.* 308:1063, 1983.
    Tufts University Diet & Nutrition Letter 1:3–5, February, 1984.
14. R. S. London, *J. Am. Med. Assn.* Sept. 5, 1980, p. 1077.
    R. S. London *et al.*, *Cancer Research* 41:3811, 1981.
    Tufts University Diet & Nutrition Letter, op. cit.
15. Half the experimental cataracts in rabbits could be arrested and in some instances reduced in size by vitamin E administration (Kailish *et al.*, 1982).
    C. B. Kailish *et al.*, *Annals of N.Y. Acad. Sci.* 393:169, 1982.
16. W. C. Willett *et al.*, *New Eng. J. Med.* 310:430, 1984.
17. P. A. Cerutti, *Science* 227:375, 1985.
18. There are two stages in cancer promotion. Vitamin E is a stage 1 inhibitor; BHA and BHT generally act as stage 2 inhibitors.
19. *Tufts University Diet & Nutrition Letter, op. cit.*
20. C. E. Melton, *Aviation, Space, and Environ. Med.* 53:105, 1982.
    R. J. Stephens *et al.*, *Chest* 5:375, 1983.
21. A. Tsai *et al.*, *Am. J. Clin. Nutr.* 31:831, 1978.
22. Bieri *et al.*, *op. cit.*
    Tufts University Diet & Nutrition Letter, op cit.

23. M. K. Horwitt, *Am. J. Clin. Nutr.* 33:1856, 1980.
24. B. Kennes *et al.*, *Gerontology*, 29:305, 1983.
25. R. Anderson *et al.*, *Am. J. Clin. Nutr.* 33:71, 1980.
26. P. J. Hornsby and J. F. Crevello, *Molecular and Cellular Endocrinology* 30:1, 1983.
27. L. H. Chen, *Am. J. Clin. Nutr.* 34:1036, 1981.
28. R. D. Lippman, *J. Gerontology* 36:550, 1981.
29. Hornsby and Crivello, *op. cit.*
Zuckerman and Geist, *op. cit.*
30. J. E. W. Davies *et al.*, *Experimental Gerontology* 12:215, 1977.
31. H. R. Massie *et al.*, *Experimental Gerontology* 11:37, 1976.
32. H. R. Massie *et al.*, *Gerontology* 30:371, 1984.
33. The addition of 0.25 to 1 percent sodium ascorbate to their diet reduced the number of rats developing colon cancer in response to a chemical carcinogenic agent from 26 percent all the way down to zero (Reddy *et al.*, 1980). The frequency of aberrations in the DNA of coal-tar workers dropped from an initial value of 5 percent to a near-normal value of 1.8 percent after 3 months' daily intake of 1 gm. of vitamin C (Sr'am *et al.*, 1983).
B. S. Reddy *et al.*, *Advances in Cancer Research* 32:237–345, 1980.
R. J. Sr'am *et al.*, *Mutation Research* 120:181, 1983.
34. C. Moertal *et al.*, *New Eng. J. Med.* 312:127, 1985.
35. Linus Pauling, quoted in *Science* 85, July/August, 1985, p. 15.
L. Pauling *et al.*, *Proceedings Natl. Acad. Sci., U.S.A.* 82:5185, 1985.
36. Pauling *et al.*, *ibid.*
37. Of additional interest: administration of 1 gm./day of vitamin C to humans has been reported to lead to a 14-percent fall in blood cholesterol after 6–12 months of administration (Dobson *et al.*, 1984).
H. M. Dobson *et al.*, *Scottish Med. J.* 29:176, 1984.

38. W. R. Thomas and P. G. Holt, *Clinical and Experimental Immunology* 32:370, 1978.

39. Some bioflavonoids antagonize the mutagenic activities of polycyclic hydrocarbons (PHC), including the metabolites produced by p-450 enzymes acting upon these hydrocarbons (Huang *et al.*, 1983). The bioflavonoid "rutin" has strong activity in this regard. Another bioflavonoid, "quercetrin," inhibits development of experimental cataracts in the degu, a type of rodent from the Andes prone to develop cataracts (Varma *et al.*, 1977). But quercetrin may also be mutagenic (Stauric, 1984). We don't know much about the possible role of bioflavonoids in nutrition in part because there are so many different kinds—more than 500 (Havsteen, 1983).

M. Huang *et al.*, *Carcinogenesis*, 4:1631, 1983.
S. D. Varma *et al.*, *Science* 195:205, 1977.
B. Stauric, *Federation Proceedings* 43:2454, 1984.
B. Havsteen, *Biochem. Pharmacol.* 32:1141, 1983.

40. Glutathione peroxidase breaks down lipid (and other) peroxides, and also hydrogen peroxide, both of which are among the damaging free radicals generated by normal metabolism. And acting together, the enzymes glutathione peroxidase and superoxide dismutase may prevent the formation of perhaps the most dangerous of all free radicals, the superoxide radical (Sunde and Hoekstra, 1980). Increasing selenium intake in the diet will increase the level of glutathione peroxidase in both rats (Scott *et al.*, 1977) and humans (Thomson *et al.*, 1982). Organically bound selenium gives a greater response in humans than the inorganic form (Thomson *et al.*, 1982).

R. A. Sunde and W. G. Hoekstra, *Nutrition Reviews* 38:265, 1980.
D. L. Scott *et al.*, *Acta Biochemica Biophysica*, 497:218, 1977.
C. D. Thomson *et al.*, *Am. J. Clin. Nutr.* 36:24, 1982.

41. A. Griffin and S. Clark, *Advances in Cancer Research* 29:419, 1979.

42. But the "p-450" system is like a two-edged sword. The enzymes sometimes "activate" the simple organic chemicals into forms that are carcinogenic. Selenium may help decrease those p-450 activities which play a role in this activation (Griffin and Clark, 1979).
Griffin and Clark, *op. cit.*

43. H. A. Schroeder and M. Mitchner, *J. Nutrition* 101:1531, 1971.

44. A small bit of additional experimental evidence and one curious piece of anecdotal evidence can be added. An experimental study showed that adding selenium to the drinking water of mice not only decreased their frequency of spontaneous breast cancer but shifted the peak incidence of the cancer to a later age (Schrauzer and Ishmael, 1974). The age-specific peak incidence of cancer is a rather good biomarker of aging, so the shift might suggest an age-retarding effect. For the anecdotal evidence: when Representative Claude Pepper asked a number of centenarians about their health habits, the only common trait was that many of them ate lots of onions. Interestingly enough, we see from the "rich soil" column of Table 7.2 (p. 169) that of the plants we do eat, onions are the best selenium accumulators.
G. Schrauzer and D. Ishmael, *Annals of Clinical and Laboratory Science* 4:441, 1974.

45. Griffin and Clark, *op. cit.*
J. A. Milner and G. A. Greeder, *Science* 209:825, 1980.
R. A. Passwater, *Selenium as Food and Medicine.* New Canaan, Conn.: Keats Pub. Co., 1980.
Schrauzer and Ishmael, *op. cit.*
L. W. Wattenberg, *Adv. Cancer Res.* 26:197, 1970.
H. J. Thompson *et al.*, *Cancer Res.* 44:2803, 1984.

46. A study from the Harvard School of Public Health

conducted in 1982 examined the effect of selenium levels in the blood on *future* cancer risk (Willett *et al.*, 1983). Frozen blood samples were available from participants in a blood-pressure study done back in 1973. One hundred eleven of the participants in the study had died of cancer. Comparing the levels of their blood selenium with levels of 210 persons from the same study who had remained healthy, the investigators found that most of those who developed cancer had low selenium levels *even before* the onset of the cancer.

W. C. Willett *et al.*, *Lancet* 2:130, 1983.

47. G. D. Schrauzer and D. A. White, *Bioinorganic Chemistry* 8:303, 1978.
48. B. Liebman, *Nutrition Action*, December, 1983, p. 5.
49. R. A. Passwater, *Selenium as Food and Medicine*. New Canaan, Conn.: Keats Pub. Co., 1980.
    K. Jaakkola *et al*, *Scandinavian J. Clin. Lab. Med.* 43:473, 1983.
50. Schroeder and Mitchner, *op. cit*.
51. H. J. Thompson *et al.*, *Cancer Res.* 44:2803, 1984.
52. Organic selenium is usually manufactured by inclusion of selenium in the food fed to yeasts, which then incorporate it during their growth cycles. But some manufacturers simply mix brewer's yeast with inorganic selenium salts and press the mixture into tablets. Read the label to make sure this is not what you are getting. If it says "organically bound," that's okay. If it says "added to" or "fortified," that's not what you want.
53. R. Peto *et al.*, *Nature* 290:201, 1981.
    R. B. Shekelle, *Lancet* 2:1185, 1981.
54. W. C. Willett and M. MacMahon, *New Eng. J. Med.* 310:633, 1984.
55. Peto *et al.*, *op cit*.
56. G. W. Burton and K. U. Ingold, *Science* 224:569, 1984.

57. Ames, *op. cit.*
58. Burton and Ingold, *op. cit.*
59. There is very little evidence, for example, that carotenes prevent *spontaneous* cancer in animals (Kolata, 1984).
G. Kolata, *Science* 223:1161, 1984.
60. R. G. Cutler, *Proceedings Natl. Acad. Sci. U.S.A.* 81:7627, 1984.
61. The National Cancer Institute is now conducting a 5-year study in which about half of 14,000 male physicians are taking excess beta-carotenes and the other half a placebo, to see if there will be a difference in their cancer incidence.
62. Ames, *op. cit.*
63. G. A. Hazelton and C. A. Lang, *Proceedings of the Society for Experimental Biology and Medicine* 176:249, 1984.
64. S. Tas and R. L. Walford, *Mechanisms of Ageing and Development* 19:73, 1982.
65. S. Oerin and E. Vochitsu, *J. Gerontol.* 20:417, 1965.
66. D. Harman, *Radiation Research* 16:753, 1962.
67. See Note 12, chart F, Chapter 6 (p. 388).
68. Cysteine is not in any case an agent of choice, being quite unstable in the presence of merely trace amounts of copper and iron. Also, it is rapidly metabolized, and its movement into cells is regulated by specific transport systems. Thus, it seems unlikely that a high cysteine intake will increase the SH glutathione levels.

Glutathione itself is not effectively transported into cells (Meister, 1984), but at least two other agents seem able to increase SH glutathione in the tissues of animals: gamma-glutamyl cysteine and several forms of thiazolidine-4-carboxylic acid, or TC (Meister, 1984). Used so far in animals only by injection, gamma-glutamylcysteine bypasses a regulated step of SH glutathione synthesis, so it could be effective in raising SH levels (Anderson and Meister, 1983). TC has been used in humans for 20 years, in treating liver and bowel disturbances (Weber *et al.*, 1982). An amino acid and a natural liver metabolite, it elevates SH levels either when added to the diet or by injection. Following injection into mice, it raises the levels by at least 100 percent, depending upon dosage (Weber *et al.*, 1982). A related compound, L-2-oxo-TC, is thought to work much better (Weber *et al.*, 1982; Meister, 1983, 1984), especially its magnesium salt (Miquel and Lindseth, 1983). It may also help to slow the rate of accumulation of age pigment in cells and decrease plasma cholesterol (Miquel and Lindseth, 1983). And it increases the average life span of flies (Fleming and Yengoyan, 1981; Miquel and Lindseth, 1983) as well as mice (Oeriu and Vochitsu, 1965). Since TC is a normal component of mammalian cells, and has already been extensively used for treatment of liver disease, clinical testing as an antiaging drug in humans has been suggested (Miquel and Lindseth, 1983).

A. Meister, *Nutrition Reviews* 42:397–410, 1984.

M. E. Anderson and A. Meister, *Proceedings Nat. Acad. Sci.* 80:707–11, 1983.

H. U. Weber *et al.*, *Archives of Gerontology and Geriatrics* 1:299–310, 1982.

A. Meister, *Science* 220:472–77, 1983.

J. Miquel and K. Lindseth, in *Intervention in the Aging Process, Part B: Basic Research and Preclinical Screening* (ed. W. Regelson and F. M. Sinex). New York: Alan R. Liss, 1983, p. 317.

Fleming and Yengoyan, *op. cit.*

Oerin and Vochitsu, *op. cit.*

69. N. P. Buu-Hoi and A. R. Ratsimamanja, *C. R. Soc. Biol.* 153:1180, 1959.

Fleming and Yengoyan, *op. cit.*

Miquel and Lindseth, *op. cit.*

M. Heidrick *et al.*, *Mechanisms of Ageing and Development* 27:341, 1984.

70. Fleming and Yengoyan, *op. cit.*
71. A. Comfort, *Nature* 229:254, 1971. (See Note 12 of Chapter 6, curve G.)
72. BHT (The full chemical name is bishydroxytoluene) has been used more than BHA (bishydroxyanisole) in attempts to influence the aging process, and—at least so far as average life span is concerned—with a bit more success than other antioxidants. One group (Sharma and Wadhwa, 1983) found that it would prolong both average and maximum life span and decrease the accumulation of age pigment in fruit flies: for males, maximum life span went from 51 days for controls to 67 days for treated flies; for females, from 57 days for controls to 71 days for flies on BHT. In one study, rats fed BHT had better survival rates than controls but also (See my comments on pages 149–50) lower body weights (Olsen *et al.*, 1983). Another study showed *no* increase in survival in rats fed BHT for 104 weeks, or even a slight *decrease* at high doses (Hirose *et al.*, 1981). In a recent study, it was shown that feeding BHA to middle-aged mice would reduce the amount of age-related damage to DNA in their liver cells (Lawson and Stohs, 1985).

    Considerable discussion has arisen as to whether BHT may be toxic to the liver and/or cause cancer. Toxic effects are much sharper in rodents than in primates like monkeys (and presumably man) (Pascal, 1974; Brennan, 1975). Even so, ingestion of BHT by rats even in amounts up to 1 percent of the food intake for 2 years (a substantial portion of their total life span) has had little or no toxic effect, and has not increased the frequency of spontaneous cancers (Hirose *et al.*, 1982). High doses in rodents do increase the size of the liver (Crampton *et al.*, 1977), owing largely to the proliferation of the cells' machinery for making enzymes involved in the liver's normal function of metabolizing and discarding organic chemicals that get into the body and don't belong there (Scully *et al.*, 1976).

BHT and BHA have been shown in a number of studies to be not mutagenic, and indeed to *decrease* the mutagenicity of numerous chemical compounds (Talalay *et al.*, 1978; Slaga and Bracken, 1977; Wattenberg, 1978; Wattenberg *et al.*, 1980). BHT suppresses the induction of cancer by excess ultraviolet light (Black *et al.*, 1978): 70 percent of the control animals subjected to ultraviolet light developed skin tumors; BHT-treated animals, only 32 percent.

In contrast to the numerous studies (many more could be cited) in which BHT or BHA has been anticarcinogenic, there are a few claims for carcinogenicity. Most but not all of these present only marginal evidence. In one study (Clapp *et al.*, 1974), for example: at 12 months of age the incidence of *lung* tumors was 18 percent in normal mice, 11 percent in BHT-fed mice (a decrease); but at 18 months of age the incidences were 24 percent and 67 percent respectively, an increase in the BHT-treated mice at the later age. The incidence of lymph-gland tumors at 12 months was 23 percent in normal mice and 29 percent in BHT-fed mice (an increase); but at 18 months of age the situation reversed to 56 percent in normal mice and only 13 percent in BHT-fed mice. This double reversal makes the study less than convincing. The amount of BHT was 0.75 percent by weight added to the food—a very large amount. Recent well-conducted studies (Witschi and Morse, 1983; Imaida *et al.*, 1983; Cohen *et al.*, 1984) noted that 12 weeks of BHT treatment significantly *promoted* the development in mice of lung tumors induced by injection of urethane benzo(a)pyrene, a carcinogen; that BHT caused proliferation of cells in the lining of the lungs; that BHT or BHA *promoted* bladder cancer induced by the carcinogen BBN, but *inhibited* precancerous changes in the liver initiated by DENA; that BHT inhibited DMBA-induced mammary cancer and DMBA-induced proliferation of adrenal cells.

We see from the above that one group could recommend BHT or BHA as being prophylactic against cancer, and another could ban it as being carcinogenic. One possible reason for this duality concerns the interaction of BHT and BHA with enzymes that metabolize simple organic chemicals and drugs in the body—chemicals like benzene, drugs like phenobarbital. Mostly, these enzymes metabolize the chemicals or drugs to an inactive form, but in *some* combinations the final product may be carcinogenic. (See Note 42 above.) Now, BHT and BHA will induce higher levels of these enzymes—for example, for the curious, glutathione-S-transferase and epoxide hydratase, but *not* aryl hydrocarbon hydroxylase (Talalay *et al.*, 1978). In the majority of cases these enzymes lead to *inactivation* of potential carcinogens; however, in a few cases they may *activate* the carcinogens. In the majority of cases BHT and BHA alter the balance between metabolic activation and inactivation of carcinogens favorably. But not in all cases. And there's the problem. These metabolic effects of BHT and BHA are *in addition to* their antioxidant properties. Finally, in some instances BHT and BHA can suppress the immune system (Ball *et al.*, 1985) and thereby alter resistance to cancer.

While BHT has received more attention, BHA would seem the drug of choice if human application were to be considered (McCarty, 1984). It is considerably less toxic (Talalay *et al.*, 1978; Wattenberg, 1978), and as a possible side benefit, it will increase the level of glutathione in the body. In its 40-year history as a food additive, it has produced no known negative health effects in humans. A recent flurry over whether at the high dose of 2 percent it causes stomach tumors in rats has been mitigated by the fact that the tumors occur only in the "forestomach"—something unique to rodents and not present in pigs, dogs, or guinea pigs, which have proved unaffected by the same doses of the chemical. On current evidence, I do not recommend supplementation with BHA or BHT. England has favored BHT as a food additive; Japan has banned BHA.

S. P. Sharma and R. Wadhwa, *Mechanisms of Ageing and Development* 23:67, 1983.

P. Olsen *et al.*, *Pharmacologica & Toxicologica* 53:433, 1983.

M. Hirose *et al.*, *Food and Cosmetics and Toxicology* 19:147, 1981.

T. Lawson and S. Stohs, *Mechanisms of Ageing and Development* 30:179. 1985.

G. Pascal, *World Rev. Nutr. Diet.* 19:q37, 1974.

A. L. Brennan, *J. Am. Oil Chemists Society* 52:59, 1975.

R. F. Crampton *et al.*, *Toxicology*, 7:289, 1977.

M. F. Scully *et al.*, *Biochemical Society Transactions* 4:526, 1976.

P. Talalay *et al.*, *Adv. Enzyme Reg.* 17:23, 1978.

T. J. Slaga and W. M. Bracken, *Cancer Research* 37:1631, 1977.

L. W. Wattenberg, *Adv. Cancer Res.* 26:197. 1978.

L. W. Wattenberg *et al.*, *Cancer Res.* 40:2820, 1980.

H.S. Black *et al.*, *Cancer Research* 38:1384, 1978.

N. K. Clapp *et al.*, *Food and Cosmetics and Toxicology* 12:367, 1974.

H. R. Witschi and C.C. Morse, *J. Nat. Cancer Inst.* 71:859, 1983.

K. Imaida *et al.*, *Carcinogenesis* 4:895, 1983.

L. A. Cohen *et al.*, *J. Nat. Cancer Inst.* 72:165, 1984.

S. Ball, R. Weindruch, and R. L. Walford, in *Free Radicals, Aging and Degenerative Diseases* (ed. J. E. Johnson and R. L. Walford). New York: Plenum Press, 1986 (in press).

M. F. McCarty, *Medical Hypotheses* 14:213, 1984.

73. E. Schneider and J. D. Reed, Jr., *New Eng. J. Med.* 312:1159, 1985.

74. Recalling that in the oxidation of fats caused by free radicals there are initiation, propagation (chain-forming), and termination stages, we might reasonably add to our diet natural antioxidants that protect at the first two stages: to inhibit initiation, selenium; to inhibit propagation, vitamin E and vitamin C (or BHA—which, however, I do not recommend; see Note 72 above). Termination occurs when two free radicals combine and cancel each other out. It cannot be influenced by outside manipulation. Finally, beta-carotene, which belongs to a less-understood class of antioxidants, may be recommended.

75. W. Regelson, in *Intervention in the Aging Process, Part A: Quantition, Epidemiology, and Clinical Research* (ed. W. Regelson and F. M. Sinex). New York: Alan R. Liss, 1983, p. 3.
76. N. Fabris *et al.*, *Internat. J. Immunopharmacol.* 1986 (in press).
77. L. Aladaheff *et al.*, *Nutrition Reviews* 42:33, 1984.
78. R. B. Pelton and R. J. Williams, *Proceedings of the Society for Experimental Biology and Medicine* 99:632, 1958.
79. K. E. Cheney *et al.*, *Exper. Gerontol.* 15:237, 1980.
80. E. P. Ralli and M. E. Dunn, *Vitamin and Hormones* 11:133, 1953.
81. *Ibid.*
82. C. Nice *et al.*, *J. Sports Med.* 24:26, 1984.
83. K. Lindseth and J. Miquel, AGE 4:133, 1981.
K. Lindseth *et al.*, *12th Ann. Meeting, Am. Aging Assn.*, Sept. 23–29, 1982, p. 18.
84. M. L. Fonda *et al.*, *Exper. Geront.* 15:473, 1980.
C. S. Rose *et al.*, *Am. J. Clin. Nutr.* 29:847, 1976.
85. Fonda *et al.*, *op. cit.*
86. H. Schaumburg *et al.*, *New Eng. J. Med.* 309:445, 1983.

87. Federal Register, *Vitamins and Mineral Drug Products for Over-the-Counter Use.* DHEW, Food and Drug Admin. 44, #53, March 16, 1979.
88. C. E. Finch. *Quarterly Rev. Biol.* 51:49, 1976.
89. Centrophenoxine (also know as Meclofenoxate and by the European trade names of Lucidril and Helfergin) has been used in Europe for a long time as a psychiatric drug. Along with other so-called nootropic drugs (piracetum is another), it is claimed to enhance energy metabolism as measured by changes in ATP turnover, glycolysis, and oxygen utilization. It may improve learning ability in mice and monkeys (Dylewski *et al.*, 1983; Dean *et al.*, 1983). Doses of 400 to 800 mg. given daily to 52 patients with various central-nervous-system problems led to improvements in their confused states (Destram, 1961). It very definitely decreases the accumulation of age pigment in the brain and heart muscle of guinea pigs (Nandi, 1968; Spoerri *et al.*, 1974), rats (Riga and Riga, 1974; Brizzee *et al.*, 1981), and mice (Dylewski *et al.*, 1983). It may act in part by elevating the levels of antioxidant enzymes in the brain (Roy *et al.*, 1983). In rats, administration of centrophenoxine in dosages of 100 mg./kg. body weight daily for 2 months increased the RNA in the brain cortex of old rats until it reached the young-adult level. This was attributed to a free-radical-scavenging activity of the drug after incorporation into nerve-cell membranes (Zs-Nagy and Senser, 1984).

    The effects of centrophenoxine and DMAE on mean and maximum life spans in fruit flies and mice have been investigated (Hochschild, 1971, 1973). In short-lived mouse strains, the drugs extended mean life spans by up to 30 percent and maximum life spans by 11–27 percent. But in long-lived mouse strains, neither mean nor maximum life spans (22 and 32 months, respectively) were altered. In another study, and starting at 6 months of age, a long-lived strain of mice was maintained on a fairly high dose of centrophenoxine. The experiment was terminated at 30 months, at which time 40 percent of treated and only 10 percent of untreated mice were surviving.

The total data on centrophenoxine and/or DMAE look promising, and centrophenoxine has been used for a long time in humans in Europe, although not primarily as an antiaging drug. It has not shown any toxicity in humans.

R. L. Dean *et al.*, in *Experimental and Clinical Intervention in Aging* (ed. R. F. Walker and R. L. Cooper). New York: Marcel Dekker, 1983, p. 279.

D. P. Dylewski *et al.*, *Neurobiol. of Aging* 4:89, 1983.

H. Destram, *Presse Medical* 69:1999, 1961.

K. Nandi, *J. Gerontology* 23:82, 1968.

P. E. Spoerri *et al.*, *Mechanisms of Ageing and Development* 3:311, 1974.

S. Riga and D. Riga, *Brain Research* 72:265, 1974.

K. R. Brizzee *et al.*, in *Age Pigments* (ed. R. S. Sohal). North Holland: Elsevier, 1982, p. 102.

D. Roy *et al.*, *Experimental Gerontology* 18:185, 1983.

I. Zs-Nagy and I. Senser, *Experimental Gerontology* 19:171, 1984.

R. Hochschild, *Experimental Gerontology* 6:133, 1971; 8:177, 1973; 8:185, 1973.

R. Hochschild, *Gerontologia* 19:271, 1973.

90. A. Goldstein *et al.*, in *Intervention in the Aging Process, Part A: Quantitation, Epidemiology and Clinical Research* (ed. W. Regelson and F. M. Sinex). New York: Alan R. Liss, 1983, p. 169.

91. Injecting the hormone into old mice does ameliorate some of the problems due to age-related failure of the immune system (Weksler, 1983; Goldstein *et al.*, 1983). The immune system can be substantially rejuvenated by grafting of a young thymus plus young bone marrow into old mice (Hirokawa *et al.*, 1982).

Russian scientists have reported that injections of crude thymus extracts 5 days per month will prolong the average life spans of mice by 28 percent and maximum life spans by 9 percent, along with a great improvement in immune-response capacity and a reduction in incidence of leukemia from 14 percent in noninjected mice to zero in injected mice, and in breast cancer from 52 percent in noninjected mice to 20 percent in injected mice (Anisimov *et al.*, 1982). Unfortunately, they used short-lived strains, with maximum life spans of only 26 months, so their results could be interpreted as influencing disease rather than the aging process. Dr. Gino Doria of Italy and Dr. Rita Effros in my laboratory at UCLA have shown that major portions of the immune decline of aging can be reversed with thymic-hormone injections.

M. Weksler, *Annals Intern. Med.* 98:105, 1983.

Goldstein *et al.*, *op. cit.*

K. Hirokawa *et al.*, *Clinical Immunology and Immunopathology* 22:297, 1982.

V. N. Anisimov *et al.*, *Mechanisms of Ageing and Development* 19:245, 1982.

92. A. Schwartz *et al.*, in *Intervention in the Aging Process*, *op. cit.* p. 267.
93. Among the several effects attributed to DHEA (Schneider and Reed, 1985), one is that it may inhibit weight gain by increasing the metabolic rate and by directing energy into a "futile cycle," thereby increasing oxygen consumption and increasing the generation of heat within fatty tissues. These combined processes could be labeled "calorie wasting." If such is the case, one would expect DHEA to increase the generation of free radicals, in which case it might *not* decelerate aging but the reverse. We must await the results of studies in truly long-lived strains of mice. Most studies to date have been conducted in mouse

strains with genetic disorders or exaggerated susceptibility to various diseases—in short, not on normal mice.
E. L. Schneider and J. D. Reed, Jr., *New Eng. J. Med.* 312:1159, 1985.

94. L. Ernster and B. D. Nelson in *Biomedical and Clinical Aspects of Coenzyme Q*, Vol. 3. Amsterdam: Elsevier, 1981, p. 159.
95. E. G. Bliznakoff, *Mechanisms of Ageing and Development* 7:189, 1978.
96. E. G. Bliznakoff in *Biomedical and Clinical Aspects of Coenzyme Q*, Vol. 3. Amsterdam: Elsevier, 1981, p. 311.
97. P. R. Borum, *Annual Rev. Nutr.* 3:233, 1983.
98. Y. Suzuki *et al.*, in *Carnitine Biosynthesis, Metabolism, and Function* (ed. R. A. Frenkel and J. D. McGarry). New York: Academic Press, 1980. p. 341.
99. O. Fanelli, *Life Sciences* 23:2563, 1978.
100. M. Maebashi *et al.*, *Lancet* 2:805, 1978.
101. C. Cavazza, *Chem. Abstracts* 100:203597f, 1984.
102. M. Lyte and M. Shinitzky, *Biochemica et Biophysica Acta* 812:133, 1985.
103. M. Shinitzky *et al.*, in *Intervention in the Aging Process, op. cit., Part B: Basic Research and Preclinical Screening*, p. 175.
104. R. Weindruch, in *Longevity Letter*, February 1985, p. 2.

Chapter 8

1. I've been actively involved in sports all my life: Southwest A. A. U. gymnastic champion (on the rings) my last year in high school; captain of the wrestling team at the University of Chicago for two years; scuba diver since the very beginning of the sport. Even now I spend three 20-minute periods a week at aerobic exercise with my heart rate at 75 percent of maximum, do about an hour of isometric bodybuilding weekly, and spend uncounted hours of pure pleasure at sports

(such as body surfing, since I live at the beach). So my criticism of the exercise mania is not that of a "sedentary" person trying to justify his laziness.

2. S. Port *et al.*, *New Eng. J. Med.* 303:1133, 1980.
3. C. Bissell and T. Samorajski, *AGE* 6:134, 1983.
4. J. W. Starnes *et al.*, *Am. J. Physiol.* 245:H560, 1983.
   E. Steinhagen-Thiessen *et al.*, *AGE* 6:143, 1983.
   A. Z. Reznick *et al.*, *Biochem. Med.* 28:347, 1982.
   J. A. Chesky *et al.*, *J. Applied Physiol.* 55:1349, 1983.
5. In another study, mice 6, 19, and 27 months old were forced to exercise on a motor-driven wheel for 30 minutes per day for 10 weeks, after which their leg muscles were examined by electron microscopy. In the 27-month-old but not in the younger mice, the exercise actually *accelerated* the regressive muscle changes normally seen with aging (Ludatscher *et al.*, 1983).
   R. Ludatscher *et al.*, *Exper. Geront.* 18:113, 1983.
6. R. Coleman *et al.*, *Biology of the Cell* 46:207, 1982.
7. A. B. K. Basson *et al.*, *Comparative Biochemistry and Physiology* 71A:369. 1982.
8. Studies in monkeys kept on high-cholesterol diets and either exercised (1 hour 3 times week on a treadmill) or not have shown rather convincingly that exercise protects against the development of arteriosclerosis (Kramsch, 1981).
   D. M. Kramsch, *New Eng. J. Med.* 305:1483, 1981.
9. E. Hietanen (ed.), *Regulation of Serum Lipids by Physical Exercise.* Boca Raton, Fla.: CRC Press, 1982.
10. L. W. Gibbons *et al.*, *Circulation* 67:977, 1983.
11. C. C. Johnson *et al.*, *J. Am. Diet. Assn.* 81:695, 1982.
12. Losing weight along with the exercise maximizes the beneficial effects on the blood fats (Tran and Weltman, 1985)..
    Z. V. Tran and A. Weltman, *J. Am. Med. Assn.* 254:914, 1985.
13. S. Port *et al.*, *New Eng. J. Med.* 303:1133, 1980.
    M. Rosenthal *et al.*, *Diabetes* 32:408, 1983.
14. S. N. Blair *et al.*, *J. Am. Med. Assn.* 252:487, 1984.

15. B. Liebman, *Nutr. Action*, November, 1981, p. 9.
16. M. Elsayad *et al.*, *J. Gerontology* 35:383, 1980.
17. W. W. Spirduso, *J. Gerontology* 35:850, 1980.
18. R. A. Bruce, *Med. and Sci. in Sports and Exercise* 16:8, 1984.
19. Treadmill time to exhaustion is equally good (Gibbons *et al.*, 1983).
    L. W. Gibbons *et al.*, *J. Am. Diet. Assn.* 81:695, 1982.
20. The age-related decline in maximum oxygen consumption may be different in longitudinal than in cross-sectional studies. Thus, for a contrary view to what I have said about the rates of decline when sedentary are compared with athletic individuals, see Bruce, 1984.
    Bruce, *op. cit.*
21. E. Hietanen (ed.), *Regulation of Serum Lipids by Physical Exercise*. Boca Raton, Fla.: CRC Press, 1982.
    Editorial, *Lancet* 2:718, 1978.
22. L. W. Shaw, *Am. J. Cardiology* 48:39, 1981.
23. R. L. Paffenbarger *et al.*, *J. Am. Med. Assn.* 252:491, 1984.
24. R. J. Barnard, M. R. Massey, *et al.*, *Diabetes Care* 6:268, 1983.
    R. J. Barnard, P. M. Guzy, *et al.*, *J. Cardiac Rehab.* 3:183, 1982.
    J. A. Hall *et al.*, *The Physician and Sports Med.* 10:90, 1982.
25. Port *et al.*, *op. cit.*
    O. Segerberg, Jr., *Living to Be 100*. New York: Scribner, 1982.

Chapter 9

1. Quoted in *Nutrition Action*, July/August, 1982.
2. W. J. Broad, *Science* 204:1060. 1979.
3. *Los Angeles Times*, Sept. 25, 1983, Part I, p. 4.
4. D. Ornish, *Stress, Diet, and Your Heart*. New York: Holt, Rinehart and Winston, 1982.
5. A. Parachini, cited by *Los Angeles Times*, Sept. 4, 1984, Part V, p. 1.

6. R. L. Walford, *Maximum Life Span*. New York: W. W. Norton, 1983.
7. R. L. Walford, *Los Angeles Times*, June 5, 1983, Travel Section.
8. I don't mean to indicate that an author's mere possession of orthodox "credentials" necessarily means his advice is sound. Dr. Berger's *The Immune Power Diet* is, in my opinion as both an immunologist and a nutritionist, merely one long clinical anecdote, and close to being fantasy—even though Dr. Berger is a regular medical doctor.
9. W. O. Spitzer, *Canadian Med. Assn. J.* 121:1193. 1979.
10. If body fat in women falls substantially below 10 to 14 percent as sometimes happens in heavy-duty exercisers, they may stop menstruating. This apparently does no harm, and they can start menstruating again by gaining a little weight. But if you are either pregnant or attempting to become pregnant, you should not be on a rigorous dietary program unless that is prescribed by your doctor.
11. K. Cheney *et al.*, *Exper. Gerontol.* 15:237, 1980.
R. Weindruch *et al.*, AGE 5:111, 1982.
12. H. N. Munro and V. R. Young, *Postgraduate Med.* 63:143, 1978.
13. H. N. Munro, in *Mammalian Protein Metabolism* (ed. H. N. Munro and J. B. Allison), Vol. 2. New York: Academic Press, 1964, p. 3.
14. *Nutrition Action*, September, 1984.
15. P. A. Crapo *et al.*, *Diabetes*, 26:1178, 1977.
P. A. Crapo, *Nutrition Today*, 19:6, 1984.
16. D. A. Jenkins *et al.*, *Am. J. Clin. Nutr.* 34:362, 1981.
17. The fact is that most people have so many amylases (enzymes that break down carbohydrates) in their gut that complex carbohydrates are broken down to simple ones almost imediately.
18. Dietary fiber is quite different from "crude fiber"—an older, narrower term which designates the part of the cell wall that is left after severe acid and base extrac-

tion. "Crude fiber" values appear in many food tables but are of little value. True dietary fiber may be 4 to 5 times as plentiful as "crude fiber."

19. According to Dr. Dennis Burkitt, the leading physician in this area, every population with a low average fiber intake has an increased frequency of heart disease, gallstones, diabetes, obesity, varicose veins, colorectal cancer, hiatus hernia, diverticulitis, and hemorrhoids.
20. M. M. Baig *et al.*, *Drug Nutrient Interactions* 3:109, 1985.
21. The food substance queuosine (found in certain transfer RNAs) may be an example. Recent experiments suggest that mice cannot synthesize it and must get it from their diet (Nishimura, 1983), but it is not yet recognized as an "essential" nutrient. Sufficient amounts are found in common plant and animal food products such as wheat germ, tomatoes, and yogurt, but might not be present in a junk-food diet supplemented with merely the RDA list of essential nutrients.
    S. Nishimura, *Progress in Nucleic Acid Research* 28:50, 1983.
22. U. Verkhoshansky, *Soviet Sports Review* 17:41, 1982.
23. C. C. Johnson *et al.*, *J. Am. Dietetic Assn.* 81:695, 1982.
24. B. F. Hurley *et al.*, *J. Am. Med. Assn.* 252:507, 1984.
    L. Goldberg *et al.*, *J. Am. Med. Assn.* 252:504, 1984.

Chapter 10

1. Ohaus #720 Triple Beam platform balance: available from (for example) Sargent-Welch Scientific Co., 7300 North Linden Ave., P.O. Box 1026, Skokie, Ill. 60077.
2. *Nutrition Action*, October, 1984, p. 12.
3. *Consumer Reports*, February, 1981, p. 68.
4. *Ibid.*
5. R. L. Walford, *Maximum Life Span*. New York: W. W. Norton, 1983.
6. I. M. Buzzard *et al.*, *Am. J. Clin. Nutr.* 36:94, 1982.

7. M. Liebman and T. L. Bazzarre, *Am. J. Clin. Nutr.* 38:612, 1983.
8. *Science News* 127:278, May 4, 1985.
9. *Nutrition Reviews* 42:374, 1984.
10. K. H. Duncan *et al.*, *Am. J. Clin. Nutr.* 37:763, 1983.
11. S. Belman, *Carcinogenesis* 4:1063, 1983.
12. B. H. S. Lau *et al.*, *Nutrition Research* 3:119, 1983.
13. Garlic also has antithrombotic effects. However, these probably cannot be gained from garlic pills, oils, extracts, or other commercial preparations because most manufacturing processes begin with steam distillation. Fresh garlic is best. Unfortunately, garlic and onions provide a lingering reminder of their ingestion because the sulfur compounds from garlic and onions, when absorbed from the intestines into the blood, find their way into expired air and sweat.
14. *Sierra Club Bulletin*, July/August, 1984.
15. F. H. Mattson, in *Dietary Fats and Health* (ed. E. G. Perkins and W. J. Visek). AOCS Monograph 10, Am. Oil Chemists Society, 1983, p. 679.
16. D. Shapcott, in *Nutrition and Killer Diseases* (ed. J. Rose), Park Ridge, N.J.: Noyes Pub., 1982, p. 30.
17. G. L. Feder, in *Aging and the Geochemical Environment*. Washington, D.C.: National Academy Press, 1981, p. 92.
18. Shapcott, *op. cit.*

Readings and Resources

Nutrition Software

Dr. Walford's Interactive Diet Planner

Designed to help you put together optimal daily food combinations to achieve highest quality and full RDA values at lowest caloric and fat intake, this software contains a 300-member best-foods total-nutrient data base. Additional high/low-diet menus are included. The *Diet Planner* is the software companion to this book. Available from The Longbrook Co., Suite 1215, 1015 Gayley Avenue, Los Angeles, CA 90024, at $48 postage paid. Available at time of writing for IBM-PC or XT with MS/DOS 2.0 or later operating system and 64 K or more of RAM, IBM Color Graphics/Interface Card with color monitor, or Enhanced Graphics Adaptor with color monitor; runs on most IBM compatibles with graphics capabilities (compaq, for example). Also for Apple II or IIe with DOS 3.3 or Pro Dos operating system (See inner flap of book jacket).

Books

Maximum Life Span by Roy L. Walford, M.D.
New York: W. W. Norton & Co., 1983 (hardcover)
New York: Avon Books (paperback)

Basic background book on the science of aging research: the history of gerontology, the different theories of aging, the sociopolitical aspects of the long-living society when it is achieved, and anecdotal stories of the author's life as a gerontologist.

Prolongevity II by Albert Rosenfeld
New York: Alfred A. Knopf, 1985 (hardcover)
Well-written survey of modern gerontology by the former science editor of *Life* and *Saturday Review*.

Jane Brody's Nutrition Book by Jane Brody
New York: W. W. Norton & Co., 1981
Simply the best available popularly written book on general nutrition. Highly recommended.

Newsletters

If you are serious about increasing your longevity, you will want to keep abreast of the latest advances. The following three newsletters make up the best combination to do this.

Longevity Letter
American Longevity Assn.
330 S. Spalding Dr., Suite 304
Beverly Hills, Calif. 90212

Written by Dr. Don Swanson, a former classmate of mine at the California Institute of Technology and now a specialist in information retrieval, this comprehensive letter presents an in-depth analysis of the developing literature of aging research, antiaging therapies, and the diseases of late life. As a rule, one subject is comprehensively covered in each issue.

Life Extension Report (formerly *Anti-Aging News*)
2835 Hollywood Blvd.
Hollywood, Fla. 33020

An excellent companion to the above, somewhat overly enthusiastic about antioxidants and other drug therapies but comprehensive, well written, and well documented. More immediately up-to-date than the *Longevity Letter*, *Life Extension Report* includes full accounts of the latest findings presented at each year's various gerontology conferences and their practical applications. Highly recommended!

Nutrition Action Health Letter
Center for Science in the Public Interest
1501 16th St., N.W.
Washington, D.C., 20036

An absolute must if you are at all concerned about the product quality of what you are putting into your stomach.

Instrumentation

Instruments for estimating body fat:

Slim Guide Skinfold Calipers—inexpensive (about $20), satisfactory, and accompanied by an easy-to-read pamphlet. Available from Sharper Image Catalogue, 680 Davis St., San Francisco, Calif. 94111.

Fat-O-Meter—least expensive (about $10), satisfactory, with well-written pamphlet. Available from Creative Engineering, Inc., 5148 Saddle Ridge Rd., Plymouth, Mich. 48170.

Skyndex Electronic Fat Calculator—expensive, with built-in calculator. Available from Sharper Image Catalogue.

Special Food Sources

Key Gourmet, Box 3691, Beverly Hills, Calif. 90212, for dried mushrooms of various types: morels, chanterelles, porcini, cèpes . . .

Willacrik Farm, P.O. Box 599, Templeton, Calif. 93465, for elephant and other forms of garlic.

Brae Beef, Inc., 100 Greyrock Pl., Stamford, Conn. 06901, for beef from cattle fed organically without artificial stimulants or antibiotics. Lean but tender, its New York strip steak contains 20 percent calories from fat (compared with the more than 40 percent in ordinary commercial beef), with saturated/unsaturated-fat ratio of about 2:1 (compared with the more than 10:1 of regular commercial beef). To my knowledge, this is the best and most healthful red meat available short of wild game.

Smith's Bay, P.O. Box 93, Vernon, Ariz. 85940—good source of fresh herbs and spices and of whole, unground spices such as allspice, nutmeg, and the like, which are far better if you grind or grate them as needed. Particularly recommended: its sage and Spanish red garlic.

Frieda's Finest/Produce Specialties, Inc., P.O. Box 58488, Los Angeles, Calif. 90058—wholesale only, but has good pamphlets such as "Squash-lover's Guide" and "Slim Line Vegetable Guide" and will tell you who carries its produce in the West or nationwide. Involved in introducing new and exotic fruits and vegetables to the American market.

Index